Medical Terminology Systems

A Body Systems Approach

FIFTH EDITION

Barbara A. Gylys, MEd, CMA-A

Professor Emerita
College of Health and Human Services
Medical Assisting Technology
University of Toledo
Toledo, Ohio

Mary Ellen Wedding, MEd, MT(ASCP), CMA, AAPC

Professor of Health Professions
College of Health and Human Services
University of Toledo
Toledo, Ohio

Medical Terminology Systems

A Body Systems Approach

 F. A. DAVIS COMPANY • Philadelphia

Medical terminology is presented in a clear and concise manner, using the classic word-building and body systems approach to learning.

What's *Inside...*

The pages of Medical Terminology Systems: A Body Systems Approach, 5th Edition

Chapter Outlines
to orient student to each chapter's content
(see page 107)

Key Terms

This section introduces important digestive system terms and their definitions. Word analyses are also provided.

Term	Definition
asymptomatic ā-simp-tō-MĂT-ĭk	Without symptoms
defecation dĕf-ĕ-KĀ-shŭn	Elimination of feces from the gastrointestinal tract through the rectum
duodenal bulb dū-ō-DĒ-năl BŬLB	Upper duodenal area just beyond the pylorus
endoscope ĔN-dō-skōp *endo-*: in, within *-scope*: instrument for examining	Instrument consisting of a rigid or flexible fiberoptic tube and optical system for observing the inside of a hollow organ or cavity
exocrine ĔKS-ō-krĭn *exo-*: outside, outward *-crine*: secrete	Pertaining to a gland that secretes outwardly through excretory ducts to the surface of an organ or tissue or into a vessel

Key Terms highlighted in the beginning of each chapter
(see page 108)

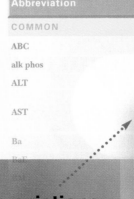

Abbreviation	Meaning
COMMON	
ABC	aspiration biopsy cytology
alk phos	alkaline phosphatase
ALT	alanine aminotransferase (elevated in liver and heart disease); formerly *SGPT*
AST	
Ba	
BaE	

Abbreviation	Meaning
COMMON	
ABC	aspiration biopsy cytology
alk phos	alkaline phosphatase
ALT	alanine aminotransferase (elevated in liver and heart disease); formerly *SGPT*

Abbreviations
for common terms
(see page 136)

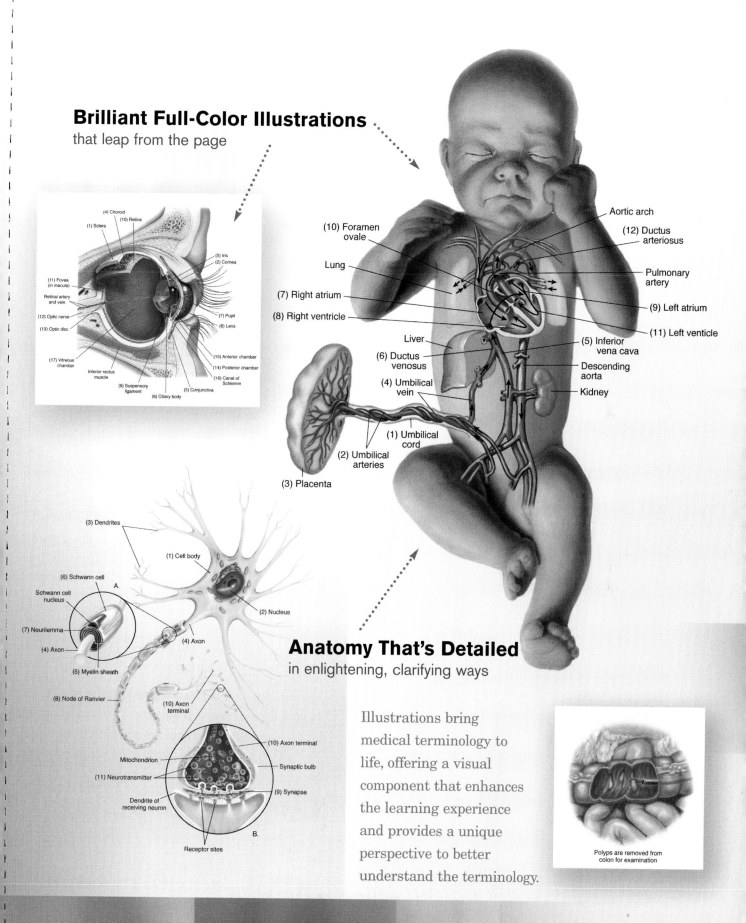

Brilliant Full-Color Illustrations
that leap from the page

(4) Choroid
(10) Retina
(1) Sclera
(5) Iris
(2) Cornea
(11) Fovea (in macula)
Retinal artery and vein
(12) Optic nerve
(7) Pupil
(13) Optic disc
(8) Lens
(17) Vitreous chamber
(15) Anterior chamber
(14) Posterior chamber
(16) Canal of Schlemm
Inferior rectus muscle
(9) Suspensory ligament
(3) Conjunctiva
(6) Ciliary body

(10) Foramen ovale
Lung
(7) Right atrium
(8) Right ventricle
Liver
(6) Ductus venosus
(4) Umbilical vein
(1) Umbilical cord
(2) Umbilical arteries
(3) Placenta

Aortic arch
(12) Ductus arteriosus
Pulmonary artery
(9) Left atrium
(11) Left venticle
(5) Inferior vena cava
Descending aorta
Kidney

(3) Dendrites
(1) Cell body
(6) Schwann cell
Schwann cell nucleus
A.
(7) Neurilemma
(2) Nucleus
(4) Axon
(4) Axon
(5) Myelin sheath
(8) Node of Ranvier
(10) Axon terminal
(10) Axon terminal
Mitochondrion
Synaptic bulb
(11) Neurotransmitter
(9) Synapse
Dendrite of receiving neuron
B.
Receptor sites

Anatomy That's Detailed
in enlightening, clarifying ways

Illustrations bring medical terminology to life, offering a visual component that enhances the learning experience and provides a unique perspective to better understand the terminology.

Polyps are removed from colon for examination

...A Unique Blend of Words and Art

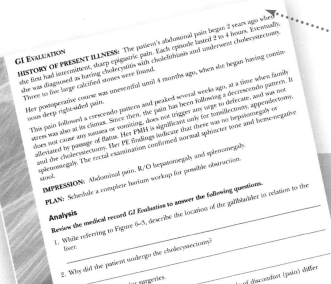

GI Evaluation

HISTORY OF PRESENT ILLNESS: The patient's abdominal pain began 2 years ago when she first had intermittent, sharp epigastric pain. Each episode lasted 2 to 4 hours. Eventually, she was diagnosed as having cholecystitis with cholelithiasis and underwent cholecystectomy. Three to five large calcified stones were found.

Her postoperative course was uneventful until 4 months ago, when she began having continuous deep right-sided pain.

This pain followed a crescendo pattern and peaked several weeks ago, at a time when family stress was also at its climax. Since then, the pain has been following a decrescendo pattern. It does not cause any nausea or vomiting, does not trigger any urge to defecate, and was not alleviated by passage of flatus. Her PMH is significant only for tonsillectomy, appendectomy, and the cholecystectomy. Her PE findings indicate that there was no hepatomegaly or splenomegaly. The rectal examination confirmed normal sphincter tone and heme-negative stool.

IMPRESSION: Abdominal pain. R/O hepatomegaly and splenomegaly.

PLAN: Schedule a complete barium workup for possible obstruction.

Analysis

Review the medical record *GI Evaluation* to answer the following questions.

1. While referring to Figure 6–3, describe the location of the gallbladder in relation to the liver.

2. Why did the patient undergo the cholecystectomy?

3. List the patient's prior surgeries.

4. How does the patient's most recent postoperative episode of discomfort (pain) differ from the initial pain she described?

Detailed Medical Records
with each body system, that provide real-life examples
(see page 146)

Fully Revised Table Format
for better retention and quick learning
(see page 128)

Procedure	Description
DIAGNOSTIC PROCEDURES	
Endoscopic	
endoscopy ĕn-DŎS-kō-pē *endo-*: in, within *-scopy*: visual examinination **upper GI** **lower GI**	Visual examination of a cavity or canal using a specialized lighted instrument called an *endoscope* The organ, cavity, or canal being examined dictates the name of the endoscopic procedure. (See Figure 4–5.) A camera and video recorder are commonly used during the procedure to provide a permanent record. Endoscopy of the esophagus (esophagoscopy), stomach (gastroscopy), and duodenum (duodenoscopy) Endoscopy of the upper GI tract is performed to identify tumors, esophagitis, gastroesophageal varices, peptic ulcers, and the source of upper GI bleeding. It is also used to confirm the presence and extent of varices in the lower esophagus and stomach in patients with liver disease. Endoscopy of the colon (colonoscopy), sigmoid colon (sigmoid-oscopy), and rectum and anal canal (proctoscopy) (See Figure 6–9.) Endoscopy of the lower GI tract is used to identify pathological conditions in the colon. It may also be used to remove polyps. When polyps are discovered in the colon, they are retrieved and tested for cancer.

Pronunciations
with all terms
(see page 116)

More Organized,
user-friendly headings

Includes Suffixes
and their meanings

Element	Meaning	Word Analysis	*(Continued)*
gingiv/o	gum(s)	gingiv/ectomy (jĭn-jĭ-VĔK-tō-mē): excision of diseased gingival tissue in surgical treatment of periodontal disease *-ectomy*: excision, removal	
sial/o	saliva, salivary gland	sial/o/lith (sī-ĂL-ō-lĭth): calculus formed in a salivary gland or duct *-lith*: stone, calculus	
Esophagus, Pharynx, and Stomach			
esophag/o	esophagus	esophag/o/scope (ē-SŎF-ă-gō-skōp): endoscope used to examine the esophagus *-scope*: instrument for examining	
pharyng/o	pharynx (throat)	pharyng/o/tonsill/itis (fă-rĭng-gō-tŏn-sĭ-LĪ-tĭs): inflammation of the pharynx and tonsils *tonsill*: tonsils *-itis*: inflammation	
gastr/o	stomach	gastr/algia (găs-TRĂL-jē-ă): pain in the stomach from any cause; also called *stomachache* *-algia*: pain	
pylor/o	pylorus	pylor/o/spasm (pī-LŌR-ō-spăzm): involuntary contraction of the pyloric sphincter of the stomach, as in pyloric stenosis *-spasm*: involuntary contraction, twitching	
Small Intestine			
duoden/o	duodenum (first part of small intestine)	duoden/o/scopy (dū-ŏd-ĕ-NŎS-kō-pē): visual examination of the duodenum *-scopy*: visual examination	
enter/o	intestine (usually small intestine)	enter/o/pathy (ĕn-tĕr-ŎP-ă-thē): any intestinal disease *-pathy*: disease	

Worksheets Containing Exercises and Activities are featured in each chapter, to help track progress and to review for quizzes and tests (see pages 142-143)

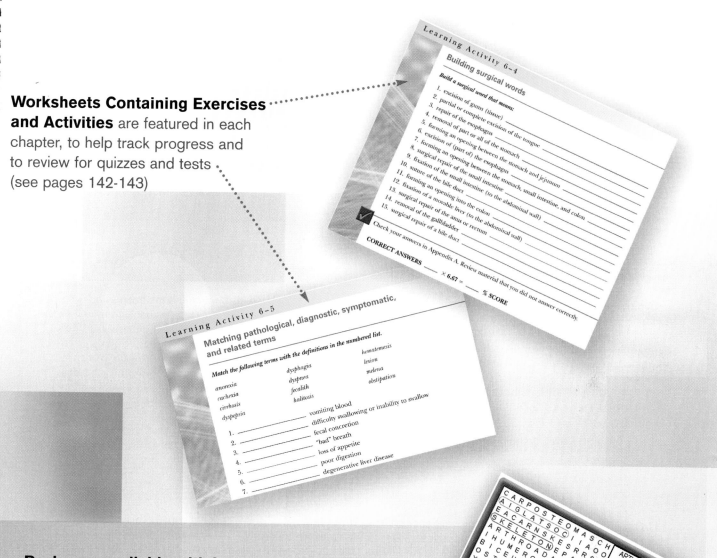

Learning Activity 6-4

Building surgical words

Build a surgical word that means:

1. excision of gums (tissue) _____
2. partial or complete excision of the tongue _____
3. repair of the esophagus _____
4. removal of part of the esophagus _____
5. forming an opening between the stomach _____
6. excision of (part of) the stomach _____
7. forming an opening between the stomach and jejunum _____
8. surgical repair of the esophagus _____
9. fixation repair of the small intestine _____
10. suture of the small intestine (to the abdominal wall) _____
11. forming an opening into the colon _____
12. fixation of the bile duct _____
13. fixation of a movable liver (to the abdominal wall) _____
14. surgical repair of the anus or rectum _____
15. removal of the gallbladder _____
    surgical repair of a bile duct _____

Check your answers in Appendix A. Review material that you did not answer correctly.

CORRECT ANSWERS _____ × 6.67 = _____ % SCORE

Learning Activity 6-5

Matching pathological, diagnostic, symptomatic, and related terms

Match the following terms with the definitions in the numbered list.

anorexia   dysphagia   hematemesis
cachexia   dyspnea   lesion
cirrhosis   fecalith   melena
dyspepsia   halitosis   obstipation

_____ vomiting blood
1. _____ difficulty swallowing or inability to swallow
2. _____ fecal concretion
3. _____ "bad" breath
4. _____ loss of appetite
5. _____ poor digestion
6. _____ degenerative liver disease
7. _____

Packages available with Interactive Medical Terminology 2.0 on CD-ROM. Designed to be used in tandem with the text, this interactive software helps students master medical terminology. IMT 2.0 includes:

- Nearly 1200 test items
- Choice of basic or advanced testing modes
- Interactive exercises such as crossword puzzles, word drag-and-drop, and word scrambles
- Comprehensive score reporting for each exercise

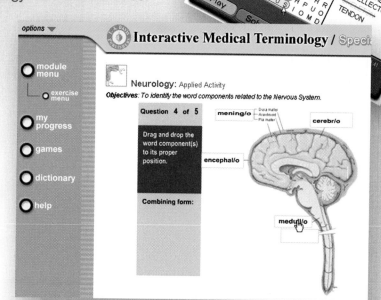

Interactive Medical Terminology / Speci

Neurology: Applied Activity

Objectives: To identify the word components related to the Nervous System.

Question 4 of 5

Drag and drop the word component(s) to its proper position.

Combining form:

mening/o   cerebr/o
encephal/o
medull/o

F. A. Davis Company
1915 Arch Street
Philadelphia, PA 19103
www.fadavis.com

Printed in the United States of America

Last digit indicates print number: 10 9 8 7 6 5 4 3 2

Acquisitions Editor: Andy McPhee
Developmental Editor: Brenna Mayer
Art and Design Manager: Joan Wendt

As new scientific information becomes available through basic and clinical research, recommended treatments and drug therapies undergo changes. The author(s) and publisher have done everything possible to make this book accurate, up to date, and in accord with accepted standards at the time of publication. The author(s), editors, and publisher are not responsible for errors or omissions or for consequences from application of the book, and make no warranty, expressed or implied, in regard to the contents of the book. Any practice described in this book should be applied by the reader in accordance with professional standards of care used in regard to the unique circumstances that may apply in each situation. The reader is advised always to check product information (package inserts) for changes and new information regarding dose and contraindications before administering any drug. Caution is especially urged when using new or infrequently ordered drugs.

Library of Congress Cataloging-in-Publication Data

0–8036–1289–3

This book is dedicated with love

■ ■ ■ ■ ■

to my best friend, colleague,
and husband, Julius A. Gylys

and

to my children,
Regina Maria
and Julius Anthony

and

to Andrew Masters,
Julia Masters, Caitlin Masters,
Anthony Mychal Bishop-Gylys,
and Matthew James Bishop-Gylys

B.A.G.

to my little ones,
Andrew Arthur Kurtz,
Katherine Louise Kurtz,
Daniel Keith Wedding, II,
Carol Ann Estelle Wedding,
Jonathan Michael Kurtz,
Donald Keith Wedding, III,
and Emily Michelle Wedding

M.E.W.

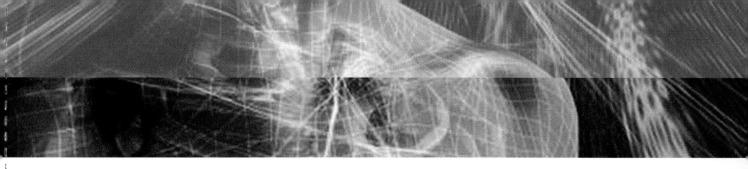

Acknowledgments

The authors would like to acknowledge the valuable contributions of F. A. Davis's editorial and production team who were responsible for this project:

- **Andy McPhee, Acquisitions Editor,** who provided the overall design and layout for the fifth edition. His vision of the work helped focus the authors at the onset of the project and his guidance throughout this endeavor provided cohesiveness.
- **Susan Rhyner, Manager of Creative Development,** whose expertise and care are evident in the quality of support staff she selected for the fifth edition. We are especially grateful for her continued support and help whenever it was needed.
- **Margaret Biblis, Publisher,** Health Professions and Medicine, whose untiring "behind-the-scenes" efforts are evident in the quality of the finished product.
- **Brenna Mayer, Developmental Editor,** whose careful and conscientious edits and suggestions for the manuscript are evident throughout the entire work. Her untiring assistance and support during this project are deeply appreciated and the authors extend their sincerest gratitude.
- **Anne Rains, Artist,** who developed high-quality illustrations throughout the textbook. Her ability to capture in line and color the words and concepts envisioned by the authors is outstanding. The authors wish to acknowledge her artistic talents and thank her for being a part of this project.

In addition, we wish to acknowledge the many, exceptionally dedicated publishing partners that helped in this publication:

- Robert Butler, Production Manager
- Mimi McGinnis, Managing Editor
- Joan Wendt, Design Manager
- Jack Brandt, Illustrations Specialist
- Kirk Pedrick, Senior Developmental Editor, Electronic Publishing
- Ralph Zickgraf, Manager, Electronic Publishing
- Melissa Reed, Assistant Editor of Development
- Kimberly Harris, Administrative Assistant.

We also extend our sincerest appreciation to Neil Kelly, Director of Sales, and his staff of sales representatives whose continued efforts have undoubtedly contributed to the success of this textbook.

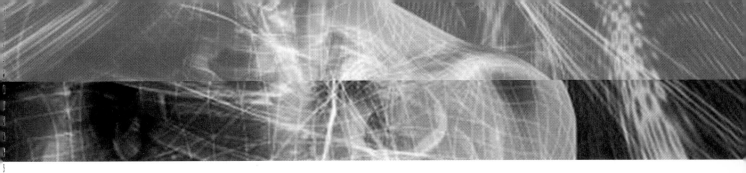

Reviewers

We sincerely thank the clinical reviewers who read and edited the manuscript and provided detailed evaluations and ideas for improving the text and illustrations:

Ann M. Barrow, MSN, RN
Coordinator of College Relations
College of Nursing
Villanova University
Villanova, Pennsylvania

Katie Barton, LPN, BA, NMCA
Medical Assistant Coordinator
Kerr Business College
Augusta, Georgia

Lisa Morris Bonsall, RN, MSN, CRNP
Independent Clinical Consultant
West Chester, Pennsylvania

John Clouse, MSR, RT(R)
Associate Professor
Department of Radiography
Owensboro Community College
Owensboro, Kentucky

Michael W. Cook, MA, RRT, RCP
Professor
Department of Respiratory Therapy
Mountain Empire Community College
Big Stone Gap, Virginia

Patti A. Fayash, CMA, CCS
Evening Adult CE Instructor
Schuykill Technology Center
Frackville, Pennsylvania
Coder
Medical Records Department
Hazleton Healthcare Alliance,
    Broad Street Campus
Hazleton, Pennsylvania

Collette Bishop Hendler, RN, BS, CCRN
Clinical Leader, Intensive Care Unit
Abington Memorial Hospital
Abington, Pennsylvania

Sue Hunt, MA, RN, CMA
Professor and Coordinator
Department of Medical Assisting
Middlesex Community College
Lowell, Massachusetts

Carol Masker
Instructor, Medical Terminology
Morris County School of Technology
Denville, New Jersey

Kay A. Nave, CMA/MRT
Program Director, Medical Assisting Program
Medical Department
Hagerstown Business College
Hagerstown, Maryland

Michelle Shipley, MS, RHIA, CCS
Director and Assistant Professor
Health Information Technology
Washburn University
Topeka, Kansas

In addition, we wish to acknowledge the following individuals who edited portions of the manuscript:

Suzanne Wambold, PhD, RN, RDCS, FASE
Director of the Cardiovascular
   Technology Program
University of Toledo
Toledo, Ohio

Craig Patrick Black, PhD, RRT-NPS
Respiratory Care Program
University of Toledo
Toledo, Ohio

Suzanne Spacek, MEd, RRT-NPS, CPFT
Director, Respiratory Care Program
University of Toledo
Toledo, Ohio

Judith A. Ruple, PhD, RN, NREMT-P
Director of the Emergency Medical
   Health Services Program
University of Toledo
Toledo, Ohio

Lastly, we feel it is only appropriate to acknowledge our deepest gratitude to Robert H. Craven, Jr., President, for his continued support of our publication efforts on this, the 125th anniversary of F. A. Davis Company, a family-owned business. In 1981 (25 years ago), Mr. Craven, through Mr. Robert Martone, Publisher, awarded these two authors an initial contract for the *Body Systems* textbook. We thank Mr. Craven and Mr. Martone for giving us the opportunity to become authors for one of the most successful and prestigious medical textbook publishing companies.

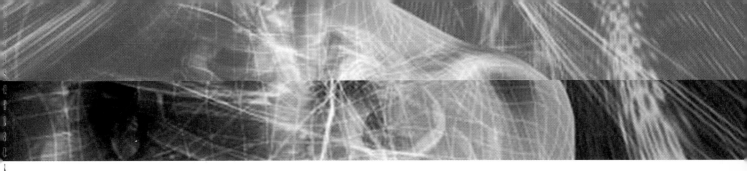

Preface

The fifth edition of *Medical Terminology Systems: A Body Systems Approach* lives up to its well-established track record of presenting medical word building principles based on a competency-based curricula. *Systems* is designed with the educational foundation of a textbook-workbook format that complements traditional lecture and classroom teaching methods. The purpose of the book is to help students learn medical terminology so they can effectively communicate with other members of the healthcare team. A variety of pedagogical features will help them develop a strong foundation in medical terminology and broaden their medical vocabulary. Although the study of medical terminology demands hard work and discipline, various self-paced activities offer interest and variety to the learning process.

All of the changes in the fifth edition are structured to make learning easier and improve retention of medical terms. Perhaps the most striking changes to this edition are the all-new, visually impressive, full-color illustrations. The artwork is specifically designed to present accurate and aesthetically pleasing representations of anatomical structures, disease conditions, and medical procedures. At the same time, the illustrations enhance course content in new and interesting ways, provide a clearer perspective for the reader, and promote long-lasting learning.

Another new feature of the fifth edition is the omission of possessive forms of all eponyms, (such as *Bowman capsule*, *Cushing syndrome*, and *Parkinson disease*). Medical dictionaries as well as the American Association for Medical Transcription and the American Medical Association support these changes. The fifth edition also contains updated, comprehensive lists of medical abbreviations and their meanings, including a "do not use" abbreviations list mandated by the Joint Commission on Accreditation of Healthcare Organizations.

Each chapter incorporates the most current technological changes in medicine. Educators and practitioners in various healthcare disciplines have provided excellent suggestions for this edition, and many of those suggestions have been integrated into the text to augment its educational effectiveness. Pharmacology information has been significantly expanded and now includes commonly used drugs, their generic and trade names, and their modes of action.

The popular, basic features of the previous edition remain intact but have been expanded and enhanced. Here's a breakdown of those features:

- **Chapter 1** explains the techniques of medical word building using basic word elements.
- **Chapter 2** categorizes major surgical, diagnostic, symptomatic, and grammatical suffixes.
- **Chapter 3** presents major prefixes of position, number and measurement, direction, and other parameters.
- **Chapter 4** introduces anatomical, physiological, and pathological terms. Combining forms denoting cellular and body structure, body position and direction, regions of the body, and additional combining forms related to body structure, diagnostic methods, and pathology are also presented. General diagnostic and therapeutic terms are described and provide a solid foundation for specific terms addressed in the body system chapters that follow.

- **Chapters 5 to 15** are organized according to specific body systems and may be taught in any sequence. These chapters include key terms; anatomy and physiology; combining forms, suffixes, and prefixes; pathology; diagnostic, symptomatic, and related terms; diagnostic and therapeutic procedures; pharmacology; abbreviations; learning activities; and medical record activities. All activities allow self-assessment and evaluation of competency.
- **Appendix A: Answer Key** contains answers to each learning activity to validate competency and provide immediate feedback for student assessment.
- **Appendix B: Abbreviations** includes an updated, comprehensive list of medical abbreviations and their meanings.
- **Appendix C: Glossary of Medical Word Elements** contains an alphabetical list of medical word elements and their meanings.
- **Appendix D: Index of Genetic Disorders** lists genetic disorders presented in the textbook.
- **Appendix E: Index of Diagnostic Imaging Procedures** lists radiographic and other diagnostic imaging procedures presented in the textbook.
- **Appendix F: Index of Pharmacology** lists medications presented in the textbook.
- **Appendix G: Index of Oncological Terms** lists terms related to oncology presented in the textbook.

Instructor's Resource Disk

The Instructor's Resource Disk (IRD) features many new and some familiar teaching aids created to make your teaching job easier and more effective. The supplemental teaching aids it provides can be used in various classroom settings—traditional classroom, distance learning, or independent studies. The IRD consists of an Activity Pack, three PowerPoint presentations, and a computerized test bank in Brownstone, a powerful test-generation program.

Activity Pack

The Activity Pack* contains a wealth of information and resources for you, including:

- *Question Bank.* The questions and answers in this popular section are taken from the *Brownstone Computerized Test Bank* found elsewhere on the IRD. These multiple-choice and true/false questions are only a small sample of the more than 1,100 test items available in the Brownstone test bank. Questions are available for each body-system chapter. The multiple-choice and true/false questions mirror the testing format used on many allied health national board examinations.
- *Suggested Course Outlines.* Course outlines are provided to help you plan the best method of covering the material presented in the textbook.
- *Student and Instructor Directed Activities.* These comprehensive teaching aids are newly developed for this edition. They provide an assortment of exercises for each body-system chapter that offers variety and interest to the course material. You can select from the various activities and determine if they are to be used as required content or supplemental material, and whether the activities are to be undertaken individually or as a group project. If group projects are selected, a Peer Evaluation Form is available.
- *Community and Internet Resources.* This section provides updated and expanded resources that offer a rich supply of technical journals, community organizations, and Internet resources to supplement classroom, Internet, and directed activities.

---

*The *Activity Pack* is available in hard copy on request for those who adopt the textbook.

- *Supplemental Medical Record Activities.* In addition to updating the medical record activities from the previous edition, we've added supplemental activities for each of the body system chapters. As in the textbook, these medical record activities use common clinical scenarios to show how medical terminology is used in the clinical area to document patient care. Activities for terminology, pronunciation, and medical record analysis are provided for each medical record, along with an answer key. In addition, each medical record focuses on a specific medical specialty. These records can be used for group activities, oral reports, medical coding activities, or individual assignments. The medical records are designed to reinforce and enhance the terminology presented in the textbook.

- *Crossword Puzzles.* These fun, educational activities are included for each body system chapter. They are designed to reinforce material covered in the chapter and can be used individually or in a group activity. They can also be used as a way of providing extra credit or "just for fun." An answer key is included for each puzzle.

- *Pronunciations and Answer Keys.* We've included in this edition a special answer key for the medical record research activities in the textbook. This key should prove to be a helpful addition when you discuss the material or correct assignments.

- *Master Transparencies.* The transparency pages offer large, clear, black-and-white anatomical illustrations perfect for making overhead transparencies and are provided for each body system.

PowerPoint Presentations

This edition of *Systems* contains not one but *three* PowerPoint presentations for your use. One, called *Lecture Notes,* provides an outline-based presentation for each body-system chapter. It consists of a chapter overview, the main functions of the body system, and selected pathology, vocabulary, and procedures for each. Full-color illustrations from the book are included. A second presentation, called *Illustrations,* contains most illustrations from the text, with one illustration per slide. The third presentation, called *Med TERMinator,* is an interactive presentation in which terms from a chapter drop into view each time you click the mouse. You can ask students to say the term aloud, define the term, or provide other feedback before moving to the next term.

Electronic Test Bank

As in the previous edition, this edition offers a powerful Brownstone test bank that allows you to create custom-generated or randomly-selected tests in a printable format from more than 1,100 multiple-choice test items. The program requires Windows 95, Windows 98, or Windows NT and is available for Macintosh on request.

Audio CD-ROM

Depending on which *Systems* version you ordered, you may find an **audio CD-ROM** in the textbook. The CD is designed to strengthen your students' ability to spell, pronounce, and understand the meaning of selected medical terms using exercises for each body system chapter. These exercises provide continuous reinforcement of correct pronunciation and usage of medical terms.

The audio CD can also be used for students in beginning transcription courses. Medical secretarial and medical transcription students can use the CD to learn beginning transcription skills by typing each word as it is pronounced. After the words are typed, spelling can be corrected by referring to either the textbook or a medical dictionary.

Interactive Medical Terminology 2.0

Interactive Medical Terminology 2.0 (IMT), a powerful interactive CD-ROM program, comes with the text, depending on which version you've chosen. IMT is a competency-based, self-paced, multimedia program that includes graphics, audio, and a dictionary culled from *Taber's Cyclopedic Medical Dictionary*. Help menus provide navigational support. The software comes with numerous interactive learning activities, including:

- word-building and word-breakdown activities
- drag-and-drop anatomical exercises
- word-search puzzles
- word scrambles
- crossword puzzles.

The exercises throughout are designed at a 90% competency level, providing immediate feedback on student competency. Students can also print their progress as they go along. The CD-ROM is especially valuable as a distance-learning tool because it provides evidence of student drill and practice in various learning activities.

Taber's Cyclopedic Medical Dictionary

The world-famous *Taber's Cyclopedic Medical Dictionary* is the recommended companion reference for this book. Virtually all terms in the new edition of *Systems* may be found in *Taber's*. In addition, *Taber's* contains etymologies for nearly all main entries presented in this textbook. We hope you enjoy this new edition as much as we enjoyed preparing it. We think you will find that it is the best edition ever.

Barbara A. Gylys
Mary Ellen Wedding

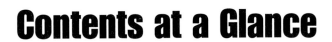

Contents at a Glance

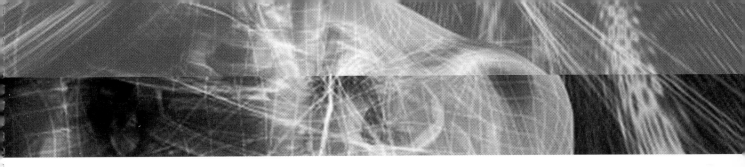

Contents

C h a p t e r   5

Integumentary System   75

Chapter 6
Digestive System   107

Chapter 9
Blood, Lymph, and Immune Systems   225

Chapter 12
Female Reproductive System   345

Chapter 13
Endocrine System   387

Appendices

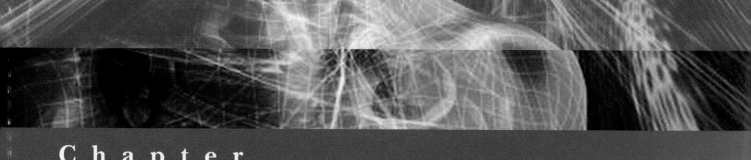

Chapter

1

Basic Elements of a Medical Word

CHAPTER OUTLINE

OBJECTIVES

Upon completion of this chapter, you will be able to:

- Identify the four basic word elements used to form medical words.
- Divide medical words into their component parts.
- Use the guidelines to define and build medical words.
- Locate the pronunciation guidelines and interpret pronunciation marks.

Medical Word Elements

The language of medicine is a specialized vocabulary used by health-care practitioners. Many medical word elements in current use had their origin as early as the 1st century B.C., when Hippocrates practiced medicine. With technological and scientific advancements in medicine, many new terms have evolved to reflect these innovations. For example, radiographic terms, such as magnetic resonance imaging (MRI) and ultrasound (US), are now used to describe current diagnostic procedures.

A medical word consists of some or all of the following elements: word root, combining form, suffix, and prefix. How you combine these elements, and whether all or some of them are present in a medical word, determines the meaning of a word. The purpose of this chapter is to help you learn to identify these elements and use them to build medical terms.

Word Roots

A **word root** is the core of a medical term and contains the fundamental meaning of the word. It is the foundation on which other elements are added to develop a complete term. Most word roots are derived from Greek or Latin. Because of this twofold origin, two different roots may have the same meaning. For example, the Greek word *derm* and the Latin word *cutane* both refer to the skin. As a general rule, Greek word roots are used to build words that describe a disease, condition, treatment, or diagnosis; Latin word roots are used to build words that describe anatomic structures. Consequently, the Greek root *derm* is used primarily in terms that describe a disease, condition, treatment, or diagnosis of the skin; the Latin root *cutane* is used primarily to describe an anatomic structure. Most medical terms contain at least one word root. (See Table 1–1.)

Table 1-1   EXAMPLES OF WORD ROOTS

This table lists examples of word roots as well as their phonetic pronunciations. Begin learning the pronunciations as you review the information below.

Greek or Latin Word	Word Root	Meaning	Word Analysis
dermatos (Gr*)	derm	skin	dermat/itis (dĕr-mă-TĪ-tĭs): inflammation of the skin *A term that describes a skin disease*
nephros (Gr)	nephr	kidney	nephr/oma (nĕ-FRŌ-mă): tumor of the kidney *A term that describes a kidney disease*
stoma (Gr)	stomat	mouth	stomat/o/pathy (stō-mă-TŎP-ă-thē): any disease of the mouth *A term that describes a mouth disease*
cutis (L)	cutane	skin	sub/cutane/ous (sŭb-kū-TĀ-nē-ŭs): beneath the skin *A term that describes the anatomic tissue layer beneath the skin*
oris (L)	or	mouth	or/al (OR-ăl): pertaining to the mouth *A term that describes an anatomic structure*
renes (L)	ren	kidney	ren/al (RĒ-năl): pertains to the kidney *A term that describes an anatomic structure*

*It is not important to know the origin of a medical word. This information is only provided to illustrate that there may be two different word roots for a single term.

Combining Forms

A combining form is a word root to which a vowel (usually an *o*) is added. The vowel has no meaning of its own, but enables two elements to be connected. Like the word root, the combining form is the basic foundation on which other elements are added to build a complete word. In this text, a combining form will be listed as *word root/vowel* (such as *gastr/o*), as illustrated in Table 1–2.

Table 1–2	**EXAMPLES OF COMBINING FORMS**

This table illustrates how word roots and vowels create combining forms. Learning combining forms rather than word roots makes pronunciation a little easier because of the terminal vowel. For example, in the table below, the word roots *gastr* and *nephr* are difficult to pronounce, whereas their combining forms *gastr/o* and *nephr/o* are easier to pronounce.

Word Root	+	Vowel	=	Combining Form	Meaning
erythr/	+	*o*	=	erythr/o	red
gastr/	+	*o*	=	gastr/o	stomach
hepat/	+	*o*	=	hepat/o	liver
immun/	+	*o*	=	immun/o	immune, immunity, safe
nephr/	+	*o*	=	nephr/o	kidney
oste/	+	*o*	=	oste/o	bone

Suffixes

A **suffix** is a word element placed at the end of a word or word root that changes the meaning of the word. In the terms tonsill/*itis*, and tonsill/*ectomy*, the suffixes are -*itis* (inflammation) and -*ectomy* (excision, removal). Changing the suffix changes the meaning of the word. In medical terminology, a suffix usually indicates a procedure, condition, disease, or part of speech. Many suffixes are derived from Greek or Latin words. (See Table 1–3.)

Prefixes

A prefix is a word element attached to the beginning of a word or word root. Adding or changing a prefix changes the meaning of the word. The prefix usually indicates a number, time, position, direction, or negation. Many of the same prefixes found in medical terminology are also found in the English language. (See Table 1–4.)

Table 1-3   EXAMPLES OF SUFFIXES

This table lists examples of suffixes as well as their phonetic pronunciations. Begin learning the pronunciations as you review the information below.

Combining Form	+	Suffix	=	Medical Word	Meaning
gastr/o (stomach)	+	*-itis* (inflammation)	=	gastritis găs-TRĪ-tĭs	inflammation of the stomach
	+	*-megaly* (enlargement)	=	gastromegaly găs-trō-MĔG-ă-lē	enlargement of the stomach
	+	*-oma* (tumor)	=	gastroma găs-TRŌ-mă	tumor of the stomach
hepat/o (liver)	+	*-itis* (inflammation)	=	hepatitis hĕp-ă-TĪ-tĭs	inflammation of the liver
	+	*-megaly* (enlargement)	=	hepatomegaly hĕp-ă-tō-MĔG-ă-lē	enlargement of the liver
	+	*-oma* (tumor)	=	hepatoma hĕp-ă-TŌ-mă	tumor of the liver

Table 1-4   EXAMPLES OF PREFIXES

This table lists examples of prefixes as well as their phonetic pronunciations. Begin learning the pronunciations as you review the information below.

Prefix	+	Word Root	+	Suffix	=	Medical Word	Meaning
a- (without)	+	*mast* (breast)	+	*-ia* (condition)	=	amastia ă-MĂS-tē-ă	without a breast
hyper- (excessive, above normal)	+	*therm* (heat)	+	*-ia* (condition)	=	hyperthermia hī-pĕr-THĔR-mē-ă	condition of excessive heat
intra- (in, within)	+	*muscul* (muscle)	+	*-ar* (relating to)	=	intramuscular ĭn-tră-MŬS-kū-lăr	within the muscle
macro- (large)	+	*card* (heart)	+	*-ia* (condition)	=	macrocardia măk-rō-KĂR-dē-ă	condition of a large heart
micro- (small)	+	*card* (heart)	+	*-ia* (condition)	=	microcardia mī-krō-KĂR-dē-ă	condition of a small heart

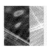

Basic Rules

Defining and building medical words are crucial skills in mastering medical terminology. Following the basic rules for each will help you master these skills.

Defining Medical Words

Here are the three basic rules for defining medical words using the example term *gastroenteritis*.

Rule #1

Define the **suffix,** or last part of the word. In this case, *-itis,* which means *inflammation.*

Rule #2

Define the first part of the word (which may be a **word root, combining form,** or **prefix**). In this case, the combining form *gastr/o* means *stomach.*

Rule #3

Define the middle parts of the word. In this case, *enter/* means *intestine.*

When you analyze *gastroenteritis* following the three previous rules, the meaning is revealed as:

1. inflammation (of)
2. stomach (and)
3. intestine

Thus, the definition of *gastroenteritis* is "inflammation (of) stomach (and) intestine." Table 1–5 further illustrates this process.

Table 1–5   DEFINING GASTROENTERITIS

This table illustrates the three rules of defining a medical word using the example *gastroenteritis.*

Combining Form	Middle	Suffix
gastr/o	**enter/**	**-itis**
stomach	intestine	inflammation
(rule 2)	(rule 3)	(rule 1)

Building Medical Words

There are three basic rules for building medical words.

Rule #1

A word root links a suffix that begins with a vowel.

Word Root	+	Suffix	=	Medical Word	Meaning
hepat/ liver	+	**-itis** inflammation	=	hepatitis hĕp-ă-TĪ-tĭs	inflammation of the liver

Rule #2

A combining form (root + *o*) links a suffix that begins with a consonant.

Combining Form	+	Suffix	=	Medical Word	Meaning
hepat/o liver	+	**-cyte** cell	=	hepatocyte HĔP-ă-tō-sīt	liver cell

Rule #3

Use a combining form to link a root to another root to form a compound word. This rule holds true even if the next root begins with a vowel, as in *osteoarthritis*. Keep in mind that the rules for linking multiple roots to each other are slightly different from the rules for linking roots and combining forms to suffixes.

Combining Form	+	Word Root	+	Suffix	=	Medical Word	Meaning
oste/o bone	+	**chondr/** cartilage	+	**-itis** inflammation	=	osteochondritis ŏs-tē-ō-kŏn-DRĪ-tĭs	inflammation of bone and cartilage
oste/o bone	+	**arthr/** joint	+	**-itis** inflammation	=	osteoarthritis ŏs-tē-ō-ăr-THRĪ-tĭs	inflammation of bone and joint

 It is time to review word building rules by completing Learning Activity 1–1, 1–2, 1–3, and 1–4.

Pronunciation Guidelines

Although the pronunciation of medical words usually follows the same rules that govern the pronunciation of English words, some medical words may be difficult to pronounce when first encountered. Therefore, selected terms in this book include phonetic pronunciation. In addition, pronunciation guidelines can be found on the inside front cover of this book. Use it whenever you need help with pronunciation of medical words. Locate and study these guidelines before proceeding with Learning Activity 1–5.

 It is time to review pronunciation guidelines by completing Learning Activity 1–5.

LEARNING ACTIVITIES

The following activities provide a review of the basic medical word elements introduced in this chapter. Complete each activity and review your answers to evaluate your understanding of this chapter.

Learning Activity 1–1

Understanding medical word elements

Fill in the following blanks to complete the sentences correctly.

1. The four elements used to form words are ___Word root, Combining form, Suffix, prefix___

2. A root is the main part or foundation of a word. In the words *teacher, teaches,* and *teach-ing,* the root is ___teach___.

Identify the following statements as true or false. If false, rewrite the statement correctly on the line provided.

3. A combining vowel is usually an *e*.   True   ~~False~~
   ___o___

4. A word root links a suffix that begins with a consonant.   True   False
   _____

5. A combining form links multiple roots to each other.   True   False
   _____

6. A combining form links a suffix that begins with a consonant. True   False
   _____

7. To define a medical word, first define the prefix.   True   False
   _____

8. A word root links a suffix that begins with a vowel.   True   False
   _____

Underline the word root in each of following combining forms.

9. splen/o (spleen)

10. hyster/o (uterus)

11. enter/o (intestine)

12. neur/o (nerve)

13. ot/o (ear)

14. dermat/o (skin)

15. hydr/o (water)

Check your answers in Appendix A. Review material that you did not answer correctly.

CORRECT ANSWERS _____ × 6.67 = _____ % **SCORE**

Learning Activity 1–2

Identifying word roots and combining forms

Underline the word roots in the following terms.

Medical Word	Meaning
1. nephritis *Suffix*	inflammation of the kidneys
2. arthrodesis	surgical fixation of a joint
3. phlebotomy	incision of a vein
4. dentist	specialist in teeth
5. gastrectomy	excision of the stomach
6. chondritis	inflammation of cartilage
7. hepatoma	tumor of the liver
8. cardiologist	specialist in the heart
9. gastria	condition of the stomach
10. osteoma	tumor of the bone

Underline the following elements that are combining forms.

11. nephr	kidney
12. cardi/o	heart
13. arthr	joint
14. oste/o/arth	bone, joint
15. cholangi/o	bile vessel

✓ Check your answers in Appendix A. Review material that you did not answer correctly.

CORRECT ANSWERS _____ × **6.67 =** _____ **% SCORE**

Learning Activity 1–3

Identifying suffixes and prefixes

Pronounce the following medical terms. Then analyze each term and write the element from each that is a suffix in the right-hand column. The first suffix is completed for you.

Term	Suffix
1. thoracotomy thō-răk-ŎT-ō-mē	*-tomy*
2. gastroscope GĂS-trō-skōp	skop
3. tonsillitis tŏn-sĭl-Ī-tĭs	itis
4. gastritis găs-TRĪ-tĭs	itis
5. tonsillectomy tŏn-sĭl-ĔK-tō-mē	ectome

Pronounce the following medical terms. Then analyze each term and write the element from each that is a prefix in the right-hand column. The first prefix is completed for you.

Term	Prefix
6. microcardia mī-krō-KĂR-dē-ă	*micro-*
7. hyperthermia hī-pĕr-THĔR-mē-ă	hiper
8. macroglossia măk-rō-GLŎS-ē-ă	makro
9. intramuscular ĭn-tră-MŬS-kū-lăr	intra
10. amastia ă-MĂS-tē-ă	amas

Check your answers in Appendix A. Review material that you did not answer correctly.

CORRECT ANSWERS _____ × 10 = _____ % **SCORE**

Learning Activity 1–4

Defining and building medical words

The three basic steps for defining medical words are:

1. Define the last part of the word, or **suffix**.
2. Define the first part of the word, or **prefix, word root**, or **combining form**.
3. Define the **middle** of the word.

Use the previous steps to define the following words. If you are not certain of a definition, refer to Appendix C, Part 1, of this textbook, which provides an alphabetical list of word elements and their definitions.

Term	Definition
1. **gastritis** găs-TRĪ-tĭs	*inflammation of*
2. **nephritis** nĕf-RĪ-tĭs	
3. **gastrectomy** găs-TRĔK-tō-mē	*excision*
4. **osteoma** ŏs-tē-Ō-mă	*tumor of the*
5. **hepatoma** hĕp-ă-TŌ-mă	*tumor of the Liver*
6. **hepatitis** hĕp-ă-TĪ-tĭs	*inflamation of the Liver*

Refer to the section "Building Medical Words" on page 5 to complete this activity. Write the number for the rule that applies to each listed term as well as a short summary of the rule. Use the abbreviation WR to designate word root, CF to designate combining form. The first one is completed for you.

Term	Rule	Summary of the Rule
7. **arthr/itis** ăr-THRĪ-tĭs	1	*A WR links a suffix that begins with a vowel.*
8. **scler/osis** sklĕ-RŌ-sĭs		
9. **arthr/o/centesis** ăr-thrō-sĕn-TĒ-sĭs		
10. **colon/o/scope** kō-LŎN-ō-skōp		
11. **chondr/itis** kŏn-DRĪ-tĭs		

Term	Rule	Summary of the Rule
12. **chondr/oma** kŏn-DRŌ-mă	___	*Humor of the*
13. **oste/o/chondr/itis** ŏs-tē-ō-kŏn-DRĪ-tĭs	___	___
14. **muscul/ar** MŬS-kū-lăr	___	*pertaining to the muscle*
15. **oste/o/arthr/itis** ŏs-tē-ō-ăr-THRĪ-tĭs	___	___

 Check your answers in Appendix A. Review material that you did not answer correctly.

CORRECT ANSWERS _____ × 10 = _____ **% SCORE**

Learning Activity 1–5

Understanding pronunciations

Review the pronunciation guidelines (located inside the front cover of this book) and then underline the correct answer in each of the following statements.

1. The diacritical mark ¯ is called a (breve, macron).

2. The diacritical mark ˘ is called a (breve, macron).

3. The ¯ indicates the (short, long) sounds of vowels.

4. The ˘ indicates the (short, long) sounds of vowels.

5. The combination *ch* is sometimes pronounced like *(k, chiy)*. Examples are *ch*olesterol, *ch*olemia.

6. When *pn* is at the beginning of a word, it is pronounced only with the sound of *(p, n)*. Examples are *pn*eumonia, *pn*eumotoxin.

7. When *pn* is in middle of a word, the *p* *(is, is not)* pronounced. Examples are ortho*pn*ea, hyper*pn*ea.

8. When *i* is at the end of a word, it is pronounced like *(eye, ee)*. Examples are bronch*i*, fung*i*, nucle*i*.

9. For *ae* and *oe*, only the (first, second) vowel is pronounced. Examples are burs*ae*, pleur*ae*.

10. When *e* and *es* form the final letter or letters of a word, they are commonly pronounced as (combined, separate) syllables. Examples are syncop*e*, systol*e*, nar*es*.

Check your answers in Appendix A. Review material that you did not answer correctly.

CORRECT ANSWERS _____ × 10 = _____ **% SCORE**

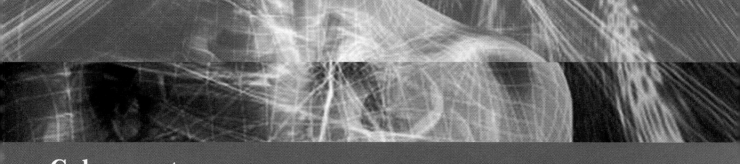

Chapter

2

Suffixes

OBJECTIVES

Upon completion of this chapter, you will be able to:

- Define and provide examples of surgical, diagnostic, pathological, and related suffixes.
- Determine the use of a combining form and word root when linking these elements to a suffix.
- Identify adjective, noun, and diminutive suffixes.
- Locate and apply guidelines for pluralizing terms.
- Demonstrate your knowledge of the chapter by completing the learning activities.

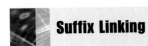

Suffix Linking

In medical words, a suffix is added to the end of a root or combining form to change its meaning. For example, the combining form *gastr/o* means stomach. The suffix *-megaly* means enlargement, and *-itis* means inflammation. *Gastr/o/megaly* is an enlargement of the stomach; *gastr/itis* is an inflammation of the stomach. Whenever you change the suffix, you change the meaning of the word. Suffixes are also used to denote singular and plural forms of a word as well as a part of speech. The following tables provide additional examples to reinforce the rules you learned in Chapter 1. (See Tables 2–1 and 2–2.)

Table 2-1 WORD ROOTS AND COMBINING FORMS WITH SUFFIXES

This table lists examples of word roots used to link a suffix that begins with a vowel. It also lists combining forms (root + o) used to link a suffix that begins with a consonant.

Element	+	Suffix	=	Medical Word	Meaning
Word Roots					
gastr (stomach)	+	*-itis* (inflammation)	=	gastritis găs-TRĪ-tĭs	inflammation of the stomach
hemat (blood)	+	*-emesis* (vomiting)	=	hematemesis hĕm-ăt-ĔM-ĕ-sĭs	vomiting of blood
arthr (joint)	+	*-itis* (inflammation)	=	arthritis ăr-THRĪ-tĭs	inflammation of a joint
Combining Forms					
gastr/o (stomach)	+	*-dynia* (pain)	=	gastrodynia găs-trō-DĬN-ē-ă	pain in the stomach
hemat/o (blood)	+	*-logy* (study of)	=	hematology hĕm-ă-TŎL-ō-jē	study of blood
arthr/o (joint)	+	*-centesis* (surgical puncture)	=	arthrocentesis ăr-thrō-sĕn-TĒ-sĭs	surgical puncture of a joint

Table 2-2 COMPOUND WORDS WITH SUFFIXES

This table lists examples of a combining form used to link a root to another root to form a compound word. This rule holds true even if the next root begins with a vowel, as in *osteoarthritis*. Recall that the rules for linking multiple roots to each other are slightly different from the rules for linking roots and combining forms to suffixes.

Combining Form	+	Word Root	+	Suffix	=	Medical Word	Meaning
gastr/o (stomach)	+	*enter* (intestine)	+	*-itis* (inflammation)	=	gastroenteritis găs-trō-ĕn-tĕr-Ī-tĭs	inflammation of stomach and intestine

Table 2–2   COMPOUND WORDS WITH SUFFIXES

Combining Form	+	Word Root	+	Suffix	=	Medical Word	Meaning
oste/o (bone)	+	*arthr* (joint)	+	*-itis* (inflammation)	=	osteoarthritis ŏs-tē-ō-ăr-THRĪ-tĭs	inflammation of bone and joint
encephal/o (brain)	+	*mening* (meninges)	+	*-itis* (inflammation)	=	encephalomeningitis ĕn-sĕf-ă-lō-mĕn-ĭn-JĪ-tĭs	inflammation of brain and meninges

Suffix Types

An effective strategy in mastering medical terminology is to learn the major types of suffixes, such as surgical, diagnostic, pathological, and related suffixes, as well as grammatical and singular and plural suffixes.

Surgical, Diagnostic, Pathological, and Related Suffixes

Surgical suffixes describe a type of invasive procedure performed on a body part. (See Table 2–3.) Diagnostic suffixes denote a procedure or test performed to identify the cause and nature of an illness. (See Table 2–4.) Pathological suffixes describe an abnormal condition or disease. (See Table 2–4.)

Table 2–3   COMMON SURGICAL SUFFIXES

This table lists commonly used surgical suffixes along with their meanings and word analyses.

Suffix	Meaning	Word Analysis
-centesis	surgical puncture	arthr/o/centesis (ăr-thrō-sĕn-TĒ-sĭs): puncture of a joint space with a needle to remove accumulated fluid from a joint *arthr/o*: joint
-clasis	to break; surgical fracture	oste/o/clasis (ŏs-tē-ŎK-lă-sĭs): surgical fracture of a bone in order to correct a deformity *oste/o*: bone
-desis	binding, fixation (of a bone or joint)	arthr/o/desis (ăr-thrō-DĒ-sĭs): binding together of a joint *arthr/o*: joint
-ectomy	excision, removal	append/ectomy (ăp-ĕn-DĔK-tō-mē): excision of the appendix *append*: appendix
-lysis	separation; destruction; loosening	thromb/o/lysis (thrŏm-BŎL-ĭ-sĭs): dissolution of a blood clot *thromb/o*: blood clot *Drug therapy is usually used to dissolve a blood clot.*

(Continued)

Table 2-3   COMMON SURGICAL SUFFIXES (Continued)

Suffix	Meaning	Word Analysis
-pexy	fixation (of an organ)	mast/o/pexy (MĂS-tō-pĕks-ē): surgical fixation of the breast(s) *mast/o*: breast *Mastopexy, an elective surgery, is performed to affix sagging breasts in a more elevated position, often improving their shape.*
-plasty	surgical repair	rhin/o/plasty (RĪ-nō-plăs-tē): surgical repair in which the structure of the nose is changed *rhin/o*: nose
-rrhaphy	suture	my/o/rrhaphy (mī-OR-ă-fē): suture of a muscle *my/o*: muscle
-stomy	forming an opening (mouth)	trache/o/stomy (trā-kē-ŎS-tō-mē): artificial opening through the neck into the trachea into which a breathing tube is inserted *trache/o*: trachea (windpipe) *A tracheostomy is usually performed to bypass an obstructed upper airway.*
-tome	instrument to cut	oste/o/tome (ŎS-tē-ō-tōm): surgical instrument for cutting through bone *oste/o*: bone
-tomy	incision	trache/o/tomy (trā-kē-ŎT-ō-mē): incision through the neck into the trachea *trache/o*: trachea (windpipe) *Tracheotomy is performed to gain access to an airway below a blockage.*
-tripsy	crushing	lith/o/tripsy (LĪTH-ō-trĭp-sē): crushing of a stone *lith/o*: stone, calculus

It is time to review surgical suffixes by completing Learning Activities 2–1, 2–2, and 2–3.

Table 2-4   COMMON DIAGNOSTIC, PATHOLOGICAL, AND RELATED SUFFIXES

This table lists commonly used diagnostic, pathological, and related suffixes along with their meanings and word analyses.

Suffix	Meaning	Word Analysis
Diagnostic		
-gram	record, writing	electr/o/cardi/o/gram (ē-lĕk-trō-KĂR-dē-ō-grăm): graphic recording of the electrical activity of the heart *electr/o*: electricity *cardi/o*: heart *An electrocardiogram allows diagnosis of specific cardiac abnormalities.*

EKG, ECG

Table 2-4   COMMON DIAGNOSTIC, PATHOLOGICAL, AND RELATED SUFFIXES

Suffix	Meaning	Word Analysis
Diagnostic		
-graph	instrument for recording	cardi/o/graph (KĂR-dē-ō-grăf): instrument used to record electrical activity of the heart *cardi/o:* heart
-graphy	process of recording	angi/o/graphy (ăn-jē-ŎG-ră-fē): radiographic image of blood vessels after injection of a contrast medium *angi/o:* vessel (usually blood or lymph)
-meter	instrument for measuring	pelv/i/meter* (pĕl-VĬM-ĕ-tĕr): instrument for measuring the pelvis *pelv/i:* pelvis
-metry	act of measuring	pelv/i/metry (pĕl-VĬM-ĕ-trē): act or process of determining the dimension of the pelvis *pelv/i:* pelvis
-scope	instrument for examining	endo/scope (ĔN-dō-skōp): flexible or rigid instrument consisting of a tube and optical system for observing the inside of a hollow organ or cavity *endo-:* in, within
-scopy	visual examination	endo/scopy (ĕn-DŎS-kō-pē): visual examination of a cavity or canal using a specialized lighted instrument called an *endo-scope* *endo-:* in, within
Pathological and Related		
-algia	pain	neur/algia (nū-RĂL-jē-ă): pain occurring along the path of a nerve *neur:* nerve
-dynia		ot/o/dynia (ō-tō-DĬN-ē-ă): pain in the ear; earache *ot/o:* ear
-cele	hernia, swelling	hepat/o/cele (hĕ-PĂT-ō-sēl): hernia of the liver *hepat/o:* liver
-ectasis	dilation, expansion	bronchi/ectasis (brŏng-kē-ĔK-tă-sĭs): abnormal dilation of one or more bronchi *bronchi:* bronchus (plural, bronchi) *Bronchiectasis is associated with various lung conditions and is commonly accompanied by chronic infection.*
-edema	swelling	lymph/edema (lĭmf-ē-DĒ-mă): swelling and accumulation of tissue fluid *lymph:* lymph *Lymphedema may be caused by a blockage of the lymph vessels.*
-emesis	vomiting	hyper/emesis (hī-pĕr-ĔM-ĕ-sĭs): excessive vomiting *hyper-:* excessive, above normal
-emia	blood condition	an/emia (ă-NĒ-mē-ă): blood condition caused by iron deficiency or decrease in red blood cells *an-:* without, not

(Continued)

Table 2-4   COMMON DIAGNOSTIC, PATHOLOGICAL, AND RELATED SUFFIXES (Continued)

Suffix	Meaning	Word Analysis
Pathological and Related		
-gen	forming, producing, origin	carcin/o/gen (kăr-SĬN-ō-jĕn): substance or agent that causes the development or increases the incidence of cancer *carcin/o: cancer*
-genesis		carcin/o/genesis (kăr-sĭ-nō-JĔN-ĕ-sĭs): the process of initiating and promoting cancer *carcin/o: cancer* *Carcinogenesis is the transformation of normal cells into cancer cells, commonly as a result of chemical, viral, or radioactive damage to genes.*
-iasis	abnormal condition (produced by something specific)	chol/e/lith/iasis* (kō-lē-lĭ-THĪ-ă-sĭs): presence or formation of gallstones in the gallbladder or common bile duct *chol/e: bile, gall* *lith: stone, calculus*
-itis	inflammation	gastr/itis (găs-TRĪ-tĭs): inflammation of the stomach *gastr: stomach*
-lith	stone, calculus	chol/e/lith* (KŌ-lē-lĭth): gallstone *chlo/e: bile, gall*
-malacia	softening	chondr/o/malacia (kŏn-drō-măl-Ā-shē-ă): softening of the articular cartilage, usually involving the patella *chondr/o: cartilage*
-megaly	enlargement	cardi/o/megaly (kăr-dē-ō-MĔG-ă-lē): enlargement of the heart *cardi/o: heart*
-oma	tumor	neur/oma (nū-RŌ-mă): tumor composed of nerve cells or swelling of a nerve that usually results from compression *neur: nerve*
-osis	abnormal condition; increase (used primarily with blood cells)	cyan/osis (sī-ă-NŌ-sĭs): dark blue or purple discoloration of the skin and mucous membrane *cyan: blue* *Cyanosis indicates a deficiency of oxygen in the blood.*
-pathy	disease	my/o/pathy (mī-ŎP-ă-thē): any disease of muscle *my/o: muscle*
-penia	decrease, deficiency	erythr/o/penia (ĕ-rĭth-rō-PĒ-nē-ă): abnormal decrease in red blood cells *erythr/o: red*
-phagia	eating, swallowing	dys/phagia (dĭs-FĀ-jē-ă): inability or difficulty in swallowing *dys-: bad; painful; difficult*
-phasia	speech	a/phasia (ă-FĀ-zē-ă): absence or impairment of speech *a-: without, not*
-phobia	fear	hem/o/phobia (hē-mō-FŌ-bē-ă): fear of blood *hem/o: blood*

Table 2–4	COMMON DIAGNOSTIC, PATHOLOGICAL, AND RELATED SUFFIXES

Suffix	Meaning	Word Analysis
Pathological and Related		
-plasia	formation, growth	dys/plasia (dĭs-PLĀ-zē-ă): abnormal development of cells, tissues, or organs *dys-:* bad; painful; difficult *Dysplasia is a general term for abnormal formation of an anatomic structure.*
-plasm		neo/plasm (NĒ-ō-plăzm): a new and abnormal formation of tissue, such as a tumor or growth *neo-:* new
-plegia	paralysis	hemi/plegia (hĕm-ē-PLĒ-jē-ă): paralysis of one side of the body *hemi-:* one half *Hemiplegia affects the right or left side of the body and is caused by a brain injury or stroke.*
-rrhage	bursting (of)	hem/o/rrhage (HĔM-ĕ-rĭj): loss of a large amount of blood within a short period, either externally or internally *hem/o:* blood
-rrhagia		men/o/rrhagia (mĕn-ō-RĀ-jē-ă): profuse discharge of blood during menstruation *men/o:* menses, menstruation
-rrhea	discharge, flow	dia/rrhea (dī-ă-RĒ-ă): abnormally frequent discharge or flow of fluid fecal matter from the bowel *dia-:* through, across
-rrhexis	rupture	arteri/o/rrhexis (ăr-tē-rē-ō-RĔK-sĭs): rupture of an artery *arteri/o:* artery
-spasm	involuntary contraction, twitching	blephar/o/spasm (BLĔF-ă-rō-spăsm): twitching of the eyelid *blephar/o:* eyelid
-stenosis	narrowing, stricture	arteri/o/stenosis (ăr-tē-rē-ō-stě-NŌ-sĭs): abnormal narrowing of an artery *arteri/o:* artery
-toxic	poison	hepat/o/toxic (HĔP-ă-tō-tŏk-sĭk): toxic to the liver *hepat/o:* liver
-trophy	nourishment, development	dys/trophy (DĬS-trō-fē): abnormal condition caused by defective nutrition or metabolism *dys-:* bad; painful; difficult

*The *i* in *pelv/i/meter* and the *e* in *chol/e/lithiasis* and *chol/e/lith* are exceptions to the rule of using the connecting vowel *o*.

 It is time to review diagnostic, pathological, and related suffixes by completing Learning Activities 2–4 and 2–5.

Grammatical Suffixes

Grammatical suffixes may be attached to word roots to form a part of speech, such as adjectives and nouns, or a singular or plural form of a medical word. They are also used to denote a diminutive form of a word that designates a smaller version of the object indicated by the root. Many of these suffixes are the same as those used in the English language. (See Table 2–5.)

Table 2–5   ADJECTIVE, NOUN, AND DIMINUTIVE SUFFIXES

This table lists adjective, noun, and diminutive suffixes along with their meanings and word analyses.

Suffix	Meaning	Word Analysis
Adjective		
-ac	pertaining to, relating to	cardi/ac (KĂR-dē-ăk): pertaining to the heart *cardi:* heart
-al		neur/al (NŪ-răl): pertaining to a nerve *neur:* nerve
-ar		muscul/ar (MŬS-kū-lăr): pertaining to muscle *muscul:* muscle
-ary		pulmon/ary (PŬL-mō-něr-ē): pertaining to the lungs *pulmon:* lung
-eal		esophag/eal (ē-sŏf-ă-JĒ-ăl): pertaining to the esophagus *esophag:* esophagus
-ic		thorac/ic (thō-RĂS-ĭk): pertaining to the chest *thorac:* chest
-ical*		path/o/log/ical (păth-ō-LŎJ-ĭ-kăl): pertaining to the study of disease *path/o:* disease *log:* study of
-ile		pen/ile (PĒ-nĭl): pertaining to the penis *pen:* penis
-ior		poster/ior (pŏs-TĒ-rē-or): pertaining to the back of the body *poster:* back (of body), behind, posterior
-ous**		cutane/ous (kū-TĀ-nē-ŭs): pertaining to the skin *cutane:* skin
-tic		acous/tic (ă-KOOS-tĭk): pertaining to hearing *acous:* hearing
Noun		
-esis	condition	di/ur/esis (dī-ū-RĒ-sĭs): abnormal secretion of large amounts of urine *di-:* double *ur:* urine
-ia		pneumon/ia (nū-MŌ-nē-ă): infection of the lung usually caused by bacteria, viruses, or diseases *pneumon:* air; lung
-ism		hyper/thyroid/ism (hī-pěr-THĪ-royd-ĭzm): condition characterized by overactivity of the thyroid gland *hyper-:* excessive, above normal *thyroid:* thyroid gland

Table 2–5   ADJECTIVE, NOUN, AND DIMINUTIVE SUFFIXES

Suffix	Meaning	Word Analysis
Noun		
-iatry	medicine; treatment	pod/iatry (pō-DĪ-ă-trē): specialty concerned with treatment and prevention of conditions of the human foot *pod:* foot
-ician	specialist	obstetr/ician (ŏb-stě-TRĬSH-ăn): physician who specializes in the branch of medicine concerned with pregnancy and childbirth *obstetr:* midwife
-ist		hemat/o/log/ist (hē-mă-TŎL-ō-jĭst): physician who specializes in the treatment of disorders of blood and blood-forming tissues *hemat/o:* blood *log:* study of
-y	condition; process	neur/o/path/y (nū-RŎP-ă-thē): disease of the nerves *neur/o:* nerve *path:* disease
Diminutive		
-icle	small, minute	ventr/icle (VĔN-trĭk-l): small cavity, as of the brain or heart *ventr:* belly, belly side
-ole		arteri/ole (ăr-TĒ-rē-ōl): the smallest of the arteries; minute artery *arteri:* artery *Arteries narrow to form arterioles (small arteries), which branch into capillaries (the smallest blood vessels).*
-ule		ven/ule (VĔN-ūl): small vein continuous with a capillary *ven:* vein

*The suffix *-ical* is a combination of *-ic* and *-al*. **The suffix *-ous* also means *composed of* or *producing*.

 It is time to review grammatical suffixes by completing Learning Activity 2–6.

Plural Suffixes

Because many medical words have Greek or Latin origins, there are a few unusual rules you need to learn to change a singular word into its plural form. Once you begin learning them, you will find that they are easy to apply. You will also find that some English endings have also been adopted for commonly used medical terms. When a word changes from a singular to a plural form, the suffix of the word is the part that changes. A summary of the rules for changing a singular word into its plural form is located on the inside back cover of this textbook. Use it to complete Learning Activity 2–7 and whenever you need help forming plural words.

 It is time to review the rules for forming plural words by completing Learning Activity 2–7.

LEARNING ACTIVITIES

The following activities provide review of the suffixes introduced in this chapter. Complete each activity and review your answers to evaluate your understanding of the chapter.

Learning Activity 2–1

Completing and building surgical words

Use the meanings in the right column to complete the surgical words in the left column. The first one is completed for you. Note: The word roots are underlined in the left column.

Incomplete Word	Meaning
1. episi /o/ _t o m y_	incision of the perineum
2. col _ec tom y_	excision (of all or part)* of the colon
3. arthr/o/ _centesis_	surgical puncture of a joint (to remove fluid)
4. splen _ectomy_	excision of the spleen
5. col/o/ _stomy_	forming an opening (mouth) into the colon
6. oste/o/ _tome_	instrument to cut bone
7. tympan/o/ _tomy_	incision of the tympanic membrane
8. trache/o/ _stomy_	forming an opening (mouth) into the trachea
9. mast _ectomy_	excision of a breast
10. lith/o/ _tripsy tomy_	incision to remove a stone or calculus
11. hemorrhoid _ectomy_	excision of hemorrhoids

*Information in parentheses is used to clarify the meaning of the word but not to build the medical term.

Build a surgical word that means:

12. forming an opening (mouth) into the colon: _Colostomy_
13. excision of the colon: _colonectomy Hemorrhoidectomy_
14. instrument to cut bone: _osteotome_
15. surgical puncture of a joint: _osteocentesis arthrocentesis_
16. incision to remove a stone: _oste lithotomy_
17. excision of a breast: _mastectomy_
18. incision of the tympanic membrane: _tympanotomy_
19. forming an opening (mouth) into the trachea: _tracheostomy_
20. excision of the spleen: _splenectomy_

CORRECT ANSWERS _____ × 5 = _____ % SCORE

Check your answers in Appendix A. Review any material that you did not answer correctly.

Note: If you are not satisfied with your level of comprehension in Learning Activity 2–1, review it and try the exercise again.

Learning Activity 2-2

Completing and building more surgical words

Use the meanings in the right column to complete the surgical words in the left column.

Incomplete Word	**Meaning**
1. arthr/o/ *desis*	fixation or binding of a joint
2. rhin/o/ *plasty*	surgical repair of the nose
3. ten/o/ *plasty*	surgical repair of tendons
4. my/o/ *rrhaphy*	suture of muscle
5. mast/o/ *pexy*	fixation of a (pendulous)* breast
6. cyst/o/ *rrhaphy*	suture of the bladder
7. oste/o/ *clasis*	surgical fracture of a bone
8. lith/o/ *tripsy*	crushing of a stone
9. enter/o/ *lysis*	separating intestinal (adhesions)
10. neur/o/ *tripsy*	crushing a nerve

*Information in parentheses is used to clarify the meaning of the word but not to build the medical term.

Build a surgical word that means:

11. surgical repair of the nose: *rhino plasty*
12. fixation of a joint: *arthrodesis*
13. suture of muscle: *myorrhaphy*
14. fixation of a (pendulous) breast: *masto pexy*
15. suture of the bladder: *cystorrhaphy*
16. repair of tendons: *teno plasty*
17. surgical fracture of a bone: *osteo clasis*
18. crushing stones: *litho tripsy*
19. separating intestinal (adhesions): *entero lysis*
20. crushing a nerve: *neuro tripsy*

✓ Check your answers in Appendix A. Review any material that you did not answer correctly.

CORRECT ANSWERS _____ × 5 = _____ **% SCORE**

Learning Activity 2–3

Selecting a surgical suffix

Use the suffixes in this list to build surgical words in the right column that reflect the meanings in the left column.

-centesis	-ectomy	-plasty	-tome
-clasis	-lysis	-rrhaphy	-tomy
-desis	-pexy	-stomy	-tripsy

1. crushing of a stone: lith/o/ _tripsy_
2. puncture of a joint (to remove fluid)*:   arthr/o/ _centesis_
3. excision of the spleen: splen/ _ectomy_
4. forming an opening (mouth) into the colon: col/o/ _stomy_
5. instrument to cut skin: derma/ _tome_
6. forming an opening (mouth) into the trachea: trache/o/ _stomy_
7. incision to remove a stone or calculus: lith/ _o_ / ~~tripsy~~ _tomy_
8. excision of a breast: mast/ _ectomy_
9. excision of hemorrhoids: hemorrhoid/ _ectomy_
10. incision of the trachea: trache/ _o_ / _tomy_
11. fixation of a breast: mast/ _o_ / _pexy_
12. excision of the colon: col/ _ectomy_
13. suture of the stomach (wall):   gastr/ _o_ / _rrhapy_
14. fixation of the uterus: hyster/ _o_ / _pexy_
15. surgical repair of the nose: rhin/ _o_ / _plasty_
16. fixation or binding of a joint: arthr/ _o_ / _desis_
17. to break or surgically fracture a bone: oste/ _o_ / _clasis_
18. loosening of nerve (tissue):   neur/ _o_ / _lysis_
19. suture of muscle: my/o/ _rrhapy_
20. incision of the tympanic membrane: tympan/ _o_ / _tomy_

*Information in parentheses is used to clarify the meaning of the word but not to build the medical term.

✓ Check your answers in Appendix A. Review any material that you did not answer correctly.

CORRECT ANSWERS _____ × 5 = _____ **% SCORE**

Learning Activity 2-4

Selecting diagnostic, pathological, and related suffixes

Use the suffixes in this list to build diagnostic, pathological, and related words in the right column that reflect the meanings in the left column.

-algia	-malacia	-phagia
-cele	-megaly	-phasia
-ectasis	-metry	-plegia
-emia	-oma	-rrhage
-genesis	-osis	-rrhea
-graph	-pathy	-rrhexis
-iasis	-penia	-spasm

1. tumor of the liver: hepat/ _____
2. pain (along the course) of a nerve: neur/ _____
3. dilation of a bronchus: bronchi/ _____
4. producing or forming cancer: carcin/o/ _____
5. abnormal condition of the skin: dermat/ _____
6. enlarged kidney: nephr/o/ _____
7. discharge or flow from the ear: ot/ _____ / _____
8. rupture of the uterus: hyster/ _____ / _____
9. spasm or twitching of the eyelid: blephar/ _____ / _____
10. herniation of the bladder: cyst/ _____ / _____
11. bursting forth (of) blood: hem/o/ _____
12. abnormal condition of a stone or calculus: lith/ _____
13. paralysis affecting one side (of the body): hemi/ _____
14. diseases of muscle (tissue):   my/ _____ / _____
15. difficult or painful eating: dys/ _____
16. softening of the bones: oste/ _____ / _____
17. without, or absence of, speech: a/ _____
18. white blood condition: leuk/ _____
19. deficiency in red (blood) cells: erythr/ _____ / _____
20. measuring the pelvis: pelv/i/ _____

✓ Check your answers in Appendix A. Review any material that you did not answer correctly.

CORRECT ANSWERS _____ × 5 = _____ **% SCORE**

Learning Activity 2-5

Building pathological and related words

Use the meanings in the right column to complete the pathological and related words in the left column.

Incomplete Word	Meaning
1. bronchi _ _ _ _ _ _ _	dilation of a bronchus
2. chole _ _ _ _	gallstone
3. carcin/o/ _ _ _ _ _ _ _	forming or producing cancer
4. oste/_/ _ _ _ _ _ _ _	softening of bone
5. hepat/_/ _ _ _ _ _ _	enlargement of the liver
6. cholelith _ _ _ _ _	abnormal condition of gallstones
7. hepat/_/ _ _ _ _	herniation of the liver
8. neur/o/ _ _ _ _ _	disease of the nerves
9. dermat _ _ _ _	abnormal condition of the skin
10. hemi _ _ _ _ _ _	paralysis of one half of the body
11. dys _ _ _ _ _ _	difficult swallowing
12. a _ _ _ _ _ _	without speech or absence of speech
13. cephal _ _ _ _ _	pain in the head; headache
14. blephar/_/ _ _ _ _ _	twitching of the eyelid
15. hyper _ _ _ _ _ _	excessive formation (of an organ or tissue)

✓ Check your answers in Appendix A. Review any material that you did not answer correctly.

CORRECT ANSWERS _ _ _ _ × **6.67 =** _ _ _ _ **% SCORE**

Learning Activity 2–6

Selecting adjective, noun, and diminutive suffixes

Use the adjective suffixes in the following list to create a medical word. The first one is completed for you. Note: When in doubt about the validity of a word, refer to a medical dictionary.

-ac	-ary	-ic	-tic
-al	-eal	-ous	-tix

Element	Medical Term	Meaning
1. thorac/	*thoracic*	pertaining to the chest
2. gastr/	_____	pertaining to the stomach
3. bacteri/	_____	pertaining to bacteria
4. aqua/	_____	pertaining to water
5. axill/	_____	pertaining to the armpit
6. cardi/	_____	pertaining to the heart
7. spin/	_____	pertaining to the spine
8. membran/	_____	pertaining to a membrane

Use the noun suffixes in the following list to create a medical word.

-er	-ism
-ia	-ist
-is	-y

Element	Medical Term	Meaning
9. intern/	_____	specialist in internal medicine
10. leuk/em/	_____	condition of "white" blood
11. sigmoid/o/scop/	_____	visual examination of the sigmoid colon
12. alcohol/	_____	condition of (excessive) alcohol
13. senil/	_____	condition associated with aging
14. allerg/	_____	specialist in treating allergic disorders
15. man/	_____	condition of madness

Use the diminutive suffixes in the following list to create a medical word.

-icle	-ole	-ule

Element	Medical Term	Meaning
16. arteri/	_____	minute artery
17. ventr/	_____	small cavity
18. ven/	_____	small vein

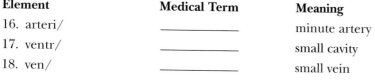

Check your answers in Appendix A. Review any material that you did not answer correctly.

CORRECT ANSWERS _____ **× 5.6 =** _____ **% SCORE**

Learning Activity 2–7

Forming plural words

Review the guidelines for plural suffixes (located inside the back cover of this book). Then write the plural form for each of the following singular terms and briefly state the rule that applies. The first one is completed for you.

Singular	Plural	Rule
1. diagnosis	*diagnoses*	*Drop the* is *and add* es.
2. fornix		
3. vertebra		
4. keratosis		
5. bronchus		
6. spermatozoon		
7. septum		
8. coccus		
9. ganglion		
10. prognosis		
11. thrombus		
12. appendix		
13. bacterium		
14. testis		
15. nevus		

✓ Check your answers in Appendix A. Review any material that you did not answer correctly.

CORRECT ANSWERS _____ × 6.67 = _____ **% SCORE**

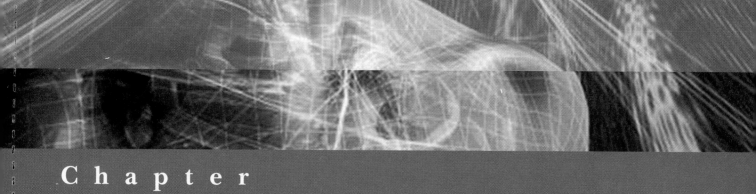

Chapter

3

Prefixes

CHAPTER OUTLINE

OBJECTIVES

Upon completion of this chapter, you will be able to:

- Explain the use of prefixes in medical terminology.
- Explain how a prefix changes the meaning of a medical word.
- Identify prefixes of position, number and measurement, and direction.
- Demonstrate your knowledge of this chapter by completing the learning activities.

Prefix Linking

Most medical words contain a root, or combining form, and a suffix. Some of them also contain prefixes. A prefix is a word element located at the beginning of a word. Substituting one prefix for another alters the meaning of the word. For example, in the term *macro/cyte*, *macro-* is a prefix meaning *large*; *-cyte* is a suffix meaning cell. A *macrocyte* is a large cell. By changing the prefix *macro-* to *micro-* (small), the meaning of the word changes. A *microcyte* is a small cell. See Table 3–1 for three other examples of how a prefix can change the meaning of a word.

Table 3–1   CHANGING PREFIXES AND MEANINGS

In this table, each word has the same root, *nat* (birth). By substituting different prefixes, a new word with a different meaning is formed.

Prefix	+	Word Root	+	Suffix	=	Medical Word	Meaning
pre- (before)	+	*nat* (birth)	+	*-al* (pertaining to, relating to)	=	prenatal prē-NĀ-tăl	pertaining to (the period) before birth
peri- (around)	+	*nat* (birth)	+	*-al* (pertaining to, relating to)	=	perinatal pĕr-ĭ-NĀ-tăl	pertaining to (the period) around birth
post- (after)	+	*nat* (birth)	+	*-al* (pertaining to, relating to)	=	postnatal pōst-NĀ-tăl	pertaining to (the period) after birth

Prefix Types

Learning the major types of prefixes, such as prefixes of position, number and measurement, and direction, as well as some others, will help you master medical terminology.

Prefixes of Position, Number and Measurement, and Direction

Prefixes are used in medical terms to denote position, number and measurement, and direction. Prefixes of position describe a place or location. (See Table 3–2.) Prefixes of number and measurement describe an amount, size, or degree of involvement. (See Table 3–3.) Prefixes of direction indicate a pathway or route. (See Table 3–4.)

Table 3–2   PREFIXES OF POSITION

This table lists commonly used prefixes of position along with their meanings and word analyses.

Prefix	Meaning	Word Analysis
epi-	above, upon	epi/derm/is (ĕp-ĭ-DĔR-mĭs): outermost layer of the skin *derm:* skin *-is:* noun ending

Table 3–2	**PREFIXES OF POSITION**	

Prefix	Meaning	Word Analysis
hypo-	under, below, deficient	hypo/derm/ic (hī-pō-DĔR-mĭk): under or inserted under the skin, as in a hypodermic injection *derm:* skin *-ic:* pertaining to, relating to
infra-	under, below	infra/cost/al (ĭn-fră-KŎS-tăl): below the ribs *cost:* ribs *-al:* pertaining to, relating to
sub-		sub/nas/al (sŭb-NĀ-săl): under the nose *nas:* nose *-al:* pertaining to, relating to
inter-	between	inter/cost/al (ĭn-tĕr-KŎS-tăl): between the ribs *cost:* ribs *-al:* pertaining to, relating to
post-	after, behind	post/nat/al (pōst-NĀ-tăl): pertaining to (the period) after birth *nat:* birth
pre-	before, in front of	pre/nat/al (prē-NĀ-tăl): pertaining to (the period) before birth *nat:* birth *-al:* pertaining to, relating to
pro-		pro/gnosis (prŏg-NŌ-sĭs): prediction of the course and end of a disease, and the estimated chance of recovery *-gnosis:* knowing
retro-	backward, behind	retro/version (rĕt-rō-VĔR-shŭn): tipping backward of an organ (such as the uterus) from its normal position *-version:* turning

Table 3–3	**PREFIXES OF NUMBER AND MEASUREMENT**	

This table lists commonly used prefixes of number and measurement along with their meanings and word analyses.

Prefix	Meaning	Word Analysis
bi-	two	bi/later/al (bī-LĂT-ĕr-ăl): pertaining to, affecting, or relating to two sides *later:* side, to one side *-al:* pertaining to, relating to
dipl-	double	dipl/opia (dĭp-LŌ-pē-ă): double vision *-opia:* vision
diplo-		diplo/bacteri/al (dĭp-lō-băk-TĒ-rē-ăl): bacterial cells linked together in pairs *bacteri:* bacteria *-al:* pertaining to, relating to
hemi-	one half	hemi/plegia (hĕm-ē-PLĒ-jē-ă): paralysis of one side of the body *-plegia:* paralysis

(Continued)

Table 3-3	PREFIXES OF NUMBER AND MEASUREMENT *(Continued)*

Prefix	Meaning	Word Analysis
hyper-	excessive, above normal	hyper/calc/emia (hī-pĕr-kăl-SĒ-mē-ă): excessive concentration of calcium in the blood *calc:* calcium *-emia:* blood condition
macro-	large	macro/cyte (MĂK-rō-sīt): abnormally large erythrocyte, such as those found in pernicious anemia *-cyte:* cell *An erythrocyte is a red blood cell.*
micro-	small	micro/scope (MĪ-krō-skōp): optical instrument that greatly magnifies minute objects *-scope:* instrument for examining
mono-	one	mono/chromat/ism (mŏn-ō-KRŌ-mă-tīzm): complete color blindness in which all colors are perceived as shades of gray *chromat:* color *-ism:* condition
uni-		uni/nucle/ar (ū-nĭ-NŪ-klē-ăr): having only one nucleus *nucle:* nucleus *-ar:* pertaining to, relating to
multi-	many, much	multi/gravida (mŭl-tĭ-GRĂV-ĭ-dă): woman who has been pregnant more than once *-gravida:* pregnant woman
poly-		poly/phobia (pŏl-ē-FŌ-bē-ă): abnormal fear of many things *-phobia:* fear
primi-	first	primi/gravida (prī-mĭ-GRĂV-ĭ-dă): woman during her first pregnancy *-gravida:* pregnant woman
quadri-	four	quadri/plegia (kwŏd-rĭ-PLĒ-jē-ă): paralysis of all four limbs *-plegia:* paralysis
tri-	three	tri/plegia (trī-PLĒ-jē-ă): hemiplegia with paralysis of one limb on the other side of the body *-plegia:* paralysis

Table 3-4	PREFIXES OF DIRECTION

This table lists commonly used prefixes of direction as well as their meanings and word analyses.

Prefix	Meaning	Word Analysis
ab-	from, away from	ab/duction (ăb-DŬK-shŭn): movement of a limb away from the body (See Figure 10–2.) *-duction:* act of leading, bringing, conducting
ad-	toward	ad/duction (ā-DŬK-shŭn): movement of a limb toward the axis of the body (See Figure 10–2.) *-duction:* act of leading, bringing, conducting

(Continued)

Table 3–4   PREFIXES OF DIRECTION

Prefix	Meaning	Word Analysis
circum-	around	circum/duction (sĕr-kŭm-DŬK-shŭn): movement of a part, such as an extremity, in a circular direction 　-duction: act of leading, bringing, conducting
peri-		peri/odont/al (pĕr-ē-ō-DŎN-tăl): located around a tooth 　odont: teeth 　-al: pertaining to, relating to
dia-	through, across	dia/rrhea (dī-ă-RĒ-ă): abnormally frequent discharge or flow of fluid fecal matter from the bowel 　-rrhea: discharge, flow
trans-		trans/vagin/al (trăns-VĂJ-ĭn-ăl): across or through the vagina 　vagin: vagina 　-al: pertaining to, relating to
ecto-	outside, outward	ecto/gen/ous (ĕk-TŎJ-ĕ-nŭs): originating outside the body or structure 　gen: forming, producing, origin 　-ous: pertaining to, relating to
exo-		exo/tropia (ĕks-ō-TRŌ-pē-ă): abnormal turning outward of one or both eyes 　-tropia: turning
extra-		extra/crani/al (ĕks-tră-KRĀ-nē-ăl): outside the skull 　crani: cranium (skull) 　-al: pertaining to, relating to
endo-	in, within	endo/crine (ĔN-dō-krĭn): secreting internally 　-crine: secrete *Endocrine refers to a gland that secretes directly into the bloodstream.*
intra-		intra/muscul/ar (ĭn-tră-MŬS-kū-lăr): within the muscle 　muscul: muscle 　-ar: pertaining to, relating to
para-*	near, beside; beyond	para/nas/al (păr-ă-NĀ-săl): beside the nose 　nas: nose 　-al: pertaining to, relating to
super-	upper, above	super/ior (soo-PĒ-rē-or): toward the head or upper portion of a structure 　-ior: pertaining to, relating to
supra-	above; excessive; superior	supra/pelv/ic (soo-pră-PĔL-vĭk): located above the pelvis 　pelv: pelvis 　-ic: pertaining to, relating to
ultra-	excess, beyond	ultra/son/ic (ŭl-tră-SŎN-ĭk): pertaining to sound frequencies too high to be perceived by the human ear 　son: sound 　-ic: pertaining to, relating to

**Para-* may also be used as a suffix meaning *to bear (offspring).*

Other Prefixes

Many other prefixes may also be used to change the meaning of a word. See Table 3–5 for a list of some other common prefixes.

Table 3–5   OTHER PREFIXES

This table lists other commonly used prefixes along with their meanings and word analyses.

Prefix	Meaning	Word Analysis

a-*	without, not	a/mast/ia (ā-MĂS-tē-ă): without a breast
		     mast: breast
		     -ia: condition
		 Amastia may be the result of a congenital defect, an endocrine disorder, or mastectomy.

an-**		an/esthesia (ăn-ĕs-THĒ-zē-ă): partial or complete loss of sensation with or without loss of consciousness *-esthesia*: feeling

anti-	against	anti/bacteri/al (ăn-tĭ-băk-TĒ-rē-ăl): pertaining to agents that destroy or stop the growth of bacteria
		     bacteri: bacteria
		     -al: pertaining to, relating to

contra-		contra/ception (kon-tră-SEP-shŭn): prevention of conception or impregnation *-ception*: conceiving
brady-	slow	brady/cardia (brăd-ē-KĂR-dē-ă): slow heart rate *-cardia*: heart
dys-	bad; painful; difficult	dys/tocia (dĭs-TŌ-sē-ă): difficult childbirth *-tocia*: childbirth, labor
eu-	good, normal	eu/pnea (ūp-NĒ-ă): normal breathing *-pnea*: breathing
hetero-	different	hetero/graft (HĔT-ē-rō-grăft): transplant of tissue from one species to a different species; *also called xenograft* *-graft*: transplantation
homo-	same	homo/graft (HŌ-mō-grăft): transplant of tissue between the same species; also called *allograft* *-graft*: transplantation
homeo-		homeo/plasia (hō-mē-ō-PLĀ-zē-ă): formation of new tissue similar to that already existing in a part *-plasia*: formation, growth
mal-	bad	mal/nutrition (măl-nū-TRĬ-shŭn): any disorder of nutrition

pan-	all	pan/arthr/itis (păn-ăr-THRĬ-tĭs): abnormal condition characterized by the inflammation of many joints of the body
		     arthr: joint
		     -itis: inflammation

pseudo-	false	pseudo/cyesis (soo-dō-si-Ē-sĭs): condition in which a woman believes she is pregnant when she is not *-cyesis*: pregnancy

Table 3–5   OTHER PREFIXES

Prefix	Meaning	Word Analysis
syn-*	union, together, joined	syn/dactyl/ism (sĭn-DĂK-tĭl-ĭzm): congenital anomaly characterized by the fusion of the fingers or toes *dactyl:* fingers; toes *-ism:* condition
tachy-	rapid	tachy/pnea (tăk-ĭp-NĒ-ă): abnormally rapid rate of breathing *-pnea:* breathing

*The prefix *a-* is usually used before a consonant. ** The prefix *an-* is usually used before a vowel. *** The prefix *syn-* appears as *sym-* before *b, p, ph,* or *m.*

 It is time to review prefixes by completing Learning Activities 3–1, 3–2, and 3–3.

LEARNING ACTIVITIES

The following activities provide review of the prefixes introduced in this chapter. Complete each activity and review your answers to evaluate your understanding of the chapter.

Learning Activity 3–1

Identifying and defining prefixes

Place a slash after each of the following prefixes and then define the prefix. The first one is completed for you.

Word	Definition of Prefix
1. inter/dental	*between*
2. hypodermic	
3. epidermis	
4. retroversion	
5. sublingual	
6. transvaginal	
7. infracostal	
8. postnatal	
9. quadriplegia	
10. hypercalcemia	
11. primigravida	
12. microscope	

13. t r i p l e g i a   _____

14. p o l y d i p s i a   _____

15. a b d u c t i o n   _____

16. a n e s t h e s i a   _____

17. m a c r o c y t e   _____

18. i n t r a m u s c u l a r   _____

19. s u p r a p e l v i c   _____

20. d i a r r h e a   _____

21. c i r c u m d u c t i o n   _____

22. a d d u c t i o n   _____

23. p e r i o d o n t a l   _____

24. b r a d y c a r d i a   _____

25. t a c h y p n e a   _____

26. d y s t o c i a   _____

27. e u p n e a   _____

28. h e t e r o g r a f t   _____

29. m a l n u t r i t i o n   _____

30. p s e u d o c y e s i s   _____

Check your answers in Appendix A. Review any material that you did not answer correctly.

CORRECT ANSWERS _____ × **3.34 =** _____ **% SCORE**

Learning Activity 3–2

Matching prefixes of position, number and measurement, and direction

Match the following terms with the definitions in the numbered list.

diarrhea	*macrocyte*	*pseudocyesis*
ectogenous	*periodontal*	*quadriplegia*
hemiplegia	*polyphobia*	*retroversion*
hypodermic	*postoperative*	*subnasal*
intercostal	*prenatal*	*suprarenal*

1. _____ tipping back of an organ

2. _____ pertaining to under the skin

3. _____ before birth

4. _____ pertaining to under the nose

5. _____ after surgery

6. _____ pertaining to between the ribs

7. _____ false pregnancy

8. _____ pertaining to around the teeth

9. _____ _____ flow through (watery bowel movement)
10. _____ pertaining to an origin outside (the body or structure)
11. _____ above the kidney
12. _____ paralysis of one half (of the body)
13. _____ paralysis of four (limbs)
14. _____ abnormally large (blood cell)
15. _____ many fears

✓ Check your answers in Appendix A. Review any material that you did not answer correctly.

CORRECT ANSWERS _____ × 6.67 = _____ **% SCORE**

Learning Activity 3–3

Matching other prefixes

Match the following terms with the definitions in the numbered list.

amastia	*dyspepsia*	*homosexual*
anesthesia	*dystocia*	*malnutrition*
antibacterial	*eupnea*	*panarthritis*
bradycardia	*heterosexual*	*syndactylism*
contraception	*homograft*	*tachycardia*

1. _____ difficult digestion
2. _____ pertaining to a different (opposite) sex
3. _____ inflammation of many joints of the body
4. _____ against bacteria
5. _____ slow heartbeat
6. _____ poor or bad nutrition
7. _____ without a breast
8. _____ without sensation
9. _____ good or normal breathing
10. _____ condition of fusion of fingers and toes
11. _____ rapid heartbeat
12. _____ against conception
13. _____ pertaining to the same sex
14. _____ difficult childbirth
15. _____ transplant (of tissue between the) same (species)

✓ Check your answers in Appendix A. Review any material that you did not answer correctly.

CORRECT ANSWERS _____ × 6.67 = _____ **% SCORE**

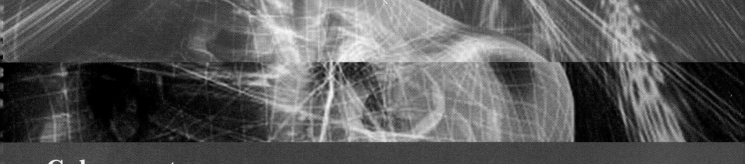

Chapter

4

Body Structure

OBJECTIVES

Upon completion of this chapter, you will be able to:

- Understand and identify levels of organization and anatomical planes of the body.
- Identify the cavities, quadrants, and regions of the body.

39

- Understand the terms related to direction, position, and planes of the body.
- Recognize, pronounce, spell, and build words related to body structure and identify common abbreviations.
- Describe diagnostic and therapeutic procedures and other terms associated with body structure.
- Demonstrate your knowledge of this chapter by completing the learning and medical record activities.

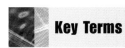 **Key Terms**

This section introduces important body structure terms and their definitions. Word analyses are also provided.

Term	Definition
cytoplasm SĪ-tō-plăzm *cyt/o:* cell *-plasm:* formation, growth	Gel-like substance that surrounds the nucleus of a cell but is contained within the cell membrane *The cytoplasm contains structures, called organelles, which carry out the essential functions of the cell.*
deoxyribonucleic acid (DNA) dē-ok-sē-ri-bō-noo-KLĒ-ĭk ĂS-ĭd	Molecule that holds genetic information and makes an exact copy of itself whenever the cell divides
diagnosis dī-ăg-NŌ-sĭs *dia-:* through, across *-gnosis:* knowing	Identification of a disease or condition by scientific evaluation of physical signs, symptoms, history, laboratory and clinical test results, and radiographic procedures
endoscope ĔN-dō-skōp *endo-:* in, within *-scope:* instrument for examining	Instrument consisting of a rigid or flexible fiberoptic tube and optical system for observing the inside of a hollow organ or cavity *Most endoscopes consist of an elongated probe fitted with a light and camera.*
etiology ē-tē-ŎL-ō-jē *eti/o:* cause *-logy:* study of	Study of the causes of disease
fluoroscope FLOO-or-ō-skōp *fluor/o:* luminous, fluorescent *-scope:* instrument for examining	Instrument, consisting of an x-ray machine and a fluorescent screen, used to view the internal organs of the body *The patient stands between the x-ray machine and the fluorescent screen, and as radiation passes through the body it produces an image. Although the regular x-ray film shows more detail, fluoroscopy is preferable when live images and movement of internal organs are required.*

Term	Definition
idiopathic ĭd-ē-ō-PĂTH-ĭk *idi/o:* unknown, peculiar *path:* disease *-ic:* pertaining to, relating to	Pertaining to conditions without clear pathogenesis, or disease without recognizable cause, as of spontaneous origin
metabolism mĕ-TĂB-ō-lĭzm	Chemical changes that take place in a cell or an organism and produce energy and basic materials needed for all life processes
prognosis prŏg-NŌ-sĭs *pro-:* before, in front of *-gnosis:* knowing	Prediction of the course and end of a disease and the estimated chance of recovery
sign SĪN	Any objective evidence or manifestation of an illness or a disordered function of the body
symptom SĬM-tŭm	Any change in the body or its functions as perceived by the patient

Introduction

This chapter provides the basic foundation for understanding the body system chapters that follow. It presents the basic structural and functional organization of the body—from the cellular level to the organism level. It also introduces terms used to describe planes of the body, body cavities, divisions of the spinal column, and quadrants and regions of the abdominal cavity. Such terms are an essential part of medical terminology and are relevant to all body systems. Pathology is also covered, as well as the terminology associated with the disease process. Finally, this chapter presents and describes terms associated with diagnostic and therapeutic procedures.

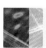

Levels of Organization

The body is composed of several levels of structure and function. Each of these levels incorporates the previous level, and contributes to the structure and function of the entire organism. The levels of organization from simplest to most complex are:

- cell
- tissue
- organ
- system
- organism

Cell

The study of the body at the cellular level is called *cytology*. The cell is the structural and functional unit of life. Body cells perform all activities associated with life, including obtaining nourishment, eliminating waste, and reproducing. Cells are composed of:

- cell membrane
- cytoplasm
- nucleus

Cell Membrane and Cytoplasm

The cell membrane acts as a barrier that encloses the entire cell. It regulates the transport of a multitude of substances to and from the cell. Within the cell membrane is a gelatinous matrix of proteins, salts, water, dissolved gases, and nutrients called **cytoplasm.** Embedded in cytoplasm are various structures called *organelles* that provide specialized functions for the cell.

Nucleus

The nucleus is responsible for metabolism, growth, and reproduction. It also carries the genetic blueprint of the organism. This blueprint is contained in a complex molecule called **deoxyribonucleic acid (DNA)** that is organized into chromatin. When the cell is ready to divide, chromatin forms chromosomes upon which approximately 31,000 genes are located. Each gene determines a unique human characteristic. Genes transmit biological information from one generation to the next and include such diverse traits as hair color, body structure, and metabolic activity. In the human, all cells except sperm cells and egg cells contain 23 pairs, or 46 chromosomes.

Tissue

The study of tissues is called *histology.* Groups of cells that perform a specialized activity are called *tissues.* Between the cells that make up tissues are varying amounts and types of nonliving, intercellular substances that provide pathways for cellular interaction. More than 200 cell types compose four major tissues of the body:

- *Epithelial tissue* covers surfaces of organs; lines cavities and canals; forms tubes, ducts, and secreting portions of glands; and makes up the epidermis of the skin. It is composed of cells arranged in a continuous sheet consisting of one or several layers.
- *Connective tissue* supports and connects other tissues and organs and is made up of diverse cell types, including fibroblasts, fat cells, and blood.
- *Muscle tissue* provides the contractile tissue of the body, which is responsible for movement.
- *Nervous tissue* transmits electrical impulses.

Organ

Organs are body structures composed of at least two or more tissue types that perform specialized functions. For example, the stomach is composed of muscle tissue, epithelial tissue, and nervous tissue. Muscle and connective tissue forms the wall of the stomach. Epithelial and connective tissue covers the internal and external surfaces of the stomach. Nervous tissue penetrates both the muscular wall and its epithelial lining to provide stimulation for the release of digestive juices and contraction of muscles in the stomach wall for digestion.

System

A body system is composed of varying numbers of organs and accessory structures that have similar or interrelated functions. For example, some of the organs of the gastrointestinal system include the esophagus, stomach, and small intestine. Some of its accessory structures include the liver, gallbladder, and pancreas. The purpose of this system is to digest food, extract nutrients from it, and eliminate waste products. Other body systems include the reproductive, respiratory, urinary, and cardiovascular systems.

Organism

The highest level of organization is the organism. An organism is a complete living entity capable of independent existence. All complex organisms, including humans, are composed of several body systems that work together to sustain life.

 ## Anatomical Position

The *anatomical position* is a body posture used as a reference when describing anatomical parts in relation to each other. In this position, the body is erect and the eyes are looking forward. The upper limbs hang to the sides, with the palms facing forward; the lower limbs are parallel, with the toes pointing straight ahead. Regardless how the body being examined or described is positioned—standing or reclining, facing forward or backward—or how the limbs are actually placed, the positions and relationships of a structure are always described as if the body were in the anatomical position. (See Figure 4–1.)

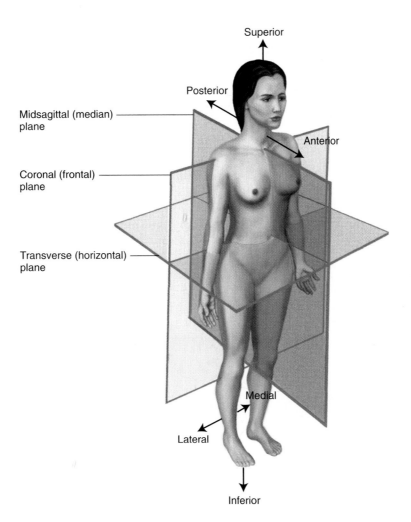

Figure 4–1   Body planes. Note that the body is in the anatomical position.

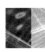

Planes of the Body

To identify various sections of the body, anatomists use an imaginary flat surface called a *plane*. Prior to the development of modern imaging techniques, conventional x-ray images were taken only on a single plane, and many body abnormalities were difficult, if not impossible, to visualize. Current imaging procedures, such as magnetic resonance imaging (MRI) and computed tomography (CT), produce three-dimensional images on more than one plane. Thus, structural abnormalities and body masses that were previously not observable with a standard x-ray taken on a single plane are currently detected using scanning devices that produce images taken in several body planes.

The most commonly used planes are midsagittal, coronal, and transverse. (See Table 4–1.) The section is named for the plane along which it is cut. Thus, a cut along a transverse plane produces a transverse, or horizontal, section. The anatomical divisions of these body planes are illustrated in Figure 4–1. Various imaging procedures are presented in this chapter and developed more extensively in the body systems chapters.

Table 4–1   PLANES OF THE BODY

This table lists planes of the body as well as the anatomical division for each.

Plane	Anatomical Division
Midsagittal (median)	Right and left halves
Coronal (frontal)	Anterior (ventral) and posterior (dorsal) aspects
Transverse (horizontal)	Superior (upper) and inferior (lower) aspects

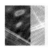

Body Cavities

The body has two major cavities: the dorsal cavity (posterior) and the ventral cavity (anterior). (See Table 4–2.) Each of these cavities has further subdivisions, as shown in Figure 4–2.

Table 4-2   BODY CAVITIES

This table lists the body cavities and some of the major organs found within them. The thoracic cavity is separated from the abdominopelvic cavity by a muscular wall called the *diaphragm*.

Cavity	Major Organ(s) in the Cavity
Dorsal	
Cranial	Brain
Spinal	Spinal cord
Ventral	
Thoracic	Heart, lungs, and associated structures
Abdominopelvic	Digestive, excretory, and reproductive organs and structures

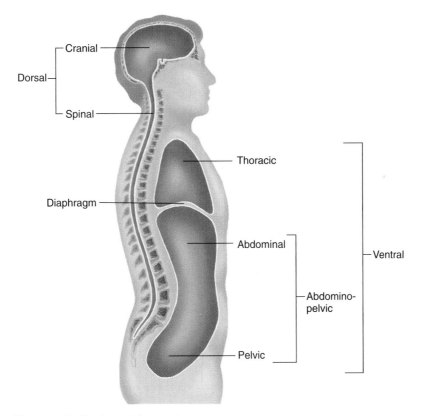

Figure 4-2   Body cavities.

Abdominopelvic Divisions

The abdominopelvic area of the body is located beneath the diaphragm. It contains the organs of digestion (abdominal area) and the organs of reproduction and excretion (pelvic area). Two anatomical methods are used to divide this area of the body for medical purposes:

- quadrants
- regions.

Quadrants

The quadrants are four divisions of the lower torso demarcated for the purpose of topographical location. They provide a means of defining specific sites for descriptive and diagnostic purposes. (See Table 4–3.) The divisions of quadrants are used in clinical examinations and medical reports. Pain, lesions, abrasions, punctures, and burns are frequently described as located in a specific quadrant. Incision sites are also identified by using body quadrants as the method of location. An imaginary cross passing through the navel identifies the four quadrants. (See Figure 4–3A.)

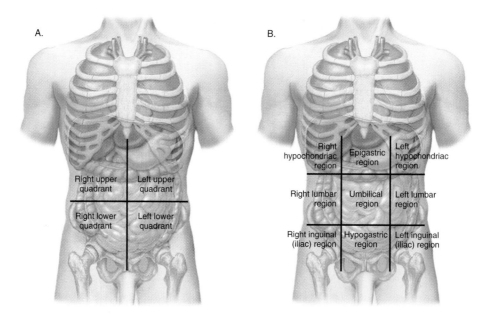

Figure 4–3 (A) Four quadrants of the abdomen. (B) Nine regions of the abdomen.

Table 4-3   BODY QUADRANTS

This table lists the quadrants of the body along with their corresponding abbreviations and identifies their major structures.

Quadrant	Abbreviation	Major Structures
Right upper	RUQ	Right lobe of liver, gallbladder, part of pancreas, part of the small and large intestines
Left upper	LUQ	Left lobe of liver, stomach, spleen, part of pancreas, part of small and large intestines
Right lower	RLQ	Part of the small and large intestines, appendix, right ovary, right fallopian tube, right ureter
Left lower	LLQ	Part of the small and large intestines, left ovary, left fallopian tube, left ureter

Regions

Whereas the quadrants of the body are used primarily to identify topographical sites, the abdominopelvic regions are used primarily to identify the location of underlying body structures and visceral organs. (See Table 4–4.) For example, the stomach is located in the left hypochondriac and epigastric region and the appendix is located in the hypogastric region. (See Figure 4–3B.)

Table 4-4   ABDOMINOPELVIC REGIONS

This table lists the names of the abdominopelvic regions and where they are located.

Region	Location
Left hypochondriac	Upper left region beneath the ribs
Epigastric	Region above the stomach
Right hypochondriac	Upper right region beneath the ribs
Left lumbar	Left middle lateral region
Umbilical	Region of the navel
Right lumbar	Right middle lateral region
Left inguinal (iliac)	Left lower lateral region
Hypogastric	Lower middle region beneath the navel
Right inguinal (iliac)	Right lower lateral region

 It is time to review the planes of the body and quadrants and regions of the abdominopelvic area by completing Learning Activities 4–1 and 4–2.

Spine

The spine is divided into sections corresponding to the vertebrae located in the spinal column. (For a more complete discussion, refer to Chapter 10, Musculoskeletal System.) These divisions are:

- cervical (neck)
- thoracic (chest)
- lumbar (loin)
- sacral (lower back)
- coccyx (tailbone).

Directional Terms

Directional terms are used to indicate the position of a structure in relation to another structure. For example, the kidneys are superior to the urinary bladder. The directional phrase *superior to* denotes *above*. This example indicates that the kidneys are located above the urinary bladder. (See Table 4–5.)

Table 4–5	DIRECTIONAL TERMS

This table lists directional terms along with their definitions. In this list, opposing terms are presented consecutively to aid memorization.

Term	Definition
Abduction	Movement away from the median plane of the body or one of its parts
Adduction	Movement toward the median plane of the body
Medial	Pertaining to the midline of the body or structure
Lateral	Pertaining to a side
Superior (cephalad)	Toward the head or upper portion of a structure
Inferior (caudal)	Away from the head, or toward the tail or lower part of a structure
Proximal	Nearer to the center (trunk of the body) or to the point of attachment to the body
Distal	Further from the center (trunk of the body) or from the point of attachment to the body
Anterior (ventral)	Near the front of the body
Posterior (dorsal)	Near the back of the body

Table 4–5   DIRECTIONAL TERMS

Term	Definition
Parietal	Pertaining to the outer wall of the body cavity
Visceral	Pertaining to the viscera, or internal organs, especially the abdominal organs
Prone	Lying horizontal with the face downward, or indicating the hand with palms turned downward
Supine	Lying on the back with the face upward, or indicating the position of the hand or foot with the palm or foot facing upward
Inversion	Turning inward or inside out
Eversion	Turning outward
Palmar	Pertaining to the palm of the hand
Plantar	Pertaining to the sole of the foot
Superficial	Toward the surface of the body
Deep	Away from the surface of the body (internal)

It is time to review body cavity, spine, and directional terms by completing Learning Activity 4–3.

Medical Word Elements

This section introduces combining forms, suffixes, and prefixes related to body structure. Word analyses are also provided.

Element	Meaning	Word Analysis
COMBINING FORMS		
Cellular Structure		
cyt/o	cell	cyt/o/logist (sĭ-TŎL-ō-jĭst): specialist in the study of the formation, structure, and function of cells *-logist:* specialist in the study of

(Continued)

Element	Meaning	Word Analysis	*(Continued)*
hist/o	tissue	hist/o/logy (hĭs-TŎL-ō-jē): study of the microscopic structures of tissues *-logy:* study of	
nucle/o	nucleus	nucle/ar (NŪ-klē-ăr): pertaining to the nucleus *-ar:* pertaining to, relating to	
kary/o		kary/o/lysis (kăr-ē-ŎL-ĭ-sĭs): destruction of the nucleus resulting in cell death *-lysis:* separation; destruction; loosening	

Position and Direction

Element	Meaning	Word Analysis	
anter/o	anterior, front	anter/ior (ăn-TĬR-ē-or): pertaining to the front of the body, organ, or structure *-ior:* pertaining to, relating to	
caud/o	tail	caud/ad (KAW-dăd): toward the tail; in a posterior direction *-ad:* toward	
crani/o	cranium (skull)	crani/al (KRĀ-nē-ăl): pertaining to the cranium *-al:* pertaining to, relating to	
dist/o	far, farthest	dist/al (DĬS-tăl): pertaining to a point further from the center (trunk of the body) or from the point of attachment to the body *-al:* pertaining to, relating to	
dors/o	back (of body)	dors/al (DOR-săl): pertaining to the back of the body *-al:* pertaining to, relating to	
infer/o	lower, below	infer/ior (ĭn-FĒ-rē-or): pertaining to the undersurface of a structure; underneath; beneath *-ior:* pertaining to, relating to	
later/o	side	later/al (LĂT-ĕr-ăl): pertaining to a side *-al:* pertaining to, relating to	
medi/o	middle	medi/ad (MĒ-dē-ăd): toward the middle or center *-ad:* toward	
poster/o	back (of body), behind, posterior	poster/ior (pŏs-TĒ-rē-or): pertaining to the back of the body *-ior:* pertaining to, relating to	

Element	Meaning	Word Analysis
proxim/o	near, nearest	proxim/al (PRŎK-sĭm-ăl): nearer to the center (trunk of the body) or to the point of attachment to the body *-al:* pertaining to, relating to
ventr/o	belly, belly side	ventr/al (VĔN-trăl): pertaining to the belly side or front of the body *-al:* pertaining to, relating to
Regions of the Body		
abdomin/o	abdomen	abdomin/al (ăb-DŎM-ĭ-năl): pertaining to the abdomen *-al:* pertaining to, relating to
cervic/o	neck; cervix uteri (neck of uterus)	cervic/al (SĔR-vĭ-kăl): pertaining to the neck *-al:* pertaining to, relating to
crani/o	cranium (skull)	crani/al (KRĀ-nē-ăl): pertaining to the cranium *-al:* pertaining to, relating to
gastr/o	stomach	hypo/gastr/ic (hī-pō-GĂS-trĭk): pertaining to beneath or below the stomach *hypo-:* under, below *-ic:* pertaining to, relating to
ili/o	ilium (lateral, flaring portion of hip bone)	ili/al (ĬL-ē-ăl): pertaining to the ilium *-al:* pertaining to, relating to
inguin/o	groin	inguin/al (ĬNG-gwĭ-năl): pertaining to the groin, the depression located between the thigh and trunk *-al:* pertaining to, relating to
lumb/o	loins, lower back	lumb/ar (LŬM-băr): pertaining to the loins, the lower back *-ar:* pertaining to, relating to
umbilic/o	navel	umbilic/al (ŭm-BĬL-ĭ-kăl): pertaining to the navel region *-al:* pertaining to, relating to
pelv/i	pelvis	pelv/i/meter* (pĕl-VĬM-ĕ-tĕr): instrument for measuring the pelvis *-meter:* instrument for measuring
pelv/o		pelv/ic (PĔL-vĭk): pertaining to the pelvis *-ic:* pertaining to, relating to

(Continued)

Element	Meaning	Word Analysis	(Continued)
spin/o	spine	spin/al (SPĪ-năl): pertaining to the spine *-al:* pertaining to, relating to	
thorac/o	chest	thorac/ic (thō-RĂS-ĭk): pertaining to the chest *-ic:* pertaining to, relating to	

Color

Element	Meaning	Word Analysis	
albin/o	white	albin/ism (ĂL-bĭn-ĭzm): partial or total lack of pigment in skin, hair, and eyes *-ism:* condition	
leuk/o		leuk/o/cyte (LOO-kō-sīt): white blood cell *-cyte:* cell	
chlor/o	green	chlor/opia (klō-RŌ-pē-ă): disorder in which viewed objects appear green *-opia:* vision *Chloropia is associated with a toxic reaction to digitalis.*	
chrom/o	color	hetero/chrom/ic (hĕt-ĕr-ō-KRŌ-mĭk): having different colors, especially of the iris or sections of the iris of both eyes *hetero-:* different *-ic:* pertaining to, relating to	
cirrh/o	yellow	cirrh/osis (sĭr-RŌ-sĭs): abnormal yellowing, especially of the skin and mucous membranes *-osis:* abnormal condition; increase (used primarily with blood cells) *Cirrhosis of the liver is usually associated with alcoholism or chronic hepatitis.*	
jaund/o		jaund/ice (JAWN-dĭs): yellow discoloration of the skin, mucous membrane, and sclera of the eye *-ice:* noun ending *Jaundice is caused by an abnormal increase of bilirubin (a yellow compound formed when red blood cells are destroyed) in the blood.*	
xanth/o		xanth/o/cyte (ZĂN-thō-sīt): cell containing yellow pigment *-cyte:* cell	
cyan/o	blue	cyan/o/tic (sī-ăn-ŎT-ĭk): pertaining to blueness, especially of the skin and mucous membranes *-tic:* pertaining to, relating to	
erythr/o	red	erythr/o/cyte (ĕ-RĬTH-rō-sīt): red blood cell *-cyte:* cell	

Element	Meaning	Word Analysis
melan/o	black	melan/oma (měl-ǎ-NŌ-mǎ): malignant tumor of melanocytes *-oma:* tumor *Melanocytes are found in the lower epidermis and are responsible for skin pigmentation.*
poli/o	gray; gray matter (of brain or spinal cord)	polio/myel/itis (pōl-ē-ō-mi-ěl-Ī-tĭs): inflammation of the gray matter of the spinal cord *myel:* bone marrow; spinal cord *-itis:* inflammation

Other

Element	Meaning	Word Analysis
acr/o	extremity	acro/o/cyan/osis (ăk-rō-sī-ǎ-NŌ-sĭs): pertaining to blueness of the extremities *cyan:* blue *-osis:* abnormal condition; increase (used primarily with blood cells)
eti/o	cause	eti/o/logy (ē-tē-ŎL-ō-jē): study of the causes of disease *-logy:* study of
fasci/o	band, fascia (fibrous membrane supporting and separating muscles)	fasci/itis (fǎs-ē-Ī-tĭs): inflammation of any fascia, the fibrous membrane that supports and separates muscles *-itis:* inflammation
idi/o	unknown, peculiar	idi/o/path/ic (ĭd-ē-ō-PĂTH-ĭk): pertaining to conditions without clear pathogenesis, or disease without recognizable cause, as of spontaneous origin *path:* disease *-ic:* pertaining to, relating to
morph/o	form, shape, structure	morph/o/logy (mor-FŎL-ō-jē): study of form, shape, and structure, especially of cells *-logy:* study of
path/o	disease	path/o/logist (pǎ-THŎL-ō-jĭst): physician specializing in examining tissues, cells, and body fluids for evidence of disease *-logist:* specialist in the study of
radi/o	radiation, x-ray; radius (lower arm bone on thumb side)	radi/o/logist (rā-dē-ŎL-ŏ-jĭst): physician specializing in imaging techniques for diagnosis and treatment of disease *-logist:* specialist in the study of

(Continued)

Element	Meaning	Word Analysis	(Continued)
somat/o	body	somat/ic (sō-MĂT-ĭk): pertaining to the body *-ic:* pertaining to, relating to	
son/o	sound	son/o/graphy (sō-NŎG-ră-fē): process of recording an image or photograph of an organ or tissue using ultrasound (inaudible sound); also called *ultrasonography* *-graphy:* process of recording *Sonography is a noninvasive imaging technique that does not use x-rays and is painless.*	
viscer/o	internal organs	viscer/al (VĬS-ĕr-ăl): pertaining to the viscera, or internal organs, in the abdominal cavity *-al:* pertaining to, relating to	
xer/o	dry	xer/osis (zē-RŌ-sĭs): abnormal dryness of the skin, mucous membranes, or conjunctiva *-osis:* abnormal condition; increase (used primarily with blood cells)	

SUFFIXES

Element	Meaning	Word Analysis	
-logy	study of	hemat/o/logy (hē-mă-TŎL-ō-jē): study of blood and its components *hemat/o:* blood	
-logist	specialist in the study of	dermat/o/logist (dĕr-mă-TŎL-ō-jĭst): physician specializing in disorders of the skin *dermat/o:* skin	
-genesis	forming, producing, origin	path/o/genesis (păth-ō-JĔN-ĕ-sĭs): source or cause of an illness or abnormal condition *path/o:* disease	
-gnosis	knowing	pro/gnosis (prŏg-NŌ-sĭs): prediction of the course and end of a disease, and the estimated chance of recovery *pro-:* before, in front of	
-gram	record, writing	arteri/o/gram (ăr-TĒ-rē-ō-grăm): record of an artery after injection of a radiopaque contrast medium *arteri/o:* artery	
-graph	instrument for recording	radi/o/graph (RĀ-dē-ō-grăf): film on which an image is produced through exposure to x-rays *radi/o:* radiation, x-rays; radius (lower arm bone on thumb side)	

Element	Meaning	Word Analysis
-graphy	process of recording	arthr/o/graphy (ăr-THRŎG-ră-fē): process of obtaining an image of a joint after injection of a radiopaque contrast medium *arthr/o:* joint
-meter	instrument for measuring	therm/o/meter (thěr-MŎM-ě-těr): instrument used for measuring heat *therm/o:* heat
-metry	act of measuring	ventricul/o/metry (věn-trĭk-ū-LŎM-ě-trē): measurement of the intraventricular cerebral pressure *ventricul/o:* ventricle (of heart or brain)
-pathy	disease	gastr/o/pathy (găs-TRŎP-ă-thē): any disease of the stomach *gastr/o:* stomach

PREFIXES

Element	Meaning	Word Analysis
ab-	from, away from	ab/duction (ăb-DŬK-shŭn): movement of a limb away from the body *-duction:* act of leading, bringing, conducting
ad-	toward	ad/duction (ă-DŬK-shŭn): movement of a limb toward the axis of the body *-duction:* act of leading, bringing, conducting
infra-	below, under	infra/cost/al (ĭn-fră-KŎS-tăl): pertaining to the area below the ribs *cost:* ribs *-al:* pertaining to, relating to
hetero-	different	hetero/morph/ous (hět-ěr-ō-MOR-fŭs): deviating from a normal type or shape *morph:* form, shape, structure *-ous:* pertaining to, relating to
homeo-	same, alike	homeo/stasis (hō-mē-ō-STĀ-sĭs): relative equilibrium in the internal environment of the body *-stasis:* standing still
peri-	around	peri/cardi/al (pěr-ĭ-KĂR-dē-ăl): pertaining to the area around the heart *cardi:* heart *-al:* pertaining to, relating to

(Continued)

Element	Meaning	Word Analysis	(Continued)
super-	upper, above	super/ior (soo-PĒ-rē-or): pertaining to the head or upper portion of a structure *-ior:* pertaining to, relating to	
trans-	across, through	trans/abdomin/al (trăns-ăb-DŎM-ĭ-năl): across the abdomen *abdomin:* abdomen *-al:* pertaining to, relating to	
ultra-	excess, beyond	ultra/son/ic (ŭl-tră-SŎN-ĭk): pertaining to sound frequencies too high to be perceived by the human ear *son:* sound *-ic:* pertaining to, relating to	

*The *i* in *pelv/i/meter* is an exception to the rule of using the connecting vowel *o.*

 It is time to review medical word elements by completing Learning Activity 4–4.

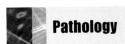

Pathology

All body cells require oxygen and nutrients for survival. They also need a stable internal environment that provides a narrow range of temperature, water, acidity, and salt concentration. This stable internal environment is called *homeostasis.* When homeostasis is significantly interrupted and cells, tissues, organs, or systems are unable to meet the challenges of everyday life, the condition is called *disease.* From a clinical point of view, disease is a *pathological* or *morbid* condition that presents a group of signs, symptoms, and clinical findings. *Signs* are objective indicators that are observable by others. A palpable mass and tissue redness are examples of signs. A *symptom* is subjective and is experienced only by the patient. Dizziness, pain, and malaise are examples of symptoms. Clinical findings are results of diagnostic and other tests performed on the patient.

Etiology is the study of the cause or origin of a disease or disorder. Here are some possible causes of disease with examples:

- metabolic (diabetes)
- infectious (measles, mumps)
- congenital (cleft lip)
- hereditary (hemophilia)
- environmental (burns, trauma)
- neoplastic (cancer).

Establishing the cause and nature of a disease is referred to as **diagnosis.** Determining a diagnosis helps in the selection of a treatment. A **prognosis** is the prediction of the course of a disease and its probable outcome. Any disease whose cause is unknown is said to be **idiopathic.** A variety of diagnostic procedures are used to identify a specific disease and determine its extent or involvement. Diagnostic tests can be uncomplicated, such as listening to chest sounds with a stethoscope, or complex, such as a biopsy. Many of the diagnostic tests listed in this text can be categorized as surgical, clinical, endoscopic, laboratory, and radiologic. Some of these tests include more than one testing modality.

Diagnostic, Symptomatic, and Related Terms

This section introduces diagnostic, symptomatic, and related terms and their meanings. Word analyses for selected terms are also provided.

Term	Definition
adhesion ăd-HĒ-zhŭn	Abnormal fibrous band that holds normally separated tissues together, usually occurring within a body cavity
analyte ĂN-ă-līt	Substance being analyzed or tested, generally by means of a chemical
contrast medium KŎN-trăst MĒD-ē-ŭm	In radiology, a substance that is injected into the body, introduced via catheter, or swallowed to facilitate radiographic imaging of internal structures that otherwise are difficult to visualize on x-ray films
dehiscence dē-HĬS-ĕns	Bursting open of a wound, especially a surgical abdominal wound
febrile FĒ-brĭl	Feverish; pertaining to a fever
homeostasis hō-mē-ō-STĀ-sĭs *homeo-:* same, alike *-stasis:* standing still	Relative constancy or equilibrium in the internal environment of the body, which is maintained by the ever-changing processes of feedback and regulation in response to external or internal changes *In homeostasis, such properties as temperature, acidity, and the concentrations of nutrients and wastes remain constant.*
inflammation ĭn-flă-MĀ-shŭn	Body defense against injury, infection, or allergy marked by redness, swelling, heat, pain and, sometimes, loss of function *Inflammation is one mechanism used by the body to protect against invasion by foreign organisms and to repair injured tissue.*

(Continued)

Term	Definition	(Continued)
morbid MOR-bĭd	Diseased; pertaining to a disease	
nuclear medicine NŪ-klē-ăr	Branch of medicine concerned with the use of radioactive substances for diagnosis, treatment, and research	
radiology rā-dē-ŎL-ō-jē *radi/o:* radiation, x-ray; radius (lower arm bone on thumb side) *-logy:* study of	Medical discipline concerned with the use of electromagnetic radiation, ultrasound, and imaging techniques for diagnosis and treatment of disease and injury (See Figure 4–4.)	
diagnostic dī-ăg-NŎS-tĭk *dia-:* through, across *gnos:* knowing *-tic:* pertaining to, relating to	Medical imaging using external sources of radiation to evaluate body structures and functions of organs	
interventional ĭn-tĕr-VĔN-shŭn-ăl	Use of imaging techniques in the nonsurgical treatment of various disorders, such as balloon angioplasty and cardiac catheterization	
therapeutic thĕr-ă-PŪ-tĭk *therapeut:* treatment *-ic:* pertaining to, relating to	Use of ionizing radiation in the treatment of malignant tumors; also called *radiation oncology*	
radionuclides rā-dē-ō-NŪ-klĭd	Substances that emit radiation spontaneously; also called *tracers* *The quantity and duration of radioactive material used in these tests are safe for humans and should not have harmful effect.*	
radiopharmaceutical rā-dē-ō-fărm-ă-SŪ-tĭ-kăl	Radionuclide attached to a protein, sugar, or other substance that travels to the organ or area of the body that will be scanned	
scan SKĂN	Term used to describe a computerized image by modality (such as computed tomography, magnetic resonance, and nuclear) or by structure (such as thyroid and bone)	
sepsis SĔP-sĭs	Pathological state, usually febrile, resulting from the presence of microorganisms or their products in the bloodstream	
suppurative SŬP-ū-rā-tĭv	Producing or associated with generation of pus	

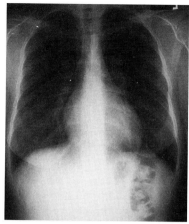

(A) Radiographic film. From McKinnis, L: *Fundamentals of Orthopedic Radiology,* page 149. F.A. Davis, 1997, with permission.

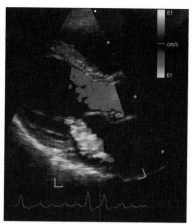

(B) Ultrasonography (Courtesy of Suzanne Wambold, PhD, University of Toledo).

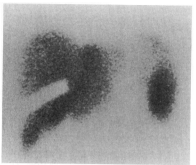

(C) Nuclear scan. From Pittiglio, DH, and Sacher, RA: *Clinical Hematology and Fundamentals of Hemostasis,* page 302, F.A. Davis, 1987, with permission.

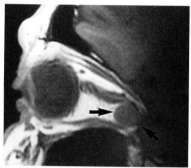

(D) CT scan. From Mazziotta, JC, and Gilman, S: *Clinical Brain Imaging: Principles and Applications,* page 27. Oxford University Press, 1992, with permission.

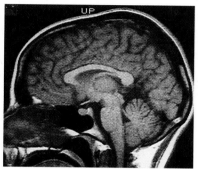

(E) MRI scan. From Mazziotta, JC, and Gilman, S: *Clinical Brain Imaging: Principles and Applications,* page 298. Oxford University Press, 1992, with permission.

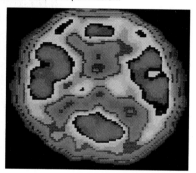

(F) PET scan of brain. From Mazziotta, JC, and Gilman, S: *Clinical Brain Imaging: Principles and Applications,* page 298. Oxford University Press, 1992, with permission.

Figure 4–4   Medical imaging.

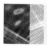 **Diagnostic and Therapeutic Procedures**

This section introduces procedures used to diagnose and treat a variety of disorders. Specific examples of these procedures are found in the body systems chapters. Descriptions are provided as well as pronunciations and word analyses for selected terms.

Procedure	Description
DIAGNOSTIC PROCEDURES	
Endoscopic	
endoscopy ĕn-DŎS-kō-pē *endo-:* in, within *-scopy:* visual examination	Visual examination of a cavity or canal using a specialized lighted instrument called an *endoscope* *Endoscopy is used for biopsy, surgery, aspirating fluids, and coagulating bleeding areas. The organ, cavity, or canal being examined dictates the name of the endoscopic procedure. (See Figure 4–5.) A camera and video recorder are commonly used during the procedure to provide a permanent record.*

(Continued)

Procedure	Description	(Continued)
laparoscopy lăp-ăr-ŎS-kō-pē *lapar/o:* abdomen *-scopy:* visual examination	Visual examination of the organs of the pelvis and abdomen through very small incisions in the abdominal wall	
thoracoscopy thor-ă-KŎS-kŏ-pē *thorac/o:* chest *-scopy:* visual examination	Examination of the lungs, pleura, and pleural space with a scope inserted through a small incision between the ribs *Thoracoscopy is an endoscopic procedure usually performed for lung biopsy, repairing perforations in the lungs, and diagnosing pleural disease.*	

Laboratory

complete blood count	Common blood test that enumerates red blood cells, white blood cells, and platelets; measures hemoglobin (the oxygen-carrying molecule in red blood cells); estimates red cell volume; and sorts white blood cells into five subtypes with their percentages	
urinalysis ū-rǐ-NĂL-ǐ-sǐs	Common urine test that evaluates the physical, chemical, and microscopic properties of urine	

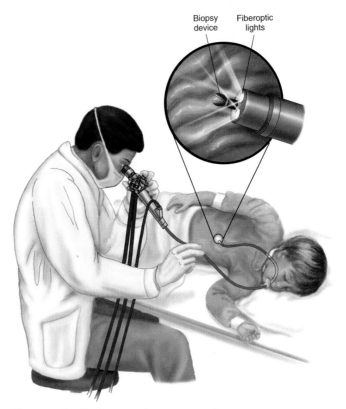

Biopsy device   Fiberoptic lights

Figure 4–5   Endoscopy (gastroscopy).

Procedure	Description
Radiographic	
computed tomography (CT) scan kŏm-PŪ-těd tō-MŎG-ră-fē *tom/o:* to cut *-graphy:* process of recording	Imaging technique achieved by rotating an x-ray emitter around the area to be scanned and measuring the intensity of transmitted rays from different angles; formerly called *computerized axial tomography* *In a CT scan, the computer generates a detailed cross-sectional image that appears as a slice. (See Figure 4–4D.) Tumor masses, bone displacement, and accumulations of fluid may be detected. During a period of two held breaths, as many as 50 continuous tomographic images can be produced in a single-slice mode. This technique may be used with or without a contrast medium.*
Doppler DŎP-lĕr	Ultrasound technique used to detect and measure blood-flow velocity and direction through the cardiac chambers, valves, and peripheral vessels by reflecting sound waves off of moving blood cells *Doppler is used to identify irregularities in blood flow through the heart and its valves as well as peripheral vascular problems, such as blood clots, venous insufficiency, and arterial blockage.*
fluoroscopy floo-or-ŎS-kō-pē *fluor/o:* luminous, fluorescent *-scopy:* visual examination	Radiographic technique in which x-rays are directed through the body to a fluorescent screen that displays continuous imaging of the motion of internal structures and immediate serial images *Fluoroscopy is used to view the motion of organs, such as the digestive tract and heart, and joints or for intervascular placement of catheters or other devices.*
magnetic resonance imaging (MRI) măg-NĔT-ĭc RĔZ-ĕn-ăns ĬM-ij-ĭng	Noninvasive imaging technique that uses radio waves and a strong magnetic field rather than an x-ray beam to produce multiplanar cross-sectional images (See Figure 4–4E.) *MRI is the method of choice for diagnosing a growing number of diseases because it provides superior soft tissue contrast, allows multiple plane views, and avoids the hazards of ionizing radiation. MRI commonly proves superior to CT scan for most central nervous system images, particularly those of the brainstem and spinal cord as well as the musculoskeletal and pelvic area. The procedure usually does not require a contrast medium.*
nuclear scan NŪ-klē-ăr	Diagnostic technique that uses a radioactive material (radiopharmaceutical) introduced into the body (inhaled, ingested, or injected) and a scanning device to determine size, shape, location, and function of various organs and structures (See Figure 4–4C.) *A nuclear scan is the reverse of a conventional radiograph. Rather than being directed into the body, radiation comes from inside the body and is then detected by the scanning device to produce an image.*

(Continued)

Procedure	Description	(Continued)
positron emission tomography (PET) PŎZ-ĭ-trŏn ē-MĬSH-ŭn tō-MŎG-ră-fē	Scan using computed tomography to record the positrons (positive charged particles) emitted from a radiopharmaceutical, producing a cross-sectional image of metabolic activity in body tissues to determine the presence of disease (See Figure 4–4F.) *PET is especially useful in scanning the brain and nervous system to diagnose disorders that involve abnormal tissue metabolism, such as schizophrenia, brain tumors, epilepsy, stroke, and Alzheimer disease as well as cardiac and pulmonary disorders.*	
radiography rā-dē-ŎG-ră-fē *radi/o:* radiation, x-ray, radius (lower arm bone on thumb side) *-graphy:* process of recording	Image produced when an x-ray is passed through the body or area and captured on a film; also called *x-ray* (See Figure 4–4A.) *On the radiograph, dense material, such as bone, appears white, and softer material, such as the stomach and liver, appears in shades of gray.*	
single photon emission computed tomography (SPECT) SĬNG-gŭl FŌ-tŏn ē-MĬ-shŭn tō-MŎG-ră-fē	Noninvasive imaging technique that provides clear, three-dimensional pictures of a major organ by injecting a radionuclide and detecting the emitted radiation using a special device called a gamma camera *A healthy organ absorbs the radionuclide at a specific rate. Overabsorption (hot spot) or underabsorption (cold spot) may be an indication of pathology.*	
tomography tō-MŎG-ră-fē *tom/o:* to cut *-graphy:* process of recording	Radiographic technique that produces an image representing a detailed cross-section or "slice" of an area, tissue, or organ at a predetermined depth *Types of tomography include computed tomography (CT), positron emission tomography (PET), and single photon emission computed tomography (SPECT).*	
ultrasonography (US) ŭl-tră-sŏn-ŎG-ră-fē *ultra-:* excess, beyond *son/o:* sound *-graphy:* process of recording	Image produced by high-frequency sound waves (ultrasound) and displaying the reflected "echoes" on a monitor; also called *ultrasound, sonography, echo,* and *echogram* (See Figure 4–4B.) *Ultrasound, unlike most other imaging methods, can create real-time moving images to view organs and functions of organs in motion. A computer analyzes the reflected echos and converts them into an image on a video monitor. Because this procedure does not use ionizing radiation (x-ray) it is used for visualizing fetuses as well as the neck, abdomen, pelvis, brain, and heart.*	

Procedure	Description
Surgical	
biopsy BĪ-ŏp-sē	Representative tissue sample removed from a body site for microscopic examination, usually to establish a diagnosis
needle	Removal of a small tissue sample for examination using a hollow needle, usually attached to a syringe
punch	Removal of a small core of tissue using a hollow instrument (punch) *An anesthetic and suturing are usually required for a punch biopsy, and minimal scarring is expected.*
shave	Removal of tissue using a surgical blade to shave elevated lesions
frozen section	Ultra-thin slice of tissue cut from a frozen specimen for immediate pathological examination *Frozen section is used for rapid diagnosis of malignancy, while the patient awaits surgery.*

THERAPEUTIC PROCEDURES

Procedure	Description
Surgical	
ablation ăb-LĀ-shŭn	Removal of a part, pathway, or function by surgery, chemical destruction, electrocautery, freezing, or radiofrequency (RF)
anastomosis ă-năs-tō-MŌ-sĭs	Surgical joining of two ducts, vessels, or bowel segments to allow flow from one to another (See Figure 4–6.)

(Continued)

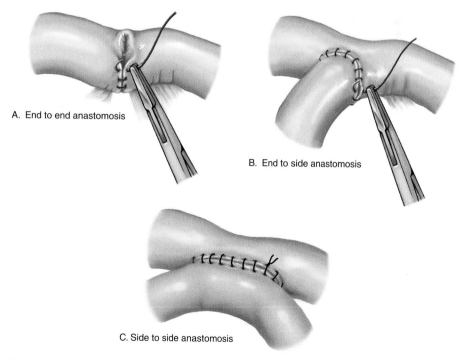

A. End to end anastomosis

B. End to side anastomosis

C. Side to side anastomosis

Figure 4–6   Anastomoses.

Procedure	Description	(Continued)
cauterize KAW-tĕr-īz	Destroy tissue by electricity, freezing, heat, or corrosive chemicals	
curettage kū-rĕ-TAZH	Scraping of a body cavity with a spoon-shaped instrument called a *curette* (curet)	
incision and drainage (I&D) ĭn-SĬZH-ŭn, DRĀN-ĭj	Incision made to allow the free flow or withdrawal of fluids from a wound or cavity	
laser surgery LĀ-zĕr SŬR-jĕr-ē	Surgical technique employing a device that emits intense heat and power at close range to cut, burn, vaporize, or destroy tissues	
radical dissection RĂD-ĭ-kăl dī-SĔK-shŭn	Surgical removal of tissue in an extensive area surrounding the surgical site in an attempt to excise all tissue that may be malignant to decrease the chance of recurrence (such as radical mastectomy)	
resection rē-SĔK-shŭn	Partial excision of a bone, organ, or other structure	

It is time to review diagnostic and therapeutic terms and procedures by completing Learning Activity 4–5.

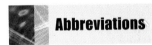

Abbreviations

This section introduces body structure abbreviations and their meanings.

Abbreviation	Meaning
ant	anterior
AP	anteroposterior
Bx, bx	biopsy
CT	computed tomography
CT scan, CAT scan	computed (axial) tomography scan

Abbreviation	Meaning
DSA	digital subtraction angiography
Dx	diagnosis
LAT, lat	lateral
LLQ	left lower quadrant
LUQ	left upper quadrant
MRI	magnetic resonance imaging
PA	posteroanterior; pernicious anemia
PET	positron emission tomography
post	posterior
RLQ	right lower quadrant
RUQ	right upper quadrant
sono	sonogram
SPECT	single photon emission computed tomography
Sx	symptom
Tx	treatment
U&L, U/L	upper and lower
US	ultrasound

LEARNING ACTIVITIES

The following activities provide review of the body structure terms introduced in this chapter. Complete each activity and review your answers to evaluate your understanding of the chapter.

Learning Activity 4–1

Identifying body planes

Label the following illustration using the terms below.

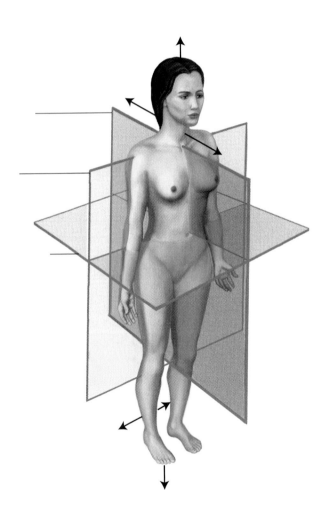

anterior	*lateral*	*posterior*
coronal (frontal) plane	*medial*	*superior*
inferior	*midsagittal (median) plane*	*transverse (horizontal) plane*

✓ Check your answers by referring to Figure 4–1 on page 43. Review material that you did not answer correctly.

Learning Activity 4–2

Identifying abdominopelvic divisions

Label the quadrants on Figure A and regions on Figure B using the terms below.

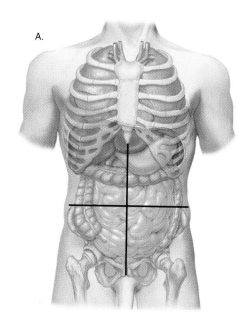

A.

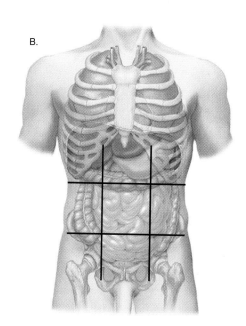

B.

epigastric region	*left lumbar region*	*right lower quadrant*
hypogastric region	*left upper quadrant*	*right lumbar region*
left hypochondriac region	*right hypochondriac region*	*right upper quadrant*
left iliac region	*right iliac region*	*umbilical region*
left lower quadrant		

✓ Check your answers by referring to Figure 4-3A and 4-3B on page 46. Review material that you did not answer correctly.

Learning Activity 4–3

Matching body cavity, spine, and directional terms

Match each term on the left with its meaning on the right.

1. _____ abdominopelvic
2. _____ adduction
3. _____ cervical

4. _____ coccyx
5. _____ deep
6. _____ eversion
7. _____ inferior (caudal)
8. _____ inversion

9. _____ lumbar
10. _____ plantar
11. _____ posterior (dorsal)
12. _____ prone

13. _____ proximal
14. _____ superficial
15. _____ thoracic

a. pertaining to the sole of the foot
b. tailbone
c. ventral cavity that contains heart, lungs, and associated structures
d. toward the surface of the body
e. lying horizontal with face downward
f. turning outward
g. nearer to the center (trunk of the body)
h. ventral cavity that contains digestive, reproductive, and excretory structures
i. turning inward or inside out
j. part of the spine known as the neck
k. movement toward the median plane
l. away from the head; toward the tail or lower part of a structure
m. away from the surface of the body; internal
n. part of the spine known as the loin
o. near the back of the body

✓ Check your answers in Appendix A. Review any material that you did not answer correctly.

CORRECT ANSWERS _____ × **6.67** = _____ **% SCORE**

Learning Activity 4–4

Matching word elements

Match the following word elements with the definitions in the numbered list.

Combining Forms		**Suffixes**	**Prefixes**
caud/o	*dist/o*	*-genesis*	*ad-*
dors/o	*eti/o*	*-gnosis*	*infra-*
hist/o	*idi/o*	*-graphy*	*ultra-*
jaund/o	*kary/o*		
leuk/o	*morph/o*		
poli/o	*somat/o*		
viscer/o	*xer/o*		

1. _____ nucleus
2. _____ far, farthest
3. _____ process of recording
4. _____ knowing
5. _____ white
6. _____ internal organs
7. _____ yellow
8. _____ tissue
9. _____ forming, producing, origin
10. _____ below, under
11. _____ excess, beyond
12. _____ tail
13. _____ back (of body)
14. _____ gray
15. _____ cause
16. _____ form, shape, structure
17. _____ dry
18. _____ unknown, peculiar
19. _____ toward
20. _____ body

Check your answers in Appendix A. Review any material that you did not answer correctly.

CORRECT ANSWERS _____ × 5 = _____ **% SCORE**

Learning Activity 4–5

Matching diagnostic and therapeutic terms and procedures

Match the following terms with the definitions in the numbered list.

ablation	*fluoroscopy*	*radionuclide*
cauterize	*morbid*	*resection*
Doppler	*nuclear scan*	*suppurative*
endoscopy	*punch biopsy*	*thoracoscopy*
febrile	*radiology*	*ultrasonography*

1. _____ medical specialty concerned with the use of electromagnetic radiation, ultrasound, and imaging techniques
2. _____ measurement of blood flow in a vessel by reflecting sound waves off moving blood cells
3. _____ image produced by using high-frequency sound waves and displaying the reflected "echoes" on a monitor

4. _____ visual examination of the lungs, pleura, and pleural space with a scope inserted through a small incision between the ribs

5. _____ excision of a core sample of tissue for examination

6. _____ visual examination of a cavity or canal using a special lighted instrument

7. _____ use of a radioactive material and scanning device to determine, size, shape, location, and function of various organs and structures

8. _____ radiographic technique that directs x-rays to a fluorescent screen and displays "live" images on a monitor

9. _____ disease, or pertaining to disease

10. _____ substance that emits radiation spontaneously; also called *tracer*

11. _____ feverish; pertaining to a fever

12. _____ partial excision of a bone, organ, or other structure

13. _____ producing or associated with generation of pus

14. _____ destruction of tissue by electricity, freezing, heat, or corrosive chemicals

15. _____ removal of a part, pathway, or function by surgery, chemical destruction, electrocautery, freezing, or radiofrequency (RF)

Check your answers in Appendix A. Review any material that you did not answer correctly.

CORRECT ANSWERS _____ × **6.67 =** _____ **% SCORE**

MEDICAL RECORD ACTIVITIES

The two medical records included in the following activities use common clinical scenarios to show how medical terminology is used to document patient care. Complete the terminology and analysis sections for each activity to help you recognize and understand terms related to body structure.

Medical Record Activity 4–1

Radiologic consultation: Cervical and lumbar spine

Terminology

The terms listed in the chart come from the medical record *Radiologic Consultation: Cervical and Lumbar Spine* that follows. Use a medical dictionary such as *Taber's Cyclopedic Medical Dictionary*, the appendices of this book, or other resources to define each term. Then review the pronunciations for each term and practice by reading the medical record aloud.

Term	Definition
AP	
atlantoaxial ăt-lăn-tō-ĂK-sē-ăl	
cervical SĔR-vĭ-kăl	
lateral LĂT-ĕr-ăl	
lumbar LŬM-băr	
lumbosacral junction lŭm-bō-SĀ-krăl	
odontoid ō-DŎN-toyd	
sacral SĀ-krăl	
scoliosis skō-lē-O-sĭs	
spasm SPĂZM	
spina bifida occulta SPĪ-nă BĬF-ĭ-dă ŏ-KŬL-tă	
vertebral bodies VĔR-tĕ-brăl	

RADIOLOGIC CONSULTATION: CERVICAL AND LUMBAR SPINE

Thank you for referring Chester Bowen to our office. Mr. Bowen presents with neck and lower back pain of more than 2 years' duration. Radiographic evaluation of June 14, 20xx, reveals the following.

AP, lateral, and odontoid views of the cervical spine demonstrate some reversal of normal cervical curvature, as seen on lateral projection. There is some right lateral scoliosis of the cervical spine. The vertebral bodies, however, appear to be well maintained in height; the intervertebral spaces are well maintained. The odontoid is visualized and appears to be intact. The atlantoaxial joint appears symmetrical.

IMPRESSION: Films of the cervical spine demonstrate some reversal of normal cervical curvature and a minimal scoliosis, possibly secondary to muscle spasm, without evidence of recent bony disease or injury. AP and lateral films of the lumbar spine, with spots of the lumbosacral junction, demonstrate an apparent minimal spina bifida occulta of the first sacral segment. The vertebral bodies, however, are well maintained in height; the intervertebral spaces appear well maintained.

PATHOLOGICAL DIAGNOSIS: Right lateral scoliosis with some reversal of normal cervical curvature.

Analysis

Review the medical record *Radiologic Consultation: Cervical and Lumbar Spine* to answer the following questions.

1. Why was the x-ray film taken of the cervical spine?

   _____

2. Did the patient appear to have experienced any type of recent injury to the spine?

   _____

3. What cervical vertebrae form the atlantoaxial joint?

   _____

4. Was the odontoid process fractured?

   _____

5. What did the radiologist believe was the possible cause of the minimal scoliosis?

   _____

Radiographic consultation: Injury of left wrist and hand

Terminology

The terms listed in the chart come from the medical record *Radiographic Consultation: Injury of Left Wrist and Hand* that follows. Use a medical dictionary such as *Taber's Cyclopedic Medical Dictionary,* the appendices of this book, or other resources to define each term. Then review the pronunciations for each term and practice by reading the medical record aloud.

Term	Definition
anterior ăn-TĬR-ē-or	
AP	
distal DĬS-tăl	
dorsal DOR-săl	
epicondyle ĕp-ĭ-KŎN-dīl	
humerus HŪ-měr-ŭs	
lucency LOO-sĕnt-sē	
medial MĒ-dē-ăl	
mm	
posterior pŏs-TĒ-rē-or	
radius RĀ-dē-ŭs	
ulna ŬL-nă	
ventral-lateral VĔN-trăl LĂT-ĕr-ăl	

RADIOGRAPHIC CONSULTATION: INJURY OF LEFT WRIST AND HAND

LEFT WRIST IMAGES: Obtained with the patient's arm taped to an arm board. There are fractures through the distal shafts of the radius and ulna. The radial fracture fragments show approximately 8 mm overlap with dorsal displacement of the distal radial fracture fragment. The distal ulnar shaft fracture shows ventral-lateral angulation at the fracture apex. There is no overriding at this fracture. No additional fracture is seen. Soft tissue deformity is present, correlating with the fracture sites.

LEFT ELBOW AND LEFT HUMERUS: Single view of the left elbow was obtained in the lateral projection. AP view of the humerus was obtained to include a portion of the elbow. A third radiograph was obtained but is not currently available for review. There is lucency through the distal humerus on the AP view along its medial aspect. It would be difficult to exclude fracture just above the medial epicondyle. On the lateral view, there is elevation of the anterior and posterior fat pad. These findings are of some concern. Repeat elbow study is recommended.

Analysis

Review the medical record *Radiographic Consultation: Injury of Left Wrist and Hand* **to answer the following questions.**

1. What is the abbreviation for anteroposterior?

   _____

2. What caused the soft tissue deformity?

   _____

3. Why was an AP view of the humerus taken?

   _____

4. Where are the left wrist fractures located?

   _____

5. Did the radiologist take any side views of the left elbow?

   _____

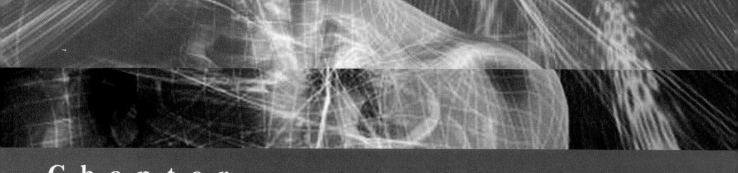

Chapter

5

Integumentary System

CHAPTER OUTLINE

OBJECTIVES

Upon completion of this chapter, you will be able to:

- Locate and describe the structures of the integumentary system.
- Recognize, pronounce, spell, and build words related to the integumentary system.
- Describe pathological conditions, diagnostic and therapeutic procedures, and other terms related to the integumentary system.
- Explain pharmacology related to the treatment of skin disorders.
- Demonstrate your knowledge of this chapter by completing the learning and medical record activities.

75

Key Terms

This section introduces important integumentary system terms and their definitions. Word analyses are also provided.

Term	Definition
adipose ĂD-ĭ-pōs *adip:* fat *-ose:* pertaining to, relating to	Fatty; pertaining to fat
androgen ĂN-drō-jĕn	Generic term for an agent, usually a hormone (testosterone) that stimulates activity of the accessory male sex organs or stimulates the development of male characteristics
dorsal DOR-săl *dors:* back (of body) *-al:* pertaining to; relating to	Indicating a position; pertaining to the back or posterior (of a structure)
ductule DŬK-tūl *duct:* to lead; carry *-ule:* small, minute	A very small duct
homeostasis hō-mē-ō-STĀ-sĭs *homeo-:* same, alike *-stasis:* standing still	Relative constancy or equilibrium in the internal environment of the body, which is maintained by the ever-changing processes of feedback and regulation in response to external or internal changes
hypodermis hi-pō-DĔR-mis *hypo-:* under, below, deficient *derm:* skin *-is:* noun ending	Subcutaneous tissue layer below the dermis
integument ĭn-TĔG-ū-mĕnt	A covering (the skin) consisting of the epidermis and dermis, or corium
systemic sĭs-TĔM-ĭk	Pertaining to the entire body rather than to one of its individual parts

Anatomy and Physiology

The integumentary system consists of the skin and its epidermal structures (integumentary glands, hair, and nails). The skin, also called *integument,* covers and protects all outer surfaces of the body and performs many vital functions. Its elaborate system of distinct tissues includes glands that produce several types of secretions, nerves that transmit impulses, and blood vessels that help regulate body temperature. (See Figure 5–1.)

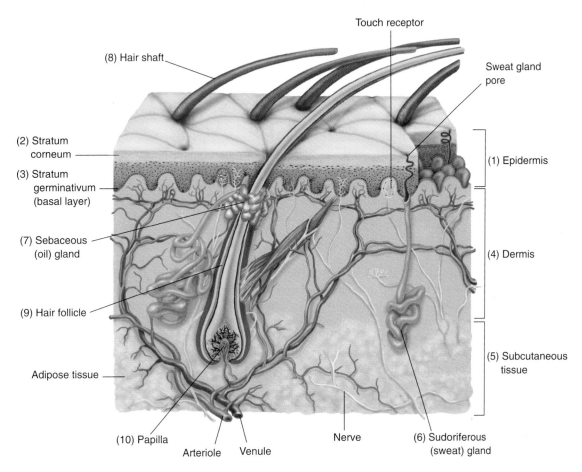

Figure 5–1 Structure of the skin and subcutaneous tissue.

Skin

The skin protects underlying structures from injury and provides sensory information to the brain. Beneath the skin's surface is an intricate network of nerve fibers that register sensations of temperature, pain, and pressure. Other important functions of the skin are protecting the body against ultraviolet rays, regulating body temperature, and preventing dehydration. The skin also acts as a reservoir for food and water and is responsible for the synthesis of vitamin D when exposed to sunlight. The skin consists of two distinct layers: the epidermis and the dermis. A subcutaneous layer of tissue binds the skin to underlying structures.

Epidermis

The outer layer, the (1) **epidermis,** is thick (comprised of five layers) on the palms of the hands and the soles of the feet but relatively thin over most other areas. Although the epidermis is composed of four or five sublayers called *strata*, the (2) **stratum corneum** and the (3) **stratum germinativum (basal layer)** are of greatest importance.

The stratum corneum is composed of dead flat cells that lack a blood supply and sensory receptors. Its thickness is correlated with normal wear of the area it covers. Only the stratum germinativum is composed of living cells and includes a basal layer where new cells are formed. As these cells move toward the stratum corneum to replace the cells that have been sloughed off, they die and become filled with a hard protein material called *keratin*. The relatively water-proof characteristic of keratin prevents body fluids from evaporating and moisture from entering the body. The entire process by which a cell forms in the basal layers, rises to the surface, becomes keratinized, and sloughs off takes about 1 month.

In the basal layer of the epidermis, specialized epithelial cells called *melanocytes* produce a dark pigment called *melanin*. Melanin filters ultraviolet radiation (light) and provides a protective barrier from the damaging effects of the sun. The number of melanocytes is about the same in all races. Differences in skin color are attributed to production of melanin. In people with dark skin, melanocytes continuously produce large amounts of melanin. In people with light skin, melanocytes produce less melanin. The activity of melanocytes is genetically regulated and, thus, inherited. Local accumulations of melanin are seen in pigmented moles and freckles. Environmental and physiological factors also play a role in skin color. An absence of pigment in the skin, eyes, and hair is most likely due to an inherited inability to produce melanin. This lack of melanin results in the condition known as *albinism*. A person with this condition is called an *albino*.

Dermis

The second layer of the skin, the (4) **dermis** (corium), lies directly beneath the epidermis. It is composed of living tissue and contains numerous capillaries, lymphatic vessels, and nerve endings. Hair follicles, sebaceous (oil) glands, and sweat glands are also located in the dermis. The **hypodermis,** or (5) **subcutaneous tissue,** is composed primarily of loose connective tissue and adipose tissue interlaced with blood vessels. It binds the dermis to underlying structures. The hypodermis stores fats, insulates and cushions the body, and regulates temperature. The amount of fat in the hypodermis varies with the region of the body and a person's sex, age, and nutritional state.

Accessory Organs of the Skin

The accessory organs of the skin consist of integumentary glands, hair, and nails. All of these structures are formed from the epidermis. The glands play an important role in body defense and maintaining homeostasis, whereas the hair and nails have more limited functional roles.

Glands

Two important glands located in the dermis produce secretions: the (6) **sudoriferous glands** produce sweat, and the (7) **sebaceous glands** produce oil. These two glands are known as *exocrine glands* because they secrete substances through ducts to an outer surface of the body rather than directly into the bloodstream.

The sudoriferous glands secrete perspiration or sweat onto the surface of the skin through pores. Pores are most plentiful on the palms, soles, forehead, and armpits (axillae). The main functions of the sudoriferous glands are to cool the body by evaporation, excrete waste products, and moisten surface cells.

The sebaceous glands are filled with cells, the centers of which contain fatty droplets. As these cells disintegrate, they yield an oily secretion called **sebum.** The acidic nature of sebum helps to destroy harmful organisms on the skin thus preventing infection. When sebaceous **ductules** become blocked, acne may result. Congested sebum causes the formation of pimples or whiteheads, and if the sebum is dark, it forms blackheads. Sex hormones, particularly **andro-**

gens, regulate the production and secretion of sebum. During adolescence, the secretions increase; as the person ages, the secretions diminish. The loss of sebum, which lubricates the skin, may be one of the reasons for the formation of wrinkles that accompany old age. Sebaceous glands are present over the entire body, except on the soles of the feet and the palms of the hands. They are especially prevalent on the scalp and face; around openings such as the nose, mouth, external ear, and anus; and on the upper back and scrotum.

Hair

Hair is found on nearly all parts of the body, except for the lips, nipples, palms of the hands, soles of the feet, and parts of the external genitalia. The visible part of the hair is the (8) **hair shaft;** the part that is embedded in the dermis is the **hair root.** The root, together with its coverings, forms the (9) **hair follicle.** At the bottom of the follicle is a loop of capillaries enclosed in a covering called the (10) **papilla.** The cluster of epithelial cells lying over the papilla reproduces and is responsible for the eventual formation of the hair shaft. As long as these cells remain alive, hair will regenerate even if it is cut, plucked, or otherwise removed. Baldness **(alopecia)** occurs when the hairs of the scalp are not replaced because of death of the papilla.

Like skin color, hair color is related to the amount of pigment produced by epidermal melanocytes. Melanocytes are found at the base of the hair follicle. Various amounts of melanin compounds of different colors (yellow, brown, and black) combine to produce hair color from blond to dark black. Both heredity and aging account for the loss of hair color due to the absence of melanin.

Nails

The nails protect the tips of the fingers and toes from bruises and injuries. (See Figure 5–2.) Each nail is formed in the (1) **nail root** and is composed of keratinized stratified squamous epithelial cells producing a very tough covering. As the nail grows, it stays attached and slides forward over the layer of epithelium called the (2) **nail bed.** This epithelial layer is continuous with the epithelium of the skin. Most of the (3) **nail body** appears pink because of the underlying vascular tissue. The half-moon shaped area at the base of the nail, the (4) **lunula,** is the region where new growth occurs. The lunula has a whitish appearance because the vascular tissue underneath does not show through.

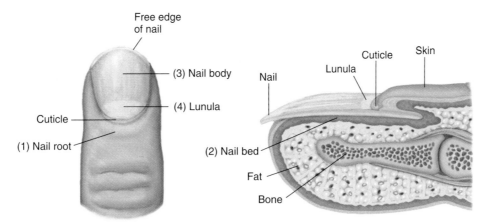

Figure 5–2   Structure of a fingernail.

 It is time to review anatomy by completing Learning Activity 5–1.

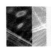 **Medical Word Elements**

This section introduces combining forms, suffixes, and prefixes related to the integumentary system. Word analyses are also provided.

Element	Meaning	Word Analysis
COMBINING FORMS		
adip/o	fat	adip/osis (ăd-ĭ-PŌ-sĭs): abnormal accumulation of fat in the body *-osis:* abnormal condition; increase (used primarily with blood cells)
lip/o		lip/o/cele (LĬP-ō-sēl): hernia containing fat or fatty tissue *-cele:* hernia, swelling
steat/o		steat/itis (stē-ă-TĪ-tĭs): inflammation of adipose (fatty) tissue *-itis:* inflammation
cutane/o	skin	sub/cutane/ous (sŭb-kū-TĀ-nē-ŭs): beneath the skin *sub-:* under, below *-ous:* pertaining to, relating to
dermat/o		dermat/o/plasty (DĔR-mă-tō-plăs-tē): plastic surgery of the skin, as in skin grafting *-plasty:* surgical repair
derm/o		hypo/derm/ic (hī-pō-DĔR-mĭk): under or inserted under the skin, as in a hypodermic injection *hypo-:* under, below *-ic:* pertaining to, relating to
hidr/o	sweat	hidr/aden/itis (hī-drăd-ĕ-NĪ-tĭs): inflammation of the sweat glands *aden:* gland *-itis:* inflammation *Do not confuse hidr/o (sweat) with hydr/o (water).*
sudor/o		sudor/esis (soo-dō-RĒ-sĭs): profuse sweating *-esis:* condition
ichthy/o	dry, scaly	ichthy/osis (ĭk-thē-Ō-sĭs): any of several dermatologic conditions in which the skin is dry and hyperkeratotic (hardened), resembling fish scales *-osis:* abnormal condition; increase (used primarily with blood cells) *A mild form called* winter itch *is commonly seen on the legs of older patients, especially during the winter months.*

Element	Meaning	Word Analysis
kerat/o	horny tissue; hard; cornea	kerat/osis (kĕr-ă-TŌ-sĭs): thickened area of the epidermis; any horny growth on the skin (such as a callus or wart) *-osis:* abnormal condition; increase (used primarily with blood cells)
melan/o	black	melan/oma (mĕl-ă-NŌ-mă): malignant tumor of melanocytes that commonly begins in a darkly pigmented mole and can metastasize widely *-oma:* tumor
myc/o	fungus (plural, fungi)	dermat/o/myc/osis (dĕr-mă-tō-mī-KŌ-sĭs): fungal infection of the skin *dermat/o:* skin *-osis:* abnormal condition; increase (used primarily with blood cells)
onych/o	nail	onych/o/malacia (ŏn-ĭ-kō-mă-LĀ-shē-ă): abnormal softening of the nails *-malacia:* softening
ungu/o		ungu/al (ŬNG-gwăl): pertaining to the nails *-al:* pertaining to, relating to
pil/o	hair	pil/o/nid/al (pī-lō-NĪ-dăl): a growth of hair in a cyst or other internal structure *nid:* nest *-al:* pertaining to, relating to *A pilonidal cyst commonly develops in the skin of the sacral region.*
trich/o		trich/o/pathy (trĭk-ŎP-ă-thē): any disease involving the hair *-pathy:* disease
scler/o	hardening; sclera (white of eye)	scler/o/derma (sklĕr-ă-DĔR-mă): chronic hardening and thickening of the skin caused by new collagen formation *-derma:* skin *Scleroderma is most common in middle-aged women and may occur in a localized form or as a systemic disease.*
seb/o	sebum, sebaceous	seb/o/rrhea (sĕb-Ō-rē-ă): excessive secretion or discharge of sebum *-rrhea:* discharge, flow *Sebum is an oil secretion of the sebaceous glands.*
squam/o	scale	squam/ous (SKWĀ-mŭs): relating to or covered with scales *-ous:* pertaining to, relating to

(Continued)

Element	Meaning	Word Analysis	(Continued)
xen/o	foreign, strange	xen/o/graft (ZEN-o-graft): surgical graft of tissue from an individual of one species to an individual of another species; also called *heterograft* *-graft:* transplantation	
xer/o	dry	xer/o/derma (zē-rō-DĔR-mă): chronic skin condition characterized by dryness and roughness *-derma:* skin *Xeroderma is a mild form of ichthyosis.*	

SUFFIXES

Element	Meaning	Word Analysis	
-cyte	cell	lip/o/cyte (LĬP-ō-sīt): fat cell *lip/o:* fat	
-derma	skin	py/o/derma (pī-ō-DĔR-mă): any pyogenic infection of the skin *py/o:* pus *Pyoderma may be primary, such as impetigo, or secondary to a previous condition.*	
-logist	specialist in the study of	dermat/o/logist (dĕr-mă-TŎL-ō-jĭst): physician specializing in treatment of skin disorders *dermat/o:* skin	
-logy	study of	dermat/o/logy (dĕr-mă-TŎL-ō-jē): study of the skin and its diseases *dermat/o:* skin	
-therapy	treatment	cry/o/therapy (krī-ō-THĔR-ă-pē): destruction of tissue by freezing with liquid nitrogen *cry/o:* cold *Cutaneous warts and actinic keratosis are common skin disorders that are responsive to cryotherapy treatment.*	

PREFIXES

Element	Meaning	Word Analysis	
an-	without, not	an/hidr/osis (ăn-hĭ-DRŌ-sĭs): diminished or complete absence of sweat *hidr:* sweat *-osis:* abnormal condition; increase (used primarily with blood cells)	
dia-	through, across	dia/phoresis (dī-ă-fă-RĒ-sĭs): condition of profuse sweating; also called *sudoresis* or *hyperhidrosis* *-phoresis:* carrying, transmission	
epi-	above, upon	epi/derm/is (ĕp-ĭ-DĔR-mĭs): outermost layer of the skin *derm:* skin *-is:* noun ending	

Element	Meaning	Word Analysis
homo-	some	homo/graft (HO-mo-graft): surgical graft of tissue from an individual of one species to an individual of the same species; also called *allograft* *-graft:* transplantation
hyper-	excessive, above normal	hyper/hidr/osis (hī-pĕr-hī-DRŌ-sĭs): excessive or profuse sweating; also called *diaphoresis* or *sudoresis* *hidr:* sweat *-osis:* abnormal condition; increase (used primarily with blood cells)
sub-	under, below	sub/ungu/al (sŭb-ŬNG-gwăl): pertaining to the area beneath the nail of a finger or toe *ungu:* nail *-al:* pertaining to, relating to

It is time to review medical word elements by completing Learning Activity 5–2.

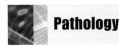

Pathology

The general appearance and condition of the skin are clinically important because they may provide clues to body conditions or dysfunctions. Pale skin may indicate shock; red, flushed, very warm skin may indicate fever and infection. A rash may indicate allergies or local infections. Even chewed fingernails may be a clue to emotional problems. For diagnosis, treatment, and management of skin disorders, the medical services of a specialist may be warranted. Dermatology is the branch of medicine concerned with skin disease, and the relationship of cutaneous lesions to **systemic** disease. The physician who specializes in the diagnosis and treatment of skin disease is known as a dermatologist.

Skin Lesions

Lesions are areas of pathologically altered tissue caused by disease, injury, or a wound due to external factors or internal disease. Evaluation of skin lesions, injuries, or changes to tissue helps establish the diagnosis of skin disorders. Lesions are described as **primary** or **secondary.** *Primary* skin lesions are the initial reaction to pathologically altered tissue and may be flat or elevated. *Secondary* skin lesions are the changes that take place in the primary lesion due to infection, scratching, trauma, or various stages of a disease. Lesions are also described by their appearance, color, location, and size as measured in centimeters. Some of the major primary and secondary skin lesions are described and illustrated in Figure 5–3.

PRIMARY LESIONS

FLAT LESIONS
Flat, discolored, circumscribed lesions of any size

Macule
Flat, pigmented, circumscribed area less than 1 cm in diameter.
Examples: freckle, flat mole, or rash that occurs in rubella.

ELEVATED LESIONS

Solid   *Fluid-filled*

Papule
Solid, elevated lesion less than 1 cm in diameter that may be the same color as the skin or pigmented.
Examples: nevus, wart, pimple, ringworm, psoriasis, eczema.

Vesicle
Elevated, circumscribed, fluid-filled lesion less than 0.5 cm in diameter.
Examples: poison ivy, shingles, chickenpox.

Nodule
Palpable, circumscribed lesion; larger and deeper than a papule (0.6 to 2 cm in diameter); extends into the dermal area.
Examples: intradermal nevus, benign or malignant tumor.

Pustule
Small, raised, circumscribed lesion that contains pus; usually less than 1 cm in diameter.
Examples: acne, furuncle, pustular psoriasis, scabies.

Tumor
Solid, elevated lesion larger than 2 cm in diameter that extends into the dermal and subcutaneous layers.
Examples: lipoma, steatoma, dermatofibroma, hemangioma.

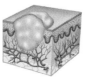

Bulla
A vesicle or blister larger than 1 cm in diameter.
Examples: second degree burns, severe poison oak, poison ivy.

Wheal
Elevated, firm, rounded lesion with localized skin edema (swelling) that varies in size, shape, and color; paler in the center than its surrounding edges; accompanied by itching.
Examples: hives, insect bites, urticaria.

SECONDARY LESIONS

DEPRESSED LESIONS
Depressed lesions caused by loss of skin surface

  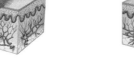

Excoriations
Linear scratch marks or traumatized abrasions of the epidermis.
Examples: scratches, abrasions, chemical or thermal burns.

Fissure
Small slit or cracklike sore that extends into the dermal layer; could be caused by continuous inflammation and drying.

Ulcer
An open sore or lesion that extends to the dermis and usually heals with scarring.
Examples: pressure sore, basal cell carcinoma.

Figure 5–3 Primary and secondary lesions.

 It is time to review skin lesions by completing Learning Activity 5–3.

Burns

Burns are tissue injuries caused by contact with thermal, chemical, electrical, or radioactive agents. Although burns generally occur on the skin, they can also involve the respiratory and digestive tract linings. Burns that have a *local* effect (local tissue destruction) are not as serious as those that have a *systemic* effect. Systemic effects are life threatening and may include dehydration, shock, and infection.

Burns are usually classified as first-, second-, or third-degree. The extent of injury and degree of severity determine a burn's classification. In *first-degree* burns, the epidermis is damaged. Symptoms are restricted to local effects, such as skin redness (erythema) and acute sensitivity to such sensory stimuli as touch, heat, or cold (hyperesthesia). A first-degree burn does not blister and heals without scar formation. Examples are damaged skin caused by sunburn or scalding with hot water. *Second-degree* burns are deep burns that damage both the epidermis and part of the dermis. They are characterized by the formation of fluid-filled blisters (vesicles or bullae), caused by the deeper penetration of heat. Second-degree burns are more painful, and recovery is usually slow but complete with no scar formation. In *third-degree* burns, both the epidermis and the dermis are destroyed and some of the underlying connective tissue is damaged, leaving the skin waxy and charred with insensitivity to touch. Because of such extensive destruction, ulcerating wounds develop and the body attempts to heal itself by forming scar tissue. Skin grafts (dermatoplasty) are frequently used to assist recovery.

An emergency method for estimating the extent of burn damage is to apply the *Rule of Nines*. This method calculates body surface involved in burns by assigning values of 9% or 18% of surface areas to specific regions. (See Figure 5–4.) Accurate estimation of damaged surface area is important for treatment with I.V. fluid, which replaces the fluids lost from tissue damage and destruction.

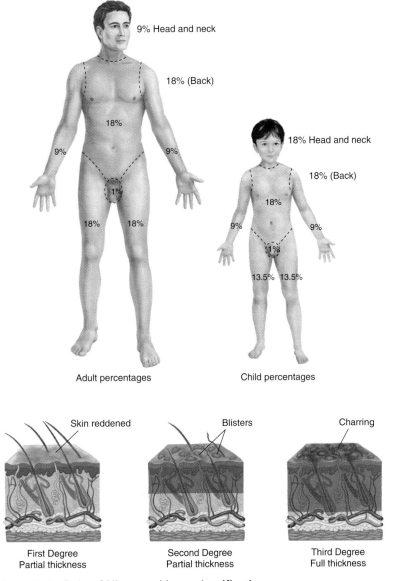

Figure 5–4 Rule of Nines and burn classification.

Oncology

Neoplasms are abnormal growths of new tissue that can be benign or malignant. *Benign* neoplasms are noncancerous growths composed of the same type of cells as the tissue in which they are growing. They harm the individual only as much as they place pressure on surrounding structures. If the benign neoplasm remains small and places no pressure on adjacent structures, it commonly is not removed. When it becomes excessively large, causes pain, or places pressure on other organs or structures, excision is necessary. *Malignant* neoplasms are composed of cancerous cells that do not necessarily resemble the tissue in which they are growing. The cells show altered function, altered appearance, and uncontrolled growth, and the malignant tumor invades the surrounding tissue. Ultimately, malignant cells break loose from the primary tumor, enter blood and lymph vessels, and travel to remote regions of the body to form secondary tumor sites, a process called *metastasis*. The ability to invade surrounding tissues and spread to remote regions of body is a distinguishing feature of malignancy. If left untreated, malignant neoplasms are usually progressive and generally fatal.

Cancer treatment includes surgery, chemotherapy, immunotherapy, and radiation therapy. Immunotherapy, also called *biotherapy*, is a recent treatment approach that stimulates the body's own immune defenses to fight tumor cells. When combined with surgery, chemotherapy, or radiation, immunotherapy may be most effective in early cancer stages.

Grading and Staging Systems

Pathologists grade and stage tumors for diagnostic and therapeutic purposes. A tumor grading system is used to evaluate the appearance and maturity of cancer cells in a tumor. Pathologists commonly describe tumors by four grades of severity based on microscopic appearance of cancer cells. (See Table 5–1.) A patient with a grade 1 tumor has the best prognosis; one with a grade 4 tumor has the worst prognosis.

The tumor, node, metastasis (TNM) system of staging is used to determine how much the cancer has spread (metastasis) within the body. The TNM system stages tumors according to three basic criteria. *T* refers to the size and extent of the primary *tumor*, *N* indicates number of area lymph *nodes* involved, *M* refers to any *metastases* of the primary tumor. A subscript number is used to indicate the size or spread of the tumor. For example, T_2 designates a small tumor; M_0 designates no metastasis. (See Table 5–2.)

Table 5–1	TUMOR GRADING

The table below defines the four tumor grades and their characteristics.

Grading	Tumor Characteristics
Grade I Tumor cells well differentiated	Close resemblance to tissue of origin, thus, retaining some specialized functions
Grade II Tumor cells moderately differentiated	Less resemblance to tissue of origin; more variation in size and shape of tumor cells; increased mitoses
Grade III Tumor cells poorly to very poorly differentiated	Does not closely resemble tissue of origin; much variation in shape and size of tumor cells; greatly increased mitoses
Grade IV Tumor cells very poorly differentiated	No resemblance to tissue of origin; great variation in size and shape of tumor cells

Table 5-2   TNM SYSTEM OF STAGING

The table below outlines the tumor, node, metastasis (TNM) system of staging, including designations, stages, and degrees of tissue involvement.

Designation	Stage	Tissue involvement
Tumor		
T_0		No evidence of primary tumor
T_{is}	Stage I	Carcinoma *in situ,* which indicates no invasion of other tissues
T_1, T_2, T_3, T_4	Stage II	Primary tumor size and extent of local invasion, where T_1 is small with minimal invasion and T_4 is large with extensive local invasion into surrounding organs and tissues
Node		
N_0		Regional lymph nodes with no abnormalities
N_1, N_2, N_3, N_4	Stage III	Degree of lymph node involvement and spread to regional lymph nodes, where N_1 is less involved with minimal spreading and N_4 is more involved with extensive spreading
Metastasis		
M_0		No evidence of metastasis
M_1	Stage IV	Indicates metastasis

The designations T_x, N_x, and M_x indicate that the tumor, node, or metastasis cannot be assessed clinically.

Basal Cell Carcinoma

Basal cell carcinoma, the most common type of skin cancer, is a malignancy of the stratum germinativum, basal cell layer of the epidermis (see Figure 5–1), or hair follicles that is commonly caused by overexposure to sunlight. (See Figure 5–5.) These tumors are locally invasive but rarely metastasize. Basal cell carcinoma is most prevalent in blond, fair-skinned men and is the most common malignant tumor affecting Caucasians. Although these tumors grow slowly, they commonly ulcerate as they increase in size and develop crusting that is firm to the touch. Metastases are uncommon with this type of cancer; however, the disease can invade the tissue sufficiently to destroy an ear, nose, or eyelid. Depending on the location, size, and depth of the lesion, treatment may include curettage and electrodesiccation, chemotherapy, surgical excision, irradiation, or chemosurgery.

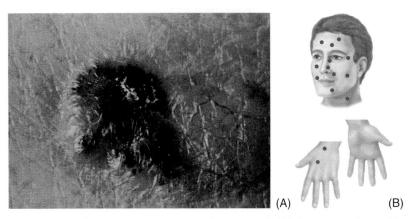

(A)   (B)

Figure 5–5   (A) Basal cell carcinoma (late stage). (B) Common sites of basal cell carcinoma. From Goldsmith, LA, Lazarus, GS, and Tharp, MD: *Adult and Pediatric Dermatology: A Color Guide to Diagnosis and Treatment*, page 144. F.A. Davis, 1997, with permission.

Squamous Cell Carcinoma

Squamous cell carcinoma of the skin arises from keratinizing epidermal cells. It is an invasive tumor with potential for metastasis and occurs most commonly in fair-skinned white men over age 60. Repeated overexposure to the sun's ultraviolet rays greatly increases the risk of squamous cell carcinoma. Other predisposing factors associated with this type of cancer include radiation therapy, chronic skin irritation and inflammation, exposure to local carcinogens (such as tar and oil), hereditary diseases (such as xeroderma pigmentosum and albinism), and the presence of premalignant lesions (such as actinic keratosis or Bowen disease).

There are two types of squamous cell carcinoma: *in situ* (confined to the original site) and *invasive*. Treatment may consist of surgical excision; curettage and electrodesiccation, which provide good cosmetic results for smaller lesions; radiation therapy, usually for older or debilitated patients; and chemotherapy, depending on the location, size, shape, degree of invasion, and condition of underlying tissue. A combination of these treatment methods may be required for a deeply invasive tumor.

Malignant Melanoma

Malignant melanoma is a neoplasm composed of abnormal melanocytes that commonly begin in a darkly pigmented mole. Although malignant melanoma is relatively rare, the incidence is rising more rapidly than any other malignancy. It is the most lethal of the skin cancers and can metastasize extensively to the liver, lungs, or brain.

Several factors may influence the development of melanoma, but the persons at greatest risk have fair complexions, blue eyes, red or blonde hair, and freckles. Excessive exposure to sunlight and severe sunburn during childhood are believed to increase the risk of melanoma in later life. Avoiding the sun and using sunscreen have proved effective in preventing the disease.

Melanomas are diagnosed by biopsy along with histologic examination. Treatment requires surgery to remove the primary cancer, along with adjuvant therapies to reduce the risk of metastasis. The extent of surgery depends on the size and location of the primary tumor and is determined by staging the disease. (See Table 5–2.)

 It is time to review burn and oncology terms by completing Learning Activity 5–4.

Diagnostic, Symptomatic, and Related Terms

This section introduces diagnostic, symptomatic, and related terms and their meanings. Word analyses for selected terms are also provided.

Term	Definition
abscess ĂB-sĕs	Walled cavity containing pus and surrounded by inflamed or necrotic tissue *If an abscess does not respond to treatment, it may require an incision to drain the purulent material.*
acne ĂK-nē	Inflammatory disease of the sebaceous glands and hair follicles of the skin
acne vulgaris	Characterized by comedones (blackheads), papules, and pustules; usually associated with seborrhea *In acne, cysts and nodules may develop and scarring is common. The face, neck, and shoulders are common sites for this condition.*
Bowen disease BŌ-ĕn dĭ-ZĒZ	Form of intraepidermal carcinoma (squamous cells) characterized by red-brown scaly or crusted lesions that resemble a patch of psoriasis or dermatitis; also called *Bowen precancerous dermatosis* *Treatment includes curettage and electrodesiccation.*
carbuncle KĂR-bŭng-kĕl	Deep-seated pyogenic infection of the skin usually involving subcutaneous tissues *A carbuncle consists of several furuncles developing in adjoining hair follicles with multiple drainage sinuses. The most common sites of these lesions are the nape of the neck, the upper back, and the buttocks. (See Figure 5–6.) See also furuncle.*

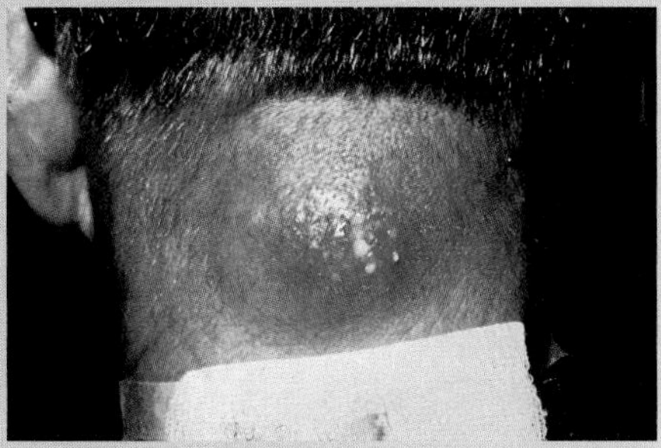

Figure 5–6 Carbuncle-furuncle. From Goldsmith, LA, Lazarus, GS, and Tharp, MD: *Adult and Pediatric Dermatology: A Color Guide to Diagnosis and Treatment,* page 364. F.A. Davis, 1997, with permission.

Term	Definition
cellulitis sĕl-ū-LĪ-tĭs	Diffuse (widespread), acute infection of the skin and subcutaneous tissue *Cellulitis is characterized by localized heat, redness, pain, swelling, and, occasionally, fever, malaise, chills, and headache.*
chloasma klō-ĂZ-mă	Pigmentary skin discoloration usually occurring in yellowish-brown patches or spots

(Continued)

Term	Definition	(Continued)
comedo KŎM-ē-dō	Typical small skin lesion of acne vulgaris caused by accumulation of keratin, bacteria, and dried sebum plugging an excretory duct of the skin *The closed form of comedo, called a* whitehead, *consists of a papule from which the contents are not easily expressed.*	
decubitus ulcer dē-KŪ-bĭ-tŭs ŬL-sĕr	Skin ulceration caused by prolonged pressure, usually in a person who is bedridden; also known as a *bedsore* *Decubitus ulcers are most commonly found in skin overlying a bony projection, such as the hip, ankle, heel, shoulder, and elbow.*	
dermatomycosis dĕr-mă-tō-mi-KŌ-sĭs *dermat/o:* skin *myc:* fungus *-osis:* abnormal condition; increase (used primarily with blood cells)	Fungal infection of the skin	
ecchymosis ĕk-ĭ-MŌ-sĭs	Skin discoloration consisting of a large, irregularly formed hemorrhagic area with colors changing from blue-black to greenish brown or yellow; commonly called a bruise (See Figure 5–7.)	

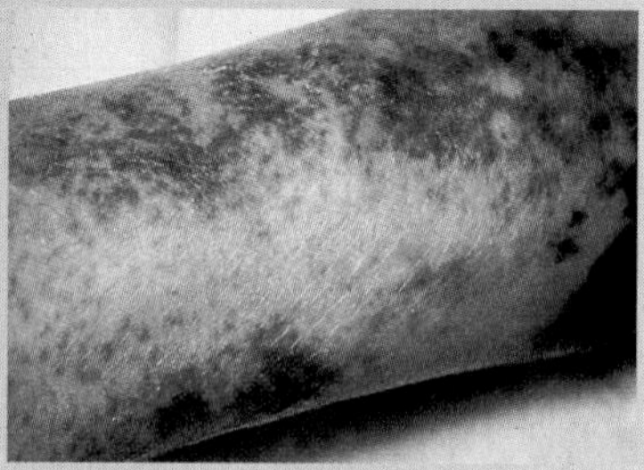

Figure 5–7 Ecchymosis. From Harmening, DM: *Clinical Hematology and Fundamentals of Hemostasis,* 4th edition, p. 489. F.A. Davis Company, 2001, with permission.

Term	Definition	
eczema ĔK-zĕ-mă	Acute or chronic skin inflammation characterized by erythema, papules, vesicles, pustules, scales, crusts, scabs and, possibly, itching *Symptoms may occur alone or in combination.*	
erythema ĕr-ĭ-THĒ-mă	Redness of the skin caused by swelling of the capillaries *An example of erythema is a mild sunburn or nervous blushing.*	
eschar ĔS-kăr	Damaged tissue following a severe burn	
furuncle FŪ-rŭng-k'l	Bacterial infection of a hair follicle or sebaceous gland that produces a pus-filled lesion commonly called a *boil* *Lesions drain a creamy pus when incised and may heal with scarring.*	
hirsutism HĔR-soot-ĭzm	Condition characterized by the excessive growth of hair or presence of hair in unusual places, especially in women	

Term	Definition
impetigo ĭm-pĕ-TĪ-gō	Inflammatory skin disease characterized by isolated pustules that become crusted and rupture
keratosis kĕr-ă-TŌ-sĭs *kerat:* horny tissue; hard; cornea *-osis:* abnormal condition; increase (used primarily with blood cells)	Thickened area of the epidermis; any horny growth on the skin (such as a callus or wart)
lentigo lĕn-TĪ-gō	Small brown macules, especially on the face and arms with lesions distributed on sun-exposed areas of the skin
pallor PĂL-or	Unnatural paleness or absence of color in the skin
pediculosis pē-dĭk-ū-LŌ-sĭs	Infestation with lice, transmitted by personal contact or common use of brushes, combs, or headgear
petechia pē-TĒ-kē-ă	Minute, pinpoint hemorrhage under the skin *A petechia is a smaller version of an ecchymosis.*
pruritus proo-RĪ-tŭs	Intense itching
psoriasis sō-RĪ-ă-sĭs	Chronic skin disease characterized by circumscribed red patches covered by thick, dry, silvery, adherent scales that are the result of excessive development of the basal layer of the epidermis *New lesions tend to appear at sites of trauma. They may be found in any location but commonly on the scalp, knees, elbows, umbilicus, and genitalia. Treatment includes topical application of various medications, keratolytics, phototherapy, and ultraviolet light therapy in an attempt to slow hyperkeratosis.*
purpura PŬR-pū-ră	Any of several bleeding disorders characterized by hemorrhage into the tissues, particularly beneath the skin or mucous membranes, producing ecchymoses or petechiae *Hemorrhage into the skin shows red darkening into purple and then brownish-yellow and finally disappearing in 2 to 3 weeks. Areas of discoloration do not disappear under pressure.*
scabies SKĀ-bēz	Contagious skin disease transmitted by the itch mite, commonly through sexual contact *Scabies manifests as papules, vesicles, pustules, and burrows and causes intense itching commonly resulting in secondary infections. The axillae, genitalia, inner aspect of the thighs, and areas between the fingers are most commonly affected.*
tinea TĬN-ē-ăh	Any fungal skin disease whose name commonly indicates the body part affected; also called *ringworm* *Examples include tinea barbae (beard), tinea corporis (body), tinea pedis (athlete's foot), tinea versicolor (skin), tinea cruris (jock itch).*

(Continued)

Term	Definition	(Continued)
urticaria ŭr-tĭ-KĀ-rē-ă	Allergic reaction of the skin characterized by the eruption of pale red elevated patches called wheals (hives)	
vitiligo vĭt-ĭl-Ī-gō	Localized loss of skin pigmentation characterized by milk-white patches	
verruca vĕr-ROO-kă	Epidermal growth caused by a virus, such as plantar warts, juvenile warts, and venereal warts *Warts may be removed by cryosurgery, electrocautery, or acids; however, they may regrow if virus remains in the skin.*	

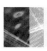 ## Diagnostic and Therapeutic Procedures

This section introduces procedures used to diagnose and treat skin disorders. Descriptions are provided as well as pronunciations and word analyses for selected terms.

Procedure	Description
DIAGNOSTIC PROCEDURES	
Clinical	
skin test (ST)	Any test in which a suspected allergen or sensitizer is applied to or injected into the skin to determine the patient's reaction to it *The most commonly used tests are the intradermal, patch, and scratch tests. The intensity of the response is determined by the wheal-and-flare reaction 10 minutes after the suspected allergen is applied. Positive and negative controls are used to verify normal skin reactivity.*
intradermal test	Identifies suspected allergens by subcutaneously injecting small amounts of extracts of the suspected allergens and observing the skin for a subsequent reaction; used to determine immunity to diphtheria (Schick test) or tuberculosis (Mantoux test)
patch test	Identifies suspected allergens by topical application of substance to be tested (e.g., food, pollen, animal fur), usually on the forearm and observing for subsequent reaction *After the patch is removed, a lack of noticeable reaction indicates a negative result; skin reddening or swelling indicates a positive result.*

Procedure	Description
scratch test	Identifies suspected allergens by placing a small quantity of suspected allergen on a lightly scratched area of the skin
	Redness or swelling at the scratch sites within 10 minutes indicates allergy to the substance indicating the test result is positive. If no reaction occurs, the test result is negative.

Surgical

biopsy BĪ-ŏp-sē	Representative tissue sample removed from a body site for microscopic examination, usually to establish a diagnosis
	Skin biopsies are used to establish or confirm a diagnosis, estimate prognosis, or follow the course of disease. Any lesion suspected of malignancy is removed and sent to the pathology laboratory.
needle	Removal of small tissue sample for examination using a hollow needle, usually attached to a syringe
punch	Removal of a small core of tissue using a hollow punch
shave	Removal of tissue using a surgical blade to shave elevated lesions
frozen section (FS)	Ultra-thin slice of tissue cut from a frozen specimen for immediate pathological examination
	Frozen section is commonly used for rapid diagnosis of malignancy after the patient has been anesthetized to determine conservative or radical approach.

THERAPEUTIC PROCEDURES

debridement dā-brēd-MŎN	Removal of foreign material and dead or damaged tissue, especially in a wound; used to promote healing and prevent infection
dermabrasion DĔRM-ă-brā-zhŭn	Removal of acne scars, nevi, tattoos, or fine wrinkles on the skin through the use of sandpaper, wire brushes, or other abrasive materials on the anesthetized epidermis
fulguration fŭl-gū-RĀ-shŭn	Tissue destruction by means of high-frequency electric sparks; also called *electrodesiccation*

Surgical

chemical peel	Chemical removal of the outer layers of skin to treat acne scarring and general keratoses; also used for cosmetic purposes to remove fine wrinkles on the face; also called *chemabrasion*
cryosurgery kri-ō-SĔR-jĕr-ē	Use of subfreezing temperature (commonly with liquid nitrogen) to destroy or eliminate abnormal tissue cells, such as tumors, warts, and unwanted, cancerous, or infected tissue
incision and drainage (I&D)	Incision in a lesion such as an abscess and drainage of its contents

Pharmacology

Various medications are available to treat skin disorders. (See Table 5–3.) Because of their superficial nature and location, many skin disorders respond well to topical drug therapy. Mild skin diseases such as contact dermatitis, acne, poison ivy, and diaper rash can be effectively treated with topical agents available as over-the-counter products. These products provide relief in mild, localized skin disorders.

Widespread or particularly severe dermatologic disorders may require systemic treatment. For example, poison ivy with large areas of open, weeping lesions may be difficult to treat with topical medication and may require a prescription-strength drug. In this case, an oral steroid or antihistamine might be prescribed to relieve inflammation and severe itching.

Table 5–3   DRUGS USED TO TREAT SKIN DISORDERS

This table lists common drug classifications used to treat skin disorders, their therapeutic actions, and selected generic and trade names.

Classification	Therapeutic Action	Generic and Trade Names
anesthetics	Block the sensation of pain by numbing the skin layers and mucous membranes *These topical drugs can be administered directly by means of sprays, creams, gargles, suppositories, and other preparations. They provide temporary symptomatic relief for minor burns, sunburns, rashes, and insect bites.*	**bupivacaine** bū-PĬV-ă-kān *Marcaine* **lidocaine** LĪ-dō-kān *Xylocaine* **procaine** PRŌ-kān *Novocain*
antifungals	Alter the cell wall of fungi or disrupt enzyme activity, resulting in cell death *Antifungals provide effective treatment for ringworm (tinea corporis), athlete's foot (tinea pedis), and fungal infection of the nail (onychomycosis). When topical antifungals are not effective, oral or intravenous antifungal drugs may be necessary.*	**clotrimazole** clō-TRĬ-mă-zōl *Lotrimin, Mycelex* **miconazole** mĭ-KŎN-ă-zōl *Micatin, Monistat-Derm* **nystatin** NĬS-tă-tĭn *Mycostatin, Nystex, Pedi-Dri* **itraconazole** ĭt-ră-KŎN-ă-zōl *Sporanox*
antihistamines	Inhibit inflammation, redness, and itching caused by allergic skin reaction and the release of histamine *In case of severe itching, antihistamines may be given orally. As a group, these drugs are also known as antipruritics.*	**diphenhydramine** di-fĕn-HĪ-dră-mēn *Benadryl* **hydroxyzine** hĭ-DRŎK-sĭ-zēn *Atarax, Vistaril*
antiseptics	Topically applied agents that inhibit the growth of bacteria, thus preventing infections in cuts, scratches, and surgical incisions	**chlorhexidine** klor-HĔKS-ĭ-dēn *Hibiclens* **ethyl or isopropyl alcohol** ĔTH-ĭl, ī-sō-PRŌ-pĭl **hydrogen peroxide** HĪ-drō-jĕn pĕ-RŎK-sid

Table 5-3 DRUGS USED TO TREAT SKIN DISORDERS

Classification	Therapeutic Action	Generic and Trade Names

corticosteroid anti-inflam-matories	Decrease inflammation and itching by suppressing the immune system's response to tissue damage
	
	Topical corticosteroids are used to treat contact dermatitis, poison ivy, insect bites, psoriasis, seborrhea, and eczema. Oral corticosteroids may be given for systemic treatment of severe or widespread inflammation or itching.
		hydrocortisone*
		hī-drō-KOR-tĭ-sōn
		  Cortaid, Dermolate, Locoid
		triamcinolone
		trī-ăm-SĬN-ō-lōn
		  Aristocort, Kenalog

keratolytics	Destroy and soften the outer layer of skin so that it is sloughed off or shed
	
	Strong keratolytics effectively remove warts and corns and aid in penetration of antifungal drugs. Milder keratolytics promote shedding of scales and crusts in eczema, psoriasis, seborrheic dermatitis, and other dry, scaly conditions. Very weak keratolytics irritate inflamed skin, acting as a tonic to accelerate healing.
		tretinoin
		TRĔT-ĭ-noyn
		  Retin-A, Vesanoid
		erythromycin
		ĕ-rĭth-rō-MĬ-sĭn
		  EryDerm, Staticin
		tetracycline
		tĕt-ră-SĪ-klēn
		  Topicycline

parasiticides	Kill insect parasites, such as mites and lice
	
	Parasiticides are used to treat scabies (mites) and pediculosis (lice). The drug is applied as a cream or lotion to the body and as a shampoo to treat the scalp (rare in scabies).
		lindane
		LĬN-dān
		  Kwell
		permethrin
		pĕr-MĔTH-rĭn
		  Nix

protectives	Cover, cool, dry, or soothe inflamed skin
	
	Protectives do not penetrate the skin or soften it; rather, they allow the natural healing process to occur by forming a long-lasting film that protects the skin from air, water, and clothing.
		lotions
		  Cetaphil moisturizing lotion
		creams
		  Neutrogena hand cream
		ointments
		  Vaseline

*The suffixes *-sone, -olone,* and *-onide* are common to generic corticosteroids.

It is time to review diagnostic, symptomatic, procedure, and pharmacology terms by completing Learning Activity 5–5.

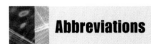

Abbreviations

This section introduces integumentary-related abbreviations and their meanings.

Abbreviation	Meaning
Bx, bx	biopsy
BCC	basal cell carcinoma
cm	centimeter
decub	decubitus (ulcer); bedsore
derm	dermatology
FS	frozen section
ID	intradermal
I&D	incision and drainage
IMP	impression (synonymous with *diagnosis*)
Sub Q, sub Q*	subcutaneous (injection)
ung	ointment
XP, XDP	xeroderma pigmentosum

*Although these abbreviations are currently found in medical records and clinical notes, the Joint Commission on Accreditation of Healthcare Organizations (JCAHO) requires their discontinuance. Instead, write out their meanings.

LEARNING ACTIVITIES

The following activities provide review of the integumentary system terms introduced in this chapter. Complete each activity and review your answers to evaluate your understanding of the chapter.

Learning Activity 5–1

Identifying integumentary structures

Label the following illustration using the terms listed below.

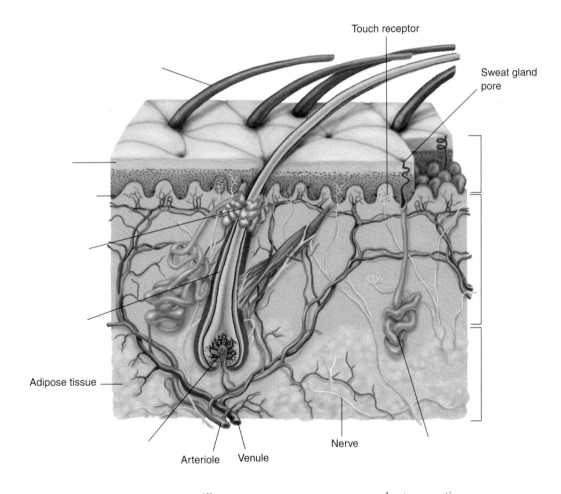

dermis   *papilla*   *subcutaneous tissue*
epidermis   *sebaceous (oil) gland* *sudoriferous (sweat) gland*
hair follicle *stratum corneum*
hair shaft   *stratum germinativum*

 Check your answers by referring to Figure 5–1 on page 77. Review material that you did not answer correctly.

Learning Activity 5–2

Building medical words

*Use **adip/o** or **lip/o** (fat) to build words that mean:*

1. tumor consisting of fat _____
2. hernia containing fat _____
3. resembling fat _____
4. fat cell _____

*Use **dermat/o** (skin) to build words that mean:*

5. inflammation of the skin _____
6. instrument to incise the skin _____

*Use **onych/o** (nail) to build words that mean:*

7. tumor of the nails _____
8. softening of the nails _____
9. abnormal condition of the nails _____
10. abnormal condition of the nails caused by a fungus _____
11. abnormal condition of a hidden (ingrown) nail _____
12. disease of the nails _____

*Use **trich/o** (hair) to build words that mean:*

13. disease of the hair _____
14. abnormal condition of hair caused by a fungus _____

*Use **-logy** or **-logist** to build words that mean:*

15. study of the skin _____
16. specialist in skin (diseases) _____

Build surgical words that mean:

17. excision of fat (adipose tissue) _____
18. removal of a nail _____
19. incision of a nail _____
20. surgical repair (plastic surgery) of the skin _____

✓ Check your answers in Appendix A. Review material that you did not answer correctly.

CORRECT ANSWERS _____ × 5 = _____ **% SCORE**

Learning Activity 5-3

Identifying skin lesions

Label the following skin lesions on the lines provided, using the terms listed below.

bulla	*macule*	*pustule*	*vesicle*
excoriations	*nodule*	*tumor*	*wheal*
fissure	*papule*	*ulcer*	

PRIMARY LESIONS

FLAT LESIONS
Flat, discolored, circumscribed lesions of any size

Flat, pigmented, circumscribed area less than 1 cm in diameter.
Examples: freckle, flat mole, or rash that occurs in rubella.

ELEVATED LESIONS

Solid   *Fluid-filled*

Solid, elevated lesion less than 1 cm in diameter that may be the same color as the skin or pigmented.
Examples: nevus, wart, pimple, ringworm, psoriasis, eczema.

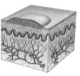

Elevated, circumscribed, fluid-filled lesion less than 0.5 cm in diameter.
Examples: poison ivy, shingles, chickenpox.

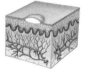

Palpable, circumscribed lesion; larger and deeper than a papule (0.6 to 2 cm in diameter); extends into the dermal area.
Examples: intradermal nevus, benign or malignant tumor.

Small, raised, circumscribed lesion that contains pus; usually less than 1 cm in diameter.
Examples: acne, furuncle, pustular psoriasis, scabies.

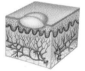

Solid, elevated lesion larger than 2 cm in diameter that extends into the dermal and subcutaneous layers.
Examples: lipoma, steatoma, dermatofibroma, hemangioma.

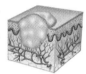

A vesicle or blister larger than 1 cm in diameter.
Examples: second degree burns, severe poison oak, poison ivy.

Elevated, firm, rounded lesion with localized skin edema (swelling) that varies in size, shape, and color; paler in the center than its surrounding edges; accompanied by itching.
Examples: hives, insect bites, urticaria.

SECONDARY LESIONS

DEPRESSED LESIONS
Depressed lesions caused by loss of skin surface

Linear scratch marks or traumatized abrasions of the epidermis.
Examples: scratches, abrasions, chemical or thermal burns.

Small slit or cracklike sore that extends into the dermal layer; could be caused by continuous inflammation and drying.

An open sore or lesion that extends to the dermis and usually heals with scarring.
Examples: pressure sore, basal cell carcinoma.

 Check your answers by referring to Figure 5–3 on page 84. Review material that you did not answer correctly.

Learning Activity 5–4

Matching burn and oncology terms

Match each term on the left with its meaning on the right.

1. _____ erythema
2. _____ T_0
3. _____ malignant
4. _____ first-degree burn
5. _____ grading
6. _____ squamous cell carcinoma
7. _____ benign
8. _____ T_1
9. _____ M_0
10. _____ third-degree burns

a. develops from keratinizing epidermal cells
b. noncancerous
c. no evidence of metastasis
d. extensive damage to underlying connective tissue
e. no evidence of primary tumor
f. determines degree of abnormal cancer cells compared with normal cells
g. heals without scar formation
h. cancerous; may be life-threatening
i. redness of skin
j. primary tumor size, small with minimal invasion

✓ Check your answers in Appendix A. Review any material that you did not answer correctly.

CORRECT ANSWERS _____ × 10 = _____ % **SCORE**

Learning Activity 5–5

Matching diagnostic, symptomatic, procedure, and pharmacology terms

Match the following terms with the definitions in the numbered list.

alopecia	*fulguration*	*petechiae*
antifungals	*impetigo*	*scabies*
autograft	*intradermal test*	*tinea*
chloasma	*keratolytics*	*urticaria*
corticosteroids	*parasiticides*	*vitiligo*
dermabrasion	*patch test*	*xenograft*
ecchymosis	*pediculosis*	

1. _____ infestation with lice
2. _____ depigmentation in areas of the skin characterized by milk-white patches
3. _____ any fungal skin disease, also called *ringworm*

4. _____ contagious skin disease transmitted by the itch mite

5. _____ skin infection characterized by vesicles that become pustular
and crusted and then rupture

6. _____ severe itching of the skin, also known as hives

7. _____ hyperpigmentation of the skin, characterized by yellowish-
brown patches or spots

8. _____ hemorrhagic spot or bruise on the skin

9. _____ minute or small hemorrhagic spots on the skin

10. _____ loss or absence of hair

11. _____ topical agents to treat athlete's foot and onychomycosis

12. _____ tissue destruction by means of high-frequency electric sparks

13. _____ agents that decrease inflammation or itching

14. _____ use of wire brushes, or other abrasive materials, to remove
scars, tattoos, or fine wrinkles

15. _____ agents that kill parasitic skin infestations

16. _____ agents that soften the outer layer of skin so that it sloughs off

17. _____ extracts of suspected allergens are subcutaneously injected

18. _____ allergens are applied topically, usually on
forearm

19. _____ graft transferred from one part of a person's body to another
part

20. _____ graft transferred from one species to a different species

Check your answers in Appendix A. Review material that you did not answer correctly.

CORRECT ANSWERS _____ × 5 = _____ **% SCORE**

MEDICAL RECORD ACTIVITIES

The two medical records included in the following activities use common clinical scenarios to show how medical terminology is used to document patient care. Complete the terminology and analysis sections for each activity to help you recognize and understand terms related to the integumentary system.

Medical Record Activity 5–1

Pathology report of skin lesion

Terminology

The terms listed in the chart come from the medical record *Pathology Report of Skin Lesion* that follows. Use a medical dictionary such as *Taber's Cyclopedic Medical Dictionary*, the appendices of this book, or other resources to define each term. Then review the pronunciations for each term and practice by reading the medical record aloud.

Term	Definition
atypia ă-TĬP-ē-ă	
atypical ā-TĬP-ĭ-kăl	
basal cell layer BĀ-săl	
Bowen disease BŌ-ĕn dĭ-ZĒZ	
carcinoma kăr-sĭ-NŌ-mă	
dermatitis dĕr-mă-TĪ-tĭs	
dermis DĔR-mĭs	
dorsum DOR-sŭm	
epidermal hyperplasia ĕp-ĭ-DĔR-măl hī-pĕr-PLĀ-zē-ă	
fibroplasia fī-brō-PLĀ-sē-ă	

Term	Definition
hyperkeratosis hī-pĕr-kĕr-ă-TŌ-sĭs	
infiltrate ĬN-fĭl-trāt	
keratinocytes kĕ-RĂT-ĭ-nō-sīts	
lymphocytic lĭm-fō-SĬT-ĭk	
neoplastic nē-ō-PLĂS-tĭk	
papillary PĂP-ĭ-lăr-ē	
pathological păth-ō-LŎJ-ĭk-ăl	
solar elastosis SŌ-lăr ĕ-lăs-TŌ-sĭs	
squamous SKWĀ-mŭs	

PATHOLOGY REPORT OF SKIN LESION

SPECIMEN: Skin on (a) dorsum left wrist and (b) left forearm, ulnar, near elbow.

CLINICAL DIAGNOSIS: Bowen disease versus basal cell carcinoma versus dermatitis.

MICROSCOPIC DESCRIPTION: (a) There is mild hyperkeratosis and moderate epidermal hyperplasia with full-thickness atypia of squamous-keratinocytes. Squamatization of the basal cell layer exists. A lymphocytic inflammatory infiltrate is present in the papillary dermis. Solar elastosis is present. (b) Nests, strands, and columns of atypical neoplastic basaloid keratinocytes grow down from the epidermis into the underlying dermis. Fibroplasia is present. Solar elastosis is noted.

PATHOLOGICAL DIAGNOSIS: (a) Bowen disease of left wrist; (b) nodular and infiltrating basal cell carcinoma of left forearm, near elbow.

Analysis

Review the medical record *Pathology Report of Skin Lesion* to answer the following questions.

1. In the specimen section, what does "skin on dorsum left wrist" mean?

2. What was the inflammatory infiltrate?

3. What was the pathologist's diagnosis for the left forearm?

4. Provide a brief description of Bowen disease, the pathologist's diagnosis for the left wrist.

Medical Record Activity 5–2

Patient referral letter: Onychomycosis

Terminology

The terms listed in the chart come from the medical record *Patient Referral Letter: Onychomycosis* that follows. Use a medical dictionary such as *Taber's Cyclopedic Medical Dictionary*, the appendices of this book, or other resources to define each term. Then review the pronunciations for each term and practice by reading the medical record aloud.

Term	Definition
alkaline phosphatase ĂL-kă-lĭn FŎS-fă-tās	
bilaterally bī-LĂT-ĕr-ăl-ē	
CA	
debridement dā-brēd-MŎN	
hypertension hī-pĕr-TĔN-shŭn	
mastectomy măs-TĔK-tŏ-mē	
neurological noor-ō-LŎJ-ĭk-ăl	
onychomycosis ŏn-ĭ-kō-mi-KŌ-sĭs	
Sporanox* SPOR-ă-nŏks	
vascular VĂS-kū-lăr	

*Refer to Table 5–3 to determine the drug classification and the generic name for Sporanox.

PATIENT REFERRAL LETTER: ONYCHOMYCOSIS

Dear Doctor Meyers:

Thank you for referring Alicia Gonzoles to my office. Mrs. Gonzoles presents to the office for evaluation and treatment of onychomycosis with no previous treatment. Past pertinent medical history does reveal hypertension and breast CA. Pertinent surgical history does reveal mastectomy.

Examination of patient's feet does reveal onychomycosis 1–5 bilaterally. Vascular and neurological examinations are intact. Previous laboratory work was within normal limits except for an elevated alkaline phosphatase of 100.

Tentative diagnosis: Onychomycosis 1–5 bilaterally

Treatment consisted of debridement of mycotic nails bilateral feet as well as dispensing a prescription for Sporanox, Pulse Pack, to be taken times three months to treat the onychomycotic infection. I have also asked her to repeat her liver enzymes in approximately 4 weeks. Mrs. Gonzoles will reappoint in 2 months for follow-up, and I will keep you informed of any changes in her progress. If you have any questions, please let me know.

Analysis

Review the medical record *Patient Referral Letter: Onychomycosis* to answer the following questions.

1. What pertinent disorders were identified in the past medical history?

2. What pertinent surgery was identified in the past surgical history?

3. Did the doctor identify any problems in the vascular system or nervous system?

4. What was the significant finding in the laboratory results?

5. What treatment did the doctor employ for the onychomycosis?

6. What did the doctor recommend regarding the abnormal laboratory finding?

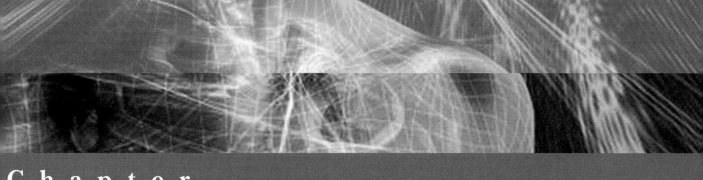

Chapter

6

Digestive System

CHAPTER OUTLINE

OBJECTIVES

Upon completion of this chapter, you will be able to:

- Locate and describe the structures of the digestive system.
- Recognize, pronounce, spell, and build words related to the digestive system.

- Describe pathological conditions, diagnostic and therapeutic procedures, and other terms related to the digestive system.
- Explain pharmacology related to the treatment of digestive disorders.
- Demonstrate your knowledge of this chapter by completing the learning and medical record activities.

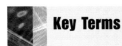 **Key Terms**

This section introduces important digestive system terms and their definitions. Word analyses are also provided.

Term	Definition
asymptomatic ā-simp-tō-MĂT-ĭk	Without symptoms
defecation dĕf-ĕ-KĀ-shŭn	Elimination of feces from the gastrointestinal tract through the rectum
duodenal bulb dū-ō-DĒ-năl BŬLB	Upper duodenal area just beyond the pylorus
endoscope ĔN-dō-skōp *endo-:* in, within *-scope:* instrument for examining	Instrument consisting of a rigid or flexible fiberoptic tube and optical system for observing the inside of a hollow organ or cavity
exocrine ĔKS-ō-krĭn *exo- :* outside, outward *-crine:* secrete	Pertaining to a gland that secretes outwardly through excretory ducts to the surface of an organ or tissue or into a vessel
friable FRĪ-ă-bŭl	Easily broken or pulverized
pepsin PĔP-sĭn	Enzyme secreted in the stomach that begins the digestion of proteins
punctate PŬNK-tāt	Having pinpoint punctures or depressions on the surface; marked with dots
varices VĂR-ĭ-sēz	Tortuous dilations of a vein
sphincter SFĪNGK-tĕr	Circular muscle constricting an orifice, such as the pyloric sphincter around the opening of the stomach into the duodenum

Anatomy and Physiology

The digestive system, also called the *gastrointestinal* (GI) system, consists of a digestive tube called the *GI tract*, or *alimentary canal*, and several accessory organs whose primary function is to break down food, prepare it for absorption, and eliminate waste. The GI tract, extending from the mouth to the anus, varies in size and structure in several distinct regions:

- mouth
- pharynx (throat)
- esophagus
- stomach
- small intestine
- large intestine
- rectum
- anus

Food passing along the GI tract is mixed with digestive enzymes and broken down into nutrient molecules, which are absorbed in the bloodstream. Undigested waste materials that cannot be absorbed in the blood are then eliminated from the body through defecation. Included in the digestive system are the accessory organs of digestion: the liver, gallbladder, and pancreas.

Mouth

The process of digestion begins in the mouth. (See Figure 6–1.) The mouth, also known as the (1) **oral cavity** or *buccal cavity*, is a receptacle for food. It is formed by the cheeks (bucca), lips, teeth, tongue, and hard and soft palates. Located around the oral cavity are three pairs of salivary glands, which secrete saliva. Saliva contains important digestive enzymes that help begin the chemical breakdown of food. In the mouth, food is broken down mechanically (by the teeth) and chemically (by saliva), and then formed into a *bolus*.

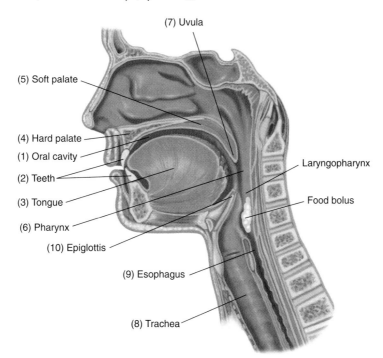

Figure 6–1 Sagittal view of the head showing oral, nasal, and pharyngeal components of the digestive system.

Teeth

The (2) **teeth** play an important role in initial stages of digestion by mechanically breaking down food (mastication) into smaller pieces as it mixes it with saliva. Teeth are covered by a hard enamel, giving them a smooth, white appearance. Beneath the enamel is the *dentin,* the main structure of the tooth. The innermost part of the tooth is the pulp, which contains nerves and blood vessels. The teeth are embedded in pink, fleshy tissue known as gums (gingiva).

Tongue

The (3) **tongue** assists in this mechanical digestion process by manipulating the bolus of food during chewing and moving it to the back of the mouth for swallowing (deglutition). The tongue also aids in speech production and taste. Rough projections on the surface of the tongue called *papillae* contain taste buds. The four basic taste sensations registered by chemical stimulation of the taste buds are sweet, sour, salty, and bitter. All other taste perceptions are combinations of these four basic flavors. In addition, sense of taste is intricately linked with sense of smell, making taste perception very complex.

Hard and Soft Palates

The two structures forming the roof of the mouth are the (4) **hard palate** (anterior portion) and the (5) **soft palate** (posterior portion). The soft palate, which forms a partition between the mouth and the nasopharynx, is continuous with the hard palate. The entire oral cavity, like the rest of the GI tract, is lined with mucous membranes.

Pharynx, Esophagus, and Stomach

As the bolus is pushed by the tongue into the (6) **pharynx** (throat), it is guided by the soft, fleshy, V-shaped structure called the (7) **uvula.** The funnel-shaped pharynx serves as a passageway to the respiratory and GI tracts and provides a resonating chamber for speech sounds. The lowest portion of the pharynx divides into two tubes: one that leads to the lungs, called the (8) **trachea,** and one that leads to the stomach, called the (9) **esophagus.** A small flap of cartilage, the (10) **epiglottis,** folds back to cover the trachea during swallowing, forcing food to enter the esophagus. At all other times, the epiglottis remains upright, allowing air to freely pass through the respiratory structures.

The **stomach,** a saclike structure located in the left upper quadrant (LUQ) of the abdominal cavity, serves as a food reservoir that continues mechanical and chemical digestion. (See Figure 6–2.) The stomach extends from the (1) **esophagus** to the first part of the small intestine, the (2) **duodenum.** The terminal portion of the esophagus, the (3) **lower esophageal (cardiac) sphincter,** is composed of muscle fibers that constrict once food has passed into the stomach. It prevents the stomach contents from regurgitating back into the esophagus. The (4) **body** of the stomach, the large central portion, together with the (5) **fundus,** the upper portion, are mainly storage areas. Most digestion takes place in the funnel-shaped terminal portion, the (6) **pylorus.** The interior lining of the stomach is composed of mucous membranes (mucosa) and contains numerous macroscopic longitudinal folds called (7) **rugae** that gradually unfold as the stomach fills. Located within the rugae, digestive glands produce hydrochloric acid (HCl) and enzymes. Secretions from these glands coupled with the mechanical churning of the stomach turn the bolus into a semiliquid form called *chyme* that slowly leaves the stomach through the (8) **pyloric sphincter** to enter the duodenum. This sphincter regulates the speed and movement of chyme into the small intestine and prohibits backflow. Food is propelled through the entire GI tract by coordinated, rhythmic muscle contractions called **peristalsis.**

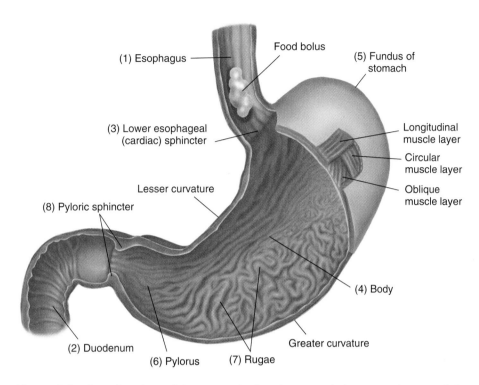

Figure 6–2   Anterior view of the stomach showing muscle layers and rugae of the mucosa.

Small Intestine

The small intestine is a coiled, 20′-long tube that begins at the pyloric sphincter and extends to the large intestine. (See Figure 6–3.) It consists of three parts:

- the (1) **duodenum,** the uppermost segment, which is about 10″ long
- the (2) **jejunum,** which is approximately 8′ long
- the (3) **ileum,** which is about 12′ long

Digestion is completed in the small intestine with the help of additional enzymes and secretions from the (4) **pancreas** and (5) **liver.** Nutrients in chyme are absorbed through microscopic, fingerlike projections called villi to enter the bloodstream and lymphatic system for distribution to the rest of the body. At the terminal end of the small intestine, a sphincter muscle called the *ileocecal valve* joins the ileum to the large intestine's cecum. When the sphincter muscle is relaxed, undigested or unabsorbed material from the small intestine is passed to the large intestine to be excreted from the body.

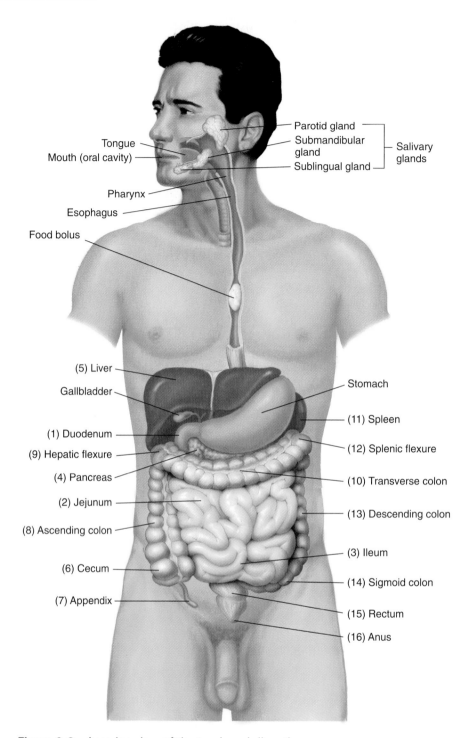

Figure 6–3   Anterior view of the trunk and digestive organs.

Large Intestine

The large intestine is about 5′ long. It begins at the ileum and extends to the anus. No digestion takes place in the large intestine. The only secretion is mucus in the colon, which lubricates fecal material so it can pass from the body. The large intestine is divided into four major regions: cecum, colon, rectum, and anus. The first 2″ or 3″ of the large intestine is called the (6) **cecum,** a pouchlike structure located below the ileocecal opening. Projecting downward from the cecum is a wormlike projection, called the (7) **appendix.** The function of the appendix is unknown; however, problems arise if it becomes infected or inflamed. The cecum merges with the colon. The main functions of the colon are to absorb water and minerals and eliminate undigested material. The colon is divided into ascending, transverse, descending, and sigmoid portions:

- The (8) **ascending colon** extends from the cecum to the lower border of the liver and turns abruptly to form the (9) **hepatic flexure.**
- The colon continues across the abdomen to the left side as the (10) **transverse colon** curving beneath the lower end of the (11) **spleen** to form the (12) **splenic flexure.**
- As the transverse colon turns downward, it becomes the (13) **descending colon.**
- The descending colon continues until it forms the (14) **sigmoid colon** and the (15) **rectum.** The rectum, the last part of the GI tract, terminates at the (16) **anus.**

 It is time to review digestive structures by completing Learning Activity 6–1.

Accessory Organs of Digestion

Although the liver, gallbladder, and pancreas lie outside the GI tract, they play a vital role in the proper digestion and absorption of nutrients. (See Figure 6–4.)

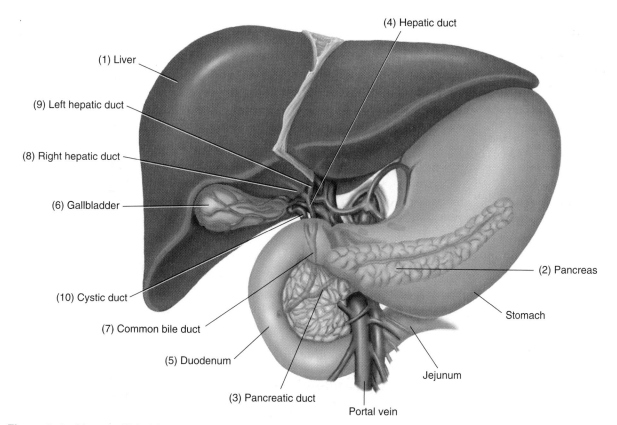

Figure 6–4 Liver, gallbladder, pancreas, and duodenum with associated ducts and blood vessels.

Liver

The (1) **liver,** the largest glandular organ in the body, weighs approximately 3 to 4 lb. It is located beneath the diaphragm in the right upper quadrant (RUQ) of the abdominal cavity. The liver performs many vital activities and death occurs if it ceases to function. Some of its important activities include:

- producing bile, used in the small intestine to emulsify and absorb fats
- removing **glucose** (sugar) from blood to synthesize glycogen (starch) and retain it for later use
- storing vitamins, such as B_{12}, A, D, E, and K
- destroying or transforming toxic products into less harmful compounds
- maintaining normal glucose levels in the blood
- destroying old erythrocytes and releasing bilirubin
- producing various blood proteins, such as prothrombin and fibrinogen, that aid in blood clotting

Pancreas

The (2) **pancreas** is an elongated, somewhat flattened organ that lies posterior and slightly inferior to the stomach. It performs both endocrine and exocrine functions. As an endocrine gland, the pancreas secretes insulin directly into the bloodstream to maintain normal blood glucose levels. For a comprehensive discussion of the endocrine function of the pancreas, review Chapter 13. As an exocrine gland, the pancreas produces digestive enzymes that pass into the duodenum through the (3) **pancreatic duct.** The pancreatic duct extends along the pancreas and, together with the (4) **hepatic duct** from the liver, enters the (5) **duodenum.** The digestive enzymes produced by the pancreas contain trypsin, which breaks down proteins; amylase, which breaks down carbohydrates; and lipase, which breaks down fat.

Gallbladder

The (6) **gallbladder,** a saclike structure on the inferior surface of the liver, serves as a storage area for bile. When bile is needed for digestion, the gallbladder releases it into the duodenum through the (7) **common bile duct.** Bile is also drained from the liver through the (8) **right hepatic duct** and the (9) **left hepatic duct.** These two structures eventually form the hepatic duct. The (10) **cystic duct** of the gallbladder merges with the hepatic duct to form the common bile duct, which leads into the duodenum. Bile production is stimulated by hormone secretions, which are produced in the duodenum, as soon as food enters the small intestine. Without bile, fat digestion is not possible.

 It is time to review anatomy of the accessory organs of digestion by completing Learning Activity 6–2.

Medical Word Elements

This section introduces combining forms, suffixes, and prefixes related to the digestive system. Word analyses are also provided.

Element	Meaning	Word Analysis
COMBINING FORMS		
Mouth		
or/o	mouth	or/al (OR-ăl): pertaining to the mouth *-al:* pertaining to, relating to
stomat/o		stomat/itis (stŏ-mă-TĪ-tĭs): inflammation of the mouth *-itis:* inflammation
gloss/o	tongue	gloss/ectomy (glŏs-ĔK-tō-mē): removal of all or part of the tongue *-ectomy:* excision, removal
lingu/o		lingu/al (LĬNG-gwăl): pertaining to the tongue *-al:* pertaining to, relating to
bucc/o	cheek	bucc/al (BŬK-ăl): pertaining to the cheek *-al:* pertaining to, relating to
cheil/o	lip	cheil/o/plasty (KĪ-lō-plăs-tē): surgical repair of a defect of the lip *-plasty:* surgical repair
labi/o		labi/al (LĀ-bē-ăl): pertaining to the lips, particularly the lips of the mouth *-al:* pertaining to, relating to
dent/o	teeth	dent/ist (DĔN-tĭst): specialist who diagnoses and treats diseases and disorders of teeth and tissues of the oral cavity *-ist:* specialist
odont/o		orth/odont/ist (or-thō-DŎN-tĭst): dentist who specializes in correcting and preventing irregularities of abnormally positioned or aligned teeth *orth:* straight *-ist:* specialist

(Continued)

Element	Meaning	Word Analysis	(Continued)
gingiv/o	gum(s)	gingiv/ectomy (jĭn-jĭ-VĔK-tō-mē): excision of diseased gingival tissue in surgical treatment of periodontal disease *-ectomy:* excision, removal	
sial/o	saliva, salivary gland	sial/o/lith (sī-ĂL-ō-lĭth): calculus formed in a salivary gland or duct *-lith:* stone, calculus	

Esophagus, Pharynx, and Stomach

Element	Meaning	Word Analysis
esophag/o	esophagus	esophag/o/scope (ē-SŎF-ă-gō-skōp): endoscope used to examine the esophagus *-scope:* instrument for examining
pharyng/o	pharynx (throat)	pharyng/o/tonsill/itis (fă-rĭng-gō-tŏn-sĭ-LĪ-tĭs): inflammation of the pharynx and tonsils *tonsill:* tonsils *-itis:* inflammation
gastr/o	stomach	gastr/algia (găs-TRĂL-jē-ă): pain in the stomach from any cause; also called *stomachache* *-algia:* pain
pylor/o	pylorus	pylor/o/spasm (pī-LOR-ō-spăzm): involuntary contraction of the pyloric sphincter of the stomach, as in pyloric stenosis *-spasm:* involuntary contraction, twitching

Small Intestine

Element	Meaning	Word Analysis
duoden/o	duodenum (first part of small intestine)	duoden/o/scopy (dū-ŏd-ĕ-NŎS-kō-pē): visual examination of the duodenum *-scopy:* visual examination
enter/o	intestine (usually small intestine)	enter/o/pathy (ĕn-tĕr-ŎP-ă-thē): any intestinal disease *-pathy:* disease
jejun/o	jejunum (second part of small intestine)	jejun/o/rrhaphy (jĕ-joo-NOR-ă-fē): suture of the jejunum *-rrhaphy:* suture

Element	Meaning	Word Analysis
ile/o	ileum (third part of small intestine)	ile/o/stomy (ĭl-ē-ŎS-tō-mē): creation of an opening between the ileum and the abdominal wall *-stomy*: forming an opening (mouth)* *An ileostomy creates an opening on the surface of the abdomen to allow feces to be discharged into a bag worn on the abdomen.*

Large Intestine

Element	Meaning	Word Analysis
append/o	appendix	append/ectomy (ăp-ĕn-DĔK-tō-mē): excision of the appendix *-ectomy: excision, removal* *Appendectomy is performed to remove a diseased appendix in danger of rupturing.*
appendic/o		appendic/itis (ă-pĕn-dĭ-SĪ-tĭs): inflammation of the appendix *-itis: inflammation*
col/o	colon	col/o/stomy (kō-LŎS-tō-mē): creation of an opening between the colon and the abdominal wall *-stomy*: forming an opening (mouth)* *A colostomy creates a place for fecal matter to exit the body other than through the anus.*
colon/o		colon/o/scopy (kō-lŏn-ŎS-kō-pē): visual examination of the colon using a colonoscope, an elongated endoscope *-scopy: visual examination*
sigmoid/o	sigmoid colon	sigmoid/o/tomy (sĭg-moyd-ŎT-ō-mē): incision of the sigmoid colon *-tomy: incision*

Terminal End of Large Intestine

Element	Meaning	Word Analysis
rect/o	rectum	rect/o/cele (RĔK-tō-sēl): herniation or protrusion of the rectum; also called *proctocele* *-cele: hernia, swelling*
proct/o	anus, rectum	proct/o/logist (prŏk-TŎL-ō-jĭst): physician who specializes in treating disorders of the colon, rectum, and anus. *-logist: specialist in the study of*
an/o	anus	peri/an/al (pĕr-ē-Ā-năl): pertaining to the area around the anus *peri-: around* *-al: pertaining to, relating to*

(Continued)

Element	Meaning	Word Analysis	(Continued)

Accessory Organs of Digestion

Element	Meaning	Word Analysis
hepat/o	liver	hepat/o/megaly (hĕp-ă-tō-MĔG-ă-lē): enlargement of the liver, usually a sign of disease *-megaly:* enlargement
pancreat/o	pancreas	pancreat/o/lysis (păn-krē-ă-TŎL-ĭ-sĭs): destruction of the pancreas by pancreatic enzymes *-lysis:* separation; destruction; loosening
cholangi/o	bile vessel	cholangi/ole (kō-LĂN-jē-ōl): small terminal portion of the bile duct *-ole:* small, minute
chol/e**	bile, gall	chol/e/lith (KŌ-lē-lĭth): gallstone *-lith:* calculus, stone *Gallstones are solid accumulations of bile and cholesterol that form in the gallbladder and common bile duct.*
cholecyst/o	gallbladder	cholecyst/ectomy (kō-lē-sĭs-TĔK-tō-mē): removal of the gallbladder by laparoscopic or open surgery *-ectomy:* excision, removal
choledoch/o	bile duct	choledoch/o/plasty (kō-LĔD-ō-kō-plăs-tē): surgical repair of the common bile duct *-plasty:* surgical repair

SUFFIXES

Element	Meaning	Word Analysis
-emesis	vomit	hyper/emesis (hī-pĕr-ĔM-ĕ-sĭs): excessive vomiting *hyper-:* excessive, above normal
-iasis	abnormal condition (produced by something specified)	chol/e/lith/iasis (kō-lē-lĭ-THĪ-ă-sĭs): presence or formation of gallstones in the gallbladder or common bile duct *chol/e:* bile, gall *lith:* stone, calculus *When gallstones form in the common bile duct, the condition is called* choledocholithiasis.
-megaly	enlargement	hepat/o/megaly (hĕp-ă-tō-MĔG-ă-lē): enlargement of the liver, usually a sign of disease *hepat/o:* liver *Hepatomegaly may be caused by hepatitis or infection, fatty infiltration (as in alcoholism), biliary obstruction, or malignancy.*

Element	Meaning	Word Analysis
-orexia	appetite	an/orexia (ăn-ō-RĔK-sē-ă): loss of appetite *an-:* without, not *Anorexia can result from various conditions, such as adverse effects of drugs or various physical or psychological causes.*
-pepsia	digestion	dys/pepsia (dĭs-PĔP-sē-ă): epigastric discomfort felt after eating; also called *indigestion* *dys-:* bad; painful; difficult
-phagia	swallowing, eating	aer/o/phagia (ĕr-ō-FĀ-jē-ă): swallowing of air *aer/o:* air
-prandial	meal	post/prandial (pōst-PRĂN-dē-ăl): following a meal *post-:* after, behind
-rrhea	discharge, flow	steat/o/rrhea (stē-ă-tō-RĒ-ă): excessive amount of fat discharged in fecal matter *-rrhea:* discharge, flow
PREFIXES		
dia-	through, across	dia/rrhea (dī-ă-RĒ-ă): abnormally frequent discharge or flow of fluid fecal matter from the bowel *-rrhea:* discharge, flow
peri-	around	peri/sigmoid/itis (pĕr-ĭ-sĭg-moy-DĪ-tĭs): inflammation of peritoneal tissue around the sigmoid colon *peri-:* around
sub-	under, below	sub/lingu/al (sŭb-LĬNG-gwăl): pertaining to the area under the tongue *lingu:* tongue *-al:* pertaining to, relating to

*When the suffix *-stomy* is used with a combining form that denotes an organ, it refers to a surgical opening to the outside of the body.

**The *e* in *chol/e* is an exception to the rule of using the connecting vowel *o*.

 It is time to review medical word elements by completing Learning Activities 6–3 and 6–4.

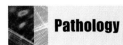

Pathology

Although some digestive disorders may be asymptomatic, many are associated with such symptoms as nausea, vomiting, bleeding, pain, and weight loss. Clinical signs, such as jaundice and edema, may indicate a hepatic disorder. Severe infection, drug toxicity, hepatic disease, and changes in fluid and electrolyte balance can cause behavioral abnormalities. Disorders of the GI tract or any of the accessory organs (liver, gallbladder, pancreas) may result in far-reaching metabolic or systemic problems that can eventually threaten life itself. Assessment of a suspected digestive disorder must include a thorough history and physical examination. A range of diagnostic tests assist in identifying abnormalities of the GI tract, liver, gallbladder, and pancreas.

For diagnosis, treatment, and management of digestive disorders, the medical services of a specialist may be warranted. Gastroenterology is the branch of medicine concerned with digestive diseases. The physician who specializes in the diagnoses and treatment of digestive disorders is known as a *gastroenterologist*. Gastroenterologists do not perform surgeries; however, under the broad classification of surgery, they do perform such procedures as liver biopsy and endoscopic examination.

Ulcer

An ulcer is a circumscribed lesion (open sore) of the skin or mucous membrane. Peptic ulcers are the most common type of ulcer that occurs in the digestive system. There are two main types of peptic ulcers: gastric ulcers, which develop in the stomach, and duodenal ulcers, which develop in the duodenum, usually in the area nearest the stomach. A third type of ulceration that affects the digestive system is associated with a disorder called colitis. As the name implies, it occurs in the colon.

Peptic Ulcer Disease

Peptic ulcer disease (PUD) develops in the parts of the GI tract that are exposed to hydrochloric acid and pepsin. Both of these products are found in gastric juice and normally act on food to begin the digestive process. The strong action of these digestive products can destroy the protective defenses of the mucous membranes of the stomach and duodenum, causing the lining to erode. Eventually, an ulcer forms. If left untreated, mucosal destruction forms a hole (perforation) in the wall lining.

Current scientific studies have identified bacterial infection with *Helicobacter pylori* as a leading cause of PUD. Its spiral shape helps the bacterium burrow into the mucosa, weakening it and making it more susceptible to the action of pepsin and stomach acid. These studies have also found that *H. pylori* releases a toxin that promotes mucosal inflammation and ulceration. Antibiotics and antacids are used to treat peptic ulcers. Patients are advised to avoid nonsteroidal anti-inflammatory drugs (NSAIDs), caffeine, smoking, and alcohol, which exacerbate the symptoms of gastric ulcers.

Ulcerative Colitis

Ulcerative colitis, a chronic inflammatory disease of the large intestine and rectum, commonly begins in the rectum or sigmoid colon and extends upward into the entire colon. It is characterized by profuse, watery diarrhea containing varying amounts of blood, mucus, and pus. Ulcerative colitis is distinguished from other closely related bowel disorders by its characteristic inflammatory pattern. The inflammation involves only the mucosal lining of the colon, and the affected portion of the colon is uniformly involved, with no patches of healthy mucosal tissue evident. Ulcerative colitis is associated with a higher risk of colon cancer. Severe cases may require surgical creation of an opening (stoma) for bowel evacuation to a bag worn on the abdomen.

Hernia

A hernia is a protrusion of any organ, tissue, or structure through the wall of the cavity in which it is naturally contained. (See Figure 6–5.) In general, though, the term is applied to the protrusion of an abdominal organ (viscus) through the abdominal wall.

An (1) **inguinal hernia** develops in the groin where the abdominal folds of flesh meet the thighs. In initial stages, it may be hardly noticeable and appears as a soft lump under the skin, no larger than a marble. In early stages, an inguinal hernia is usually reducible; that is, it can be pushed gently back into its normal place. With this type of hernia, pain may be minimal. As time passes, pressure of the abdomen against the weak abdominal wall may increase the size of the opening as well as the size of the hernia lump. If the blood supply to the hernia is cut off because of pressure, a (2) **strangulated hernia** with gangrene (necrosis) may develop. An (3) **umbilical hernia** is a protrusion of part of the intestine at the navel. It occurs more commonly in obese women and among those who have had several pregnancies. Hernias also occur in newborn infants (congenital) or during early childhood. If the defect has not corrected itself by age 2, the deformity can be surgically corrected. Treatment consists of surgical repair of the hernia (hernioplasty) with suture of the abdominal wall (herniorrhaphy).

Although hernias most commonly occur in the abdominal region, they may develop in the diaphragm. Two forms of hernia of the diaphragm include (4) **diaphragmatic hernia,** a congenital disorder, and (5) **hiatal hernia,** in which the lower part of the esophagus and the top of the stomach slides through an opening (hiatus) in the diaphragm into the thorax. With hiatal hernia, stomach acid backs up into the esophagus causing heartburn, chest pain, and swallowing difficulty. Although many hiatal hernias are asymptomatic, if the disease continues for a prolonged period, it may cause gastroesophageal reflux disease (GERD).

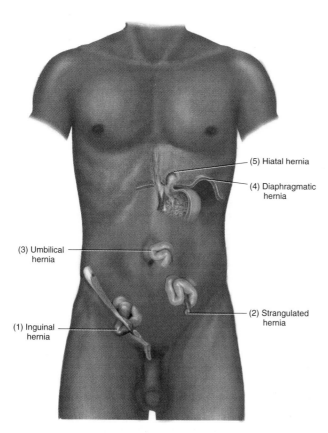

Figure 6–5 Common locations of hernia.

Bowel Obstruction

A life-threatening obstruction in which the bowel twists on itself (volvulus) with occlusion of the blood supply occurs most frequently in middle-aged and elderly men. The accumulation of gas and fluid coupled with loss of blood supply (ischemia) in the trapped bowel eventually leads to tissue death (necrosis), perforation, and an inflammation of the peritoneum (peritonitis). Surgery is required to untwist the bowel.

Telescoping of the intestine within itself (intussusception) occurs when one part of the intestine slips into another part located below it, much as a telescope is shortened by pushing one section into the next. This is a rare type of intestinal obstruction more common in infants 10 to 15 months of age than in adults. Surgery is usually necessary to correct this obstruction.

Hemorrhoids

Enlarged veins in the mucous membrane of the anal canal are called *hemorrhoids*—especially when they bleed, hurt, or itch. They may occur inside (internal) or outside (external) the rectal area. Hemorrhoids are usually caused by abdominal pressure, such as from straining during bowel movement, pregnancy, and standing or sitting for long periods. They may also be associated with some disorders of the liver or the heart.

A high-fiber diet as well as drinking plenty of water and juices plays a pivotal role in hemorrhoid prevention. Temporary relief from hemorrhoids can usually be obtained by cold compresses, sitz baths, stool softeners, or analgesic ointments. Treatment of an advanced hemorrhoidal condition involves surgical removal (hemorrhoidectomy).

Liver Disorders

A growing public health concern is the increasing incidence of viral **hepatitis.** Even though its mortality rate is low, the disease is easily transmitted and can cause significant morbidity and prolonged loss of time from school or employment. The two most common forms of hepatitis are hepatitis A, also called *infectious hepatitis,* and hepatitis B, also called *serum hepatitis.* The most common causes of hepatitis A are ingestion of contaminated food, water, or milk. Hepatitis B is usually transmitted by routes other than the mouth (parenteral), such as from blood transfusions and sexual contact. Because of patient exposure, health-care personnel are at increased risk for contracting hepatitis B, but a vaccine that provides immunity to hepatitis B is available.

One of the major symptoms of many liver disorders, including hepatitis and cirrhosis, is a yellowing of the skin (jaundice). Because the liver is no longer able to remove bilirubin, a yellow product formed when erythrocytes are destroyed, bilirubin appears in the skin and mucous membranes. This condition is also known as *icterus.* Jaundice may also result when the bile duct is blocked, causing bile to enter the bloodstream.

Diverticulosis

Diverticulosis is a condition in which small, blisterlike pockets (diverticula) develop in the inner lining of the large intestine and may balloon through the intestinal wall. These pockets occur most commonly in the sigmoid colon. They commonly do not cause any problem unless they become inflamed (diverticulitis). (See Figure 6–6.) Signs and symptoms of diverticulitis include pain, usually in the left lower quadrant (LLQ) of the abdomen; extreme constipation **(obstipation)** or diarrhea; fever; abdominal swelling; and occasional blood in bowel movements. The usual treatment for diverticulitis consists of bed rest, antibiotics, and a soft diet. In severe cases, however, excision of the diverticulum (diverticulectomy) may be advised.

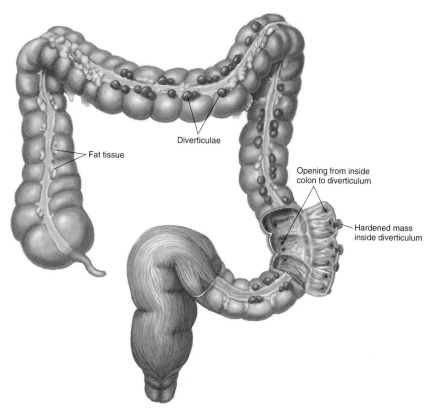

Figure 6–6   Diverticula of the colon.

Oncology

Although stomach cancer is rare in the United States, it is common in many parts of the world where food preservation is problematic. It is an important medical problem because of its high mortality rate. Men are more susceptible to stomach cancer than women. The neoplasm nearly always develops from the epithelial or mucosal lining of the stomach in the form of a cancerous glandular tumor (gastric adenocarcinoma). Persistent indigestion is one of the important warning signs of stomach cancer. Other types of GI carcinomas include esophageal carcinomas, hepatocellular carcinomas, and pancreatic carcinomas.

Colorectal cancer arises from the epithelial lining of the large intestine. Signs and symptoms, which depend largely on the location of the malignancy, include changes in bowel habits, passage of blood and mucus in stools, rectal or abdominal pain, anemia, weight loss, obstruction, and perforation. A suddenly developing obstruction may be the first symptom of cancer involving the colon between the cecum and the sigmoid because in this region, where bowel contents are liquid, a slowly developing obstruction will not become evident until the lumen is almost closed. Cancer of the sigmoid and rectum causes earlier symptoms of partial obstruction with constipation alternating with diarrhea, lower abdominal cramping pain, and distention.

Diagnostic, Symptomatic, and Related Terms

This section introduces diagnostic, symptomatic, and related terms and their meanings. Word analyses for selected terms are also provided.

Term	Definition
anorexia ăn-ō-RĔK-sē-ă *an-:* without, not *-orexia:* appetite	Lack or loss of appetite, resulting in the inability to eat *Anorexia should not be confused with anorexia nervosa, which is a complex psychogenic eating disorder characterized by an all-consuming desire to remain thin. Anorexia nervosa and a similar eating disorder called bulimia nervosa are discussed in Chapter 14.*
appendicitis ă-pĕn-dĭ-SĪ-tĭs *appendic:* appendix *-itis:* inflammation	Inflammation of the appendix, usually due to obstruction or infection *If left undiagnosed, appendicitis rapidly leads to perforation and peritonitis. Treatment is appendectomy within 24 to 48 hours of the first symptoms because delay usually results in rupture and peritonitis as fecal matter is released into the peritoneal cavity. (See Figure 6–7.)*
ascites ă-SĪ-tēz	Accumulation of serous fluid in the abdomen *Ascites is associated primarily with cirrhosis of the liver, venous hypertension (high blood pressure), cancer, and heart failure.*
borborygmus bor-bō-RĬG-mŭs	Rumbling or gurgling noises that are audible at a distance and caused by passage of gas through the liquid contents of the intestine
cachexia kă-KĔKS-ē-ă	General lack of nutrition and wasting occurring in the course of a chronic disease or emotional disturbance

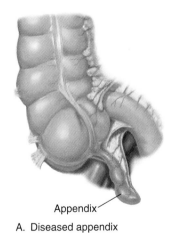

Appendix

A. Diseased appendix

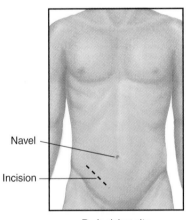

Navel

Incision

B. Incision site

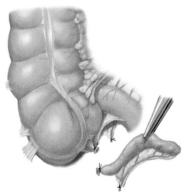

C. Excision of diseased appendix

Figure 6–7 Appendectomy.

Term	Definition
cholelithiasis kō-lē-lĭ-THĪ-ă-sĭs *chol/e:* bile, gall *lith:* stone, calculus *-iasis:* abnormal condition (produced by something specified)	Presence or formation of gallstones in the gallbladder or common bile duct *Cholelithiasis may or may not produce symptoms. (See Figure 6–8.)*
Crohn disease, regional enteritis KRŌN dĭ-ZĒZ, RĒ-jŭn-ăl ĕn-tĕr-Ī-tĭs	Chronic inflammation, usually of the ileum, but possibly affecting any portion of the intestinal tract *Crohn disease is a chronic disease distinguished from closely related bowel disorders by its inflammatory pattern that causes fever, cramping, diarrhea, and weight loss.*
cirrhosis sĭr-RŌ-sĭs	Chronic, irreversible, degenerative disease of the liver *Cirrhosis is most commonly caused by chronic alcoholism but may also be caused by toxins, infectious agents, metabolic diseases, and circulatory disorders. In this disorder, hepatic cells are replaced by fibrous tissue that impairs the flow of blood and lymph within the liver, resulting in hepatic insufficiency.*
colic KŎL-ĭk	Spasm in any hollow or tubular soft organ accompanied by pain, especially in the colon
deglutition dē-gloo-TĬSH-ŭn	Act of swallowing

(Continued)

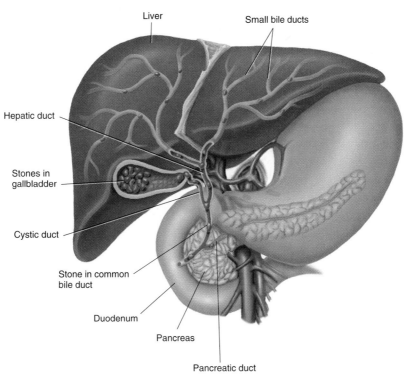

Figure 6–8   Sites of gallstones.

Term	Definition	(Continued)
dysentery DĬS-ĕn-tĕr-ē	Inflammation of the intestine, especially the colon, possibly caused by ingesting water or food containing chemical irritants, bacteria, protozoa, or parasites, that results in bloody diarrhea *Dysentery is common in underdeveloped countries and in times of disaster when sanitary living conditions, clean food, and safe water are not available.*	
dyspepsia dĭs-PĔP-sē-ă *dys-:* bad; painful; difficult *-pepsia:* digestion	Epigastric discomfort felt after eating; also called *indigestion*	
dysphagia dĭs-FĀ-jē-ă *dys-:* bad; painful; difficult *-phagia:* swallowing, eating	Inability or difficulty in swallowing; also called *aphagia*	
eructation ĕ-rŭk-TĀ-shŭn	Producing gas from the stomach, usually with a characteristic sound; also called *belching*	
fecalith FĒ-kă-lĭth	Fecal concretion	
flatus FLĀ-tŭs	Gas in the GI tract; expelling of air from a body orifice, especially the anus	
gastroesophageal reflux disease (GERD) găs-trō-ĕ-sŏf-ă-JĒ-ăl RĒ-flŭks dĭ-ZĔZ *gastr/o:* stomach *esophag:* esophagus *-eal:* pertaining to, relating to	Backflow of gastric contents into the esophagus due to a malfunction of the sphincter muscle at the inferior portion of the esophagus *GERD may occur whenever pressure in the stomach is greater than that in the esophagus and may be associated with heartburn, esophagitis, or chest pain.*	
halitosis hăl-ĭ-TŌ-sĭs	Offensive or "bad" breath	
hematemesis hĕm-ăt-ĔM-ĕ-sĭs *hemat:* blood *-emesis:* vomiting	Vomiting of blood *The vomiting of bright red blood, indicating upper GI bleeding, is commonly associated with esophageal varices or peptic ulcer.*	
irritable bowel syndrome (IBS)	Symptom complex marked by abdominal pain and altered bowel function (typically constipation, diarrhea, or alternating constipation and diarrhea) for which no organic cause can be determined; also called *spastic colon* *Contributing or aggravating factors of IBS include anxiety and stress.*	
obstipation ŏb-stĭ-PĀ-shŭn	Intestinal obstruction; also called *severe constipation*	

Term	Definition
malabsorption syndrome măl-ăb-SORP-shŭn SĬN-drōm	Symptom complex of the small intestine characterized by the impaired passage of nutrients, minerals, or fluids through intestinal villi into the blood or lymph *Malabsorption syndrome may be associated with or due to a number of diseases, including those affecting the intestinal mucosa. It may also be due to surgery, such as gastric resection and ileal bypass, or antibiotic therapy.*
melena MĔL-ĕ-nă	Passage of dark-colored, tarry stools, due to the presence of blood altered by intestinal juices
oral leukoplakia OR-ăl loo-kō-PLĀ-kē-ă *leuk/o:* white *-plakia:* plaque	Formation of white spots or patches on the mucous membrane of the tongue, lips, or cheek caused primarily by irritation *This precancerous condition is usually associated with pipe or cigarette smoking or ill-fitting dentures.*
peristalsis pĕr-ĭ-STĂL-sĭs	Progressive, wavelike movement that occurs involuntarily in hollow tubes of the body, especially the GI tract
pyloric stenosis pi-LOR-ĭk stĕ-NO-sĭs *pylor:* pylorus *-ic:* pertaining to, relating to *sten:* narrowing, stricture *-osis:* abnormal condition; increase (used primarily with blood cells)	Stricture or narrowing of the pyloric orifice, possibly due to excessive thickening of the pyloric sphincter (circular muscle of the pylorus) *Treatment for pyloric stenosis involves surgical section of the thickened muscle around the pyloric orifice.*
regurgitation rē-gŭr-jĭ-TĀ-shŭn	Backward flowing, as in the return of solids or fluids to the mouth from the stomach or the backward flow of blood through a defective heart valve
steatorrhea stē-ă-tō-RĒ-ă *steat/o:* fat *-rrhea:* discharge, flow	Passage of fat in large amounts in the feces due to failure to digest and absorb it *Steatorrhea may occur in pancreatic disease when pancreatic enzymes are not sufficient. It also occurs in malabsorption syndrome.*

 It is time to review pathological, diagnostic, symptomatic, and related terms by completing Learning Activity 6–5.

Diagnostic and Therapeutic Procedures

This section introduces procedures used to diagnose and treat digestive system disorders. Descriptions are provided as well as pronunciations and word analyses for selected terms.

Procedure	Description
DIAGNOSTIC PROCEDURES	
Endoscopic	
endoscopy ĕn-DŎS-kō-pē	Visual examination of a cavity or canal using a specialized lighted instrument called an *endoscope*
endo-: in, within *-scopy:* visual examinination	*The organ, cavity, or canal being examined dictates the name of the endoscopic procedure. (See Figure 4–5.) A camera and video recorder are commonly used during the procedure to provide a permanent record.*
upper GI	Endoscopy of the esophagus (esophagoscopy), stomach (gastroscopy), and duodenum (duodenoscopy)
	Endoscopy of the upper GI tract is performed to identify tumors, esophagitis, gastroesophageal varices, peptic ulcers, and the source of upper GI bleeding. It is also used to confirm the presence and extent of varices in the lower esophagus and stomach in patients with liver disease.
lower GI	Endoscopy of the colon (colonoscopy), sigmoid colon (sigmoidoscopy), and rectum and anal canal (proctoscopy) (See Figure 6–9.)
	Endoscopy of the lower GI tract is used to identify pathological conditions in the colon. It may also be used to remove polyps. When polyps are discovered in the colon, they are retrieved and tested for cancer.

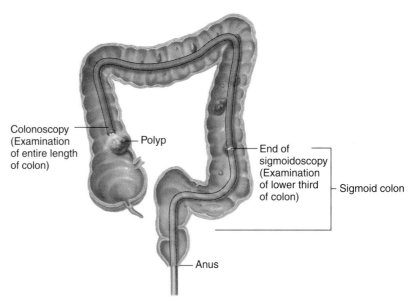

Colonoscopy (Examination of entire length of colon)

Polyp

End of sigmoidoscopy (Examination of lower third of colon)

Sigmoid colon

Anus

Figure 6–9   Colonoscopy and sigmoidoscopy.

Procedure	Description
Laboratory	
hepatitis panel hĕp-ă-TĪ-tis *hepat:* liver *-itis:* inflammation	Panel of blood tests that identify the specific virus—hepatitis A (HAV), hepatitis B (HBV), or hepatitis C (HCV)—causing hepatitis by testing serum using antibodies to each of these antigens
liver function tests (LFTs) LĬV-ĕr FŬNGK-shŭn tĕsts	Tests involving measurement of the levels of certain enzymes, bilirubin, and various proteins *LFTs are used to evaluate metabolism, storage, filtration, and excretory functions.*
serum bilirubin SĒ-rŭm bĭl-ĭ-ROO-bĭn	Measurement of the level of bilirubin in the blood *Elevated serum bilirubin indicates excessive destruction of erythrocytes, liver disease, or biliary tract obstruction. Bilirubin is a breakdown product of hemoglobin and is normally excreted from the body as bile. Excessive bilirubin causes yellowing of the skin and mucous membranes, a condition called* jaundice.
stool culture	Microbiological procedure in which microorganisms in feces are grown on media or nutrient material to identify specific pathogens
stool guaiac GWĪ-ăk	Applying a substance called guaiac to a stool sample to detect the presence of blood in the feces; also called *Hemoccult* (trade name of a modified guaiac test) *This stool test is performed to detect the presence of blood in the feces that is not apparent on visual inspection (obscure, hidden, or occult blood). It also helps detect colon cancer and determine bleeding in digestive disorders.*

(Continued)

Procedure	Description	(Continued)

Radiographic

barium enema
BĂ-rē-ŭm ĔN-ĕ-mă

Radiographic examination of the rectum and colon following enema administration of barium sulfate (contrast medium) into the rectum; also called *lower GI series*

Barium sulfate is used as the contrast medium in a barium enema. It is retained in the lower GI tract during fluoroscopic and radiographic studies. Barium enema is used for diagnosing obstructions, tumors, or other abnormalities of the colon. (See Figure 6–10.)

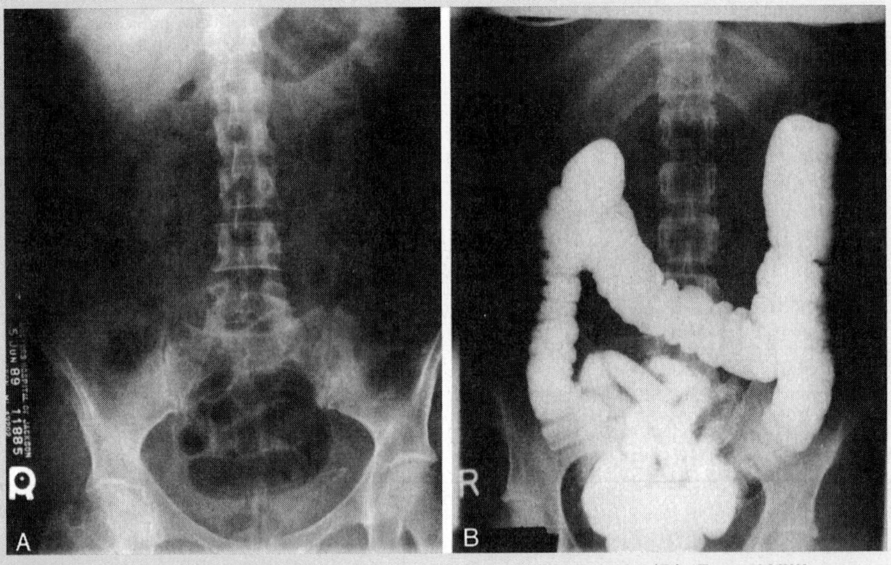

Figure 6–10 Barium enema done poorly (A) and correctly (B). From Williams, LS, and Hopper, PD: *Understanding Medical-Surgical Nursing,* 2nd edition, page 540 (Courtesy of Russell Tobe, MD). F.A. Davis, 2003, with permission.

barium swallow
BĂ-rē-ŭm SWĂL-ō

Radiographic examination of the esophagus, stomach, and small intestine following oral administration of barium sulfate (contrast medium); also called *esophagram* and *upper GI series*

Barium swallow is used to diagnose structural defects of the esophagus and vessels, such as esophageal varices. It may also be used to locate swallowed objects.

cholecystography
kō-lē-sĭs-TŎG-ră-fē

chol/e: bile, gall
cyst/o: bladder
-graphy: process of recording

Radiographic images taken of the gallbladder after administration of a contrast material containing iodine, usually in the form of a tablet

Cholecystography is used to evaluate gallbladder function and determine the presence of disease or gallstones.

Procedure	Description
computed tomography (CT) scan kŏm-PŪ-tĕd tō-MŎG-ră-fē *tom/o:* to cut *-graphy:* process of recording	Imaging technique achieved by rotating an x-ray emitter around the area to be scanned and measuring the intensity of transmitted rays from different angles; formerly called *computerized axial tomography* *In CT scanning, a computer is used to generate a detailed cross-sectional image that appears as a slice. (See Figure 4–4D.) In the digestive system, CT scans are used to view the gallbladder, liver, bile ducts, and pancreas. It is used to diagnose tumors, cysts, inflammation, abscesses, perforation, bleeding, and obstructions.*
endoscopic retrograde cholangiopancreatography (ERCP) ĕn-dō-SKŎ-pĭk RĔT-rō-grād kŏ-lăn-jē-ō-păn-krē-ă-TŎG-ră-fē *cholangi/o:* bile vessel *pancreat/o:* pancreas *-graphy:* process of recording	Endoscopic procedure that provides radiographic visualization of the bile and pancreatic ducts *A flexible fiberoptic duodenoscope is placed into the common bile duct. A radiopaque substance is instilled directly into the duct and serial x-ray films are taken. ERCP is useful in identifying partial or total obstruction of these ducts as well as stones, cysts, and tumors.*
percutaneous transhepatic cholangiography pĕr-kū-TA-nē-ŭs trăns-hĕ-PĂT-ĭk kō-lăn-jē-ŎG-ră-fē *per-:* through *cutane:* skin *-ous:* pertaining to, relating to *trans-:* through, across *hepat:* liver *-ic:* pertaining to, relating to *cholangi/o:* bile vessel *-graphy:* process of recording	Radiographic examination of the structure of the bile ducts *A contrast medium is injected through a needle passed directly into the hepatic duct. The bile duct structure can be viewed for obstructions, anatomic variations, and cysts.*
sialography sī-ă-LŎG-ră-fē *sial/o:* saliva, salivary glands *-graphy:* process of recording	Radiologic examination of the salivary glands and ducts *Sialography may be performed with or without a contrast medium.*

(Continued)

Procedure	Description	(Continued)
ultrasonography (US) ŭl-tră-sŏn-ŎG-ră-fē *ultra-:* excess, beyond *son/o:* sound *-graphy:* process of recording	Image produced by using high-frequency sound waves (ultrasound) and displaying the reflected "echoes" on a monitor (A computer analyzes the reflected echos and converts them into an image on a video monitor.); also called *ultrasound, sonography, echo,* and *echogram* *US is used to detect diseases and deformities in digestive organs, such as the gallbladder, liver, and pancreas. It is also used to locate abdominal masses outside the digestive organs.*	
abdominal ăb-DŎM-ĭ-năl *abdomin:* abdomen *-al:* pertaining to, relating to	Ultrasound visualization of the abdominal aorta, liver, gallbladder, bile ducts, pancreas, kidneys, ureters, and bladder *Abdominal ultrasound is used to diagnose and locate cysts, tumors, and malformations. It is also used to document the progression of various diseases and guide the insertion of instruments during surgical procedures.*	

Surgical

biopsy BĬ-ŏp-sē	Representative tissue sample removed from a body site for microscopic examination, usually to establish a diagnosis	
liver	Use of a large-bore needle to remove a core of liver tissue for histological examination	

THERAPEUTIC PROCEDURES

nasogastric intubation nā-zō-GĂS-trĭk ĭn-tū-BĀ-shŭn *nas/o:* nose *gastr:* stomach *-ic:* pertaining to, relating to	Insertion of a nasogastric tube through the nose into the stomach to relieve gastric distention by removing gas, gastric secretions, or food; to instill medication, food, or fluids; or to obtain a specimen for laboratory analysis	

Surgical

anastomosis ă-năs-tō-MŌ-sĭs	Surgical joining of two ducts, vessels, or bowel segments to allow flow from one to another	
ileorectal ĭl-ē-ō-RĔK-tăl *ile/o:* ileum *rect:* rectum *-al:* pertaining to, relating to	Surgical connection of the ileum and rectum after total colectomy, as is sometimes performed in the treatment of ulcerative colitis	
intestinal ĭn-TĔS-tĭ-năl	Surgical connection of two portions of the intestines; also called *enteroenterostomy*	

Procedure	Description
colostomy kō-LŎS-tō-mē *col/o:* colon *-stomy:* forming an opening (mouth)	Creation of an opening of some portion of the colon through the abdominal wall to its outside surface in order to divert fecal flow to a colostomy bag (See Figure 6–11.)
lithotripsy LĬTH-ō-trĭp-sē *lith/o:* stone, calculus *-tripsy:* crushing	Procedure for eliminating a stone within the urinary system or gallbladder by crushing the stone surgically or using a noninvasive method, such as ultrasonic shock waves, to shatter it
extracorporeal shockwave ĕks-tră-kor-POR-ē-ăl SHŎK-wāv	Use of shock waves as a noninvasive method to break up stones in the gallbladder or biliary ducts *In extracorporeal shockwave lithotripsy (ESWL), ultrasound is used to locate the stone or stones and to monitor the destruction of the stones. The patient is usually placed on a course of oral dissolution drugs to ensure complete removal of all stones and stone fragments.*

(Continued)

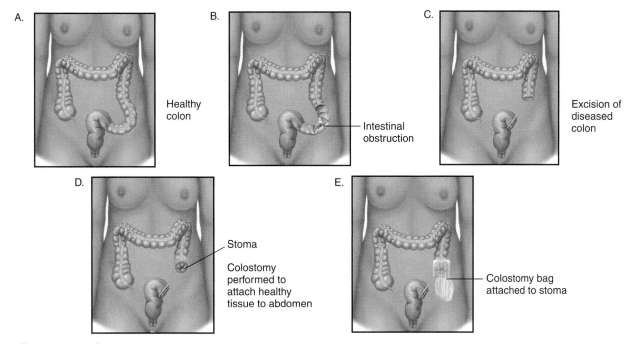

A. Healthy colon

B. Intestinal obstruction

C. Excision of diseased colon

D. Stoma — Colostomy performed to attach healthy tissue to abdomen

E. Colostomy bag attached to stoma

Figure 6–11   Colostomy.

Procedure	Description	(Continued)
polypectomy pŏl-ĭ-PĔK-tō-mē *polyp:* small growth *-ectomy:* excision, removal	Excision of a polyp *When polyps are discovered during sigmoidoscopy or colonoscopy, polypectomy is used to retrieve them to test for cancer. (See Figure 6–12.)*	
pyloromyotomy pī-lō-rō-mī-ŎT-ō-mē *pylor/o:* pylorus *my/o:* muscle *-tomy:* incision	Incision of the longitudinal and circular muscles of the pylorus; used to treat hypertrophic pyloric stenosis	

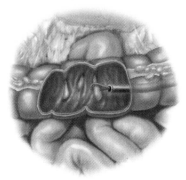

Polyps are removed from
colon for examination

Figure 6–12   Polypectomy.

Pharmacology

Various pharmaceutical agents are available to counteract abnormal conditions that occur in the GI tract. Antacids counteract or decrease excessive stomach acid, which is responsible for heartburn, gastric discomfort, and gastric reflux. Antidiarrheals and antiemetics are used to preserve water and electrolytes, which are essential for body hydration because they control the rapid elimination of digestive materials from the body. Medications that increase or decrease peristalsis are used to regulate the speed at which food passes through the GI tract. These drugs include agents that relieve "cramping" (antispasmodics) and those that help in the movement of material through a sluggish bowel (laxatives). (See Table 6–1.)

Table 6-1   DRUGS USED TO TREAT DIGESTIVE DISORDERS

This table lists common drug classifications use to treat digestive disorders, their therapeutic actions, and selected generic and trade names.

Classification	Therapeutic Action	Generic and Trade Names

antacids	Neutralize stomach acid
	
	Antacids are used for the treatment and prevention of heartburn and acid reflux and for short-term treatment of active duodenal ulcers and benign gastric ulcers.
		cimetidine
		sĭ-MĔT-ĭ-dēn
		  Tagamet, Tagamet HB
		famotidine
		fă-MŌ-tĭ-dēn
		  Mylanta AR, Pepcid, Pepcid AC

antidiarrheals	Control loose stools; relieve diarrhea
	
	Antidiarrheals produce a therapeutic effect by absorbing excess water in the stool or slowing peristalsis in the intestinal tract.
		loperamide
		lō-PĔR-ă-mĭd
		  Imodium, Imodium A-D, Kaopectate II Caplets, Maalox Antidiarrheal Caplets, Pepto Diarrhea Control
		kaolin/pectin
		KĀ-ō-lĭn/PĔK-tĭn
		  Donnagel-MB, Kao-Spen, Kapectolin, K-P

antiemetics	Control nausea and vomiting
	
	The majority of antiemetics block nerve impulses to the vomiting center in the brain.
		prochlorperazine
		prō-klor-PĔR-ă-zēn
		  Compazine, Ultrazine
		trimethobenzamide
		trī-mĕth-ō-BĔN-ză-mĭd
		  T-Gen, Ticon, Tigan, Trimazide

antispasmodics	Decrease gastrointestinal spasms
	
	Antispasmodics are anticholinergics that decrease spasms by slowing peristalsis and motility throughout the GI tract. They are used in the treatment of irritable bowel syndrome (IBS), spastic colon, and diverticulitis.
		glycopyrrolate
		glĭ-kō-PĬR-rō-lāt
		  Robinul, Robinul-Forte
		propantheline
		prō-PĂN-thĕ-lēn
		  Pro-Banthine

laxatives	Treat constipation
	
	Laxatives produce a therapeutic effect by increasing peristaltic activity in the large intestine or increasing water and electrolyte secretion into the bowel to induce defecation.
		senna, sennosides
		SĔN-ă, SĔN-ō-sĭdz
		  Dosaflex, Senna-Gen, Senokot, Senolax
		psyllium
		SĬL-ē-ŭm
		  Fiberall, Hydrocil, Metamucil, Mylanta Natural Fiber Supplement

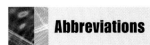

Abbreviations

This section introduces digestive-related abbreviations and their meanings.

Abbreviation	Meaning
COMMON	
ABC	aspiration biopsy cytology
alk phos	alkaline phosphatase
ALT	alanine aminotransferase (elevated in liver and heart disease); formerly *SGPT*
AST	angiotensin sensitivity test; aspartate aminotransferase (cardiac enzyme, formerly called *SGOT*)
Ba	barium
BaE	barium enema
BM	bowel movement
CT	computed tomography
CT scan, CAT scan	computed tomography scan
EGD	esophagogastroduodenoscopy
ERCP	endoscopic retrograde cholangiopancreatography
GB	gallbladder
GBS	gallbladder series
GER	gastroesophageal reflux
GERD	gastroesophageal reflux disease
GI	gastrointestinal
HAV	hepatitis A virus
HBV	hepatitis B virus
HCV	hepatitis C virus
HDV	hepatitis D virus
HEV	hepatitis E virus
IBS	irritable bowel syndrome
NG	nasogastric
PUD	peptic ulcer disease
R/O	rule out

Abbreviation	Meaning
DOSAGE SCHEDULES*	
ac	before meals
bid	twice a day
npo	nothing by mouth
pc, pp	after meals (postprandial)
po	by mouth (per os)
prn	as required
qam, qm	every morning
qh	every hour *This abbreviation may also contain a number to indicate the number of hours between administration of medication or therapy, as in q8h.*
q2h	every 2 hours
qid	four times a day
qod**	every other day
qpm, qn	every night
stat	immediately
tid	three times a day

*Because many of these abbreviations deal with pharmacology and the administration of medication, they are not unique to the digestive system.

**Although this abbreviation is currently found in medical records and clinical notes, the Joint Commission on Accreditation of Healthcare Organizations (JCAHO) requires its discontinuance. Instead, write out its meaning.

 It is time to review procedures, pharmacology, and abbreviations by completing Learning Activity 6–6.

LEARNING ACTIVITIES

The following activities provide review of the digestive system terms introduced in this chapter. Complete each activity and review your answers to evaluate your understanding of the chapter.

Learning Activity 6–1

Identifying digestive structures

Label the illustration on page 139 using the terms listed below.

anus	*hepatic flexure*	*rectum*
appendix	*ileum*	*sigmoid colon*
ascending colon	*jejunum*	*spleen*
cecum	*liver*	*splenic flexure*
descending colon	*pancreas*	*transverse colon*
duodenum		

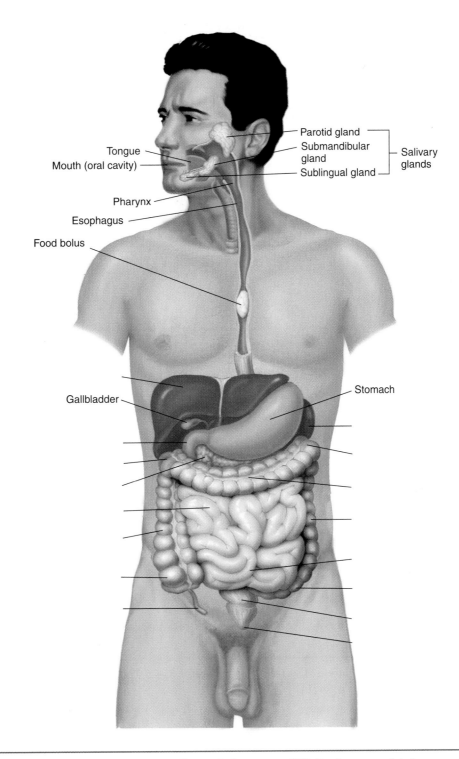

Parotid gland

Submandibular
gland

Sublingual gland

Salivary
glands

Tongue

Mouth (oral cavity)

Pharynx

Esophagus

Food bolus

Gallbladder

Stomach

Check your answers by referring to Figure 6–3 on page 112. Review material that you did not answer correctly.

Learning Activity 6–2

Identifying accessory organs of digestion

Label the following illustration using the terms listed below.

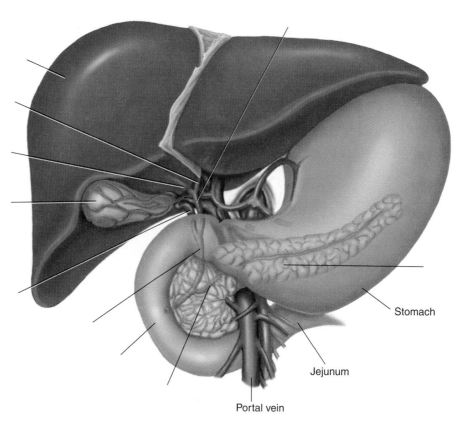

common bile duct   hepatic duct   pancreas

cystic duct   left hepatic duct   pancreatic duct

duodenum   liver   right hepatic duct

gallbladder

Check your answers by referring to Figure 6–4 on page 113. Review material that you did not answer correctly.

Learning Activity 6-3

Building medical words

Use **esophag/o** *(esophagus) to build words that mean:*

1. pain in the esophagus _____
2. spasm of the esophagus _____
3. stricture or narrowing of the esophagus _____

Use **gastr/o** *(stomach) to build words that mean:*

4. inflammation of the stomach _____
5. pain in the stomach _____
6. disease of the stomach _____

Use **duoden/o** *(duodenum),* **jejun/o** *(jejunum), or* **ile/o** *(ileum) to build words that mean:*

7. excision of all or part of the jejunum _____
8. relating to the duodenum _____
9. inflammation of the ileum _____
10. concerning the jejunum and ileum _____

Use **enter/o** *(usually small intestine) to build words that mean:*

11. inflammation of the small intestine _____
12. disease of the small intestine _____

Use **col/o** *(colon) to build words that mean:*

13. inflammation of the colon _____
14. pertaining to the colon and rectum _____
15. inflammation of the small intestine and colon _____
16. prolapse or downward displacement of the colon _____
17. disease of the colon _____

Use **proct/o** *(anus, rectum) or* **rect/o** *(rectum) to build words that mean:*

18. narrowing or constriction of the rectum _____
19. herniation of the rectum _____
20. paralysis of the anus (anal muscles) _____

Use **chol/e** *(bile, gall) to build words that mean:*

21. inflammation of the gallbladder _____
22. abnormal condition of a gallstone _____

Use **hepat/o** *(liver) or* **pancreat/o** *(pancreas) to build words that mean:*

23. tumor of the liver _____
24. enlargement of the liver _____
25. inflammation of the pancreas _____

✓ Check your answers in Appendix A. Review material that you did not answer correctly.

CORRECT ANSWERS _____ × 4 = _____ **% SCORE**

Learning Activity 6–4

Building surgical words

Build a surgical word that means:

1. excision of gums (tissue) _____

2. partial or complete excision of the tongue _____

3. repair of the esophagus _____

4. removal of part or all of the stomach _____

5. forming an opening between the stomach and jejunum _____

6. excision of (part of) the esophagus _____

7. forming an opening between the stomach, small intestine, and colon _____

8. surgical repair of the small intestine _____

9. fixation of the small intestine (to the abdominal wall) _____

10. suture of the bile duct _____

11. forming an opening into the colon _____

12. fixation of a movable liver (to the abdominal wall) _____

13. surgical repair of the anus or rectum _____

14. removal of the gallbladder _____

15. surgical repair of a bile duct _____

✓ Check your answers in Appendix A. Review material that you did not answer correctly.

CORRECT ANSWERS _____ × **6.67** = _____ **% SCORE**

Learning Activity 6–5

Matching pathological, diagnostic, symptomatic, and related terms

Match the following terms with the definitions in the numbered list.

anorexia	*dysphagia*	*hematemesis*
cachexia	*dyspnea*	*lesion*
cirrhosis	*fecalith*	*melena*
dyspepsia	*halitosis*	*obstipation*

1. _____ vomiting blood
2. _____ difficulty swallowing or inability to swallow
3. _____ fecal concretion
4. _____ "bad" breath
5. _____ loss of appetite
6. _____ poor digestion
7. _____ degenerative liver disease
8. _____ state of ill health, malnutrition, and wasting
9. _____ intractable constipation
10. _____ open sore

Check your answers in Appendix A. Review any material that you did not answer correctly.

CORRECT ANSWERS _____ × 10 = _____ **% SCORE**

Learning Activity 6–6

Matching procedures, pharmacology, and abbreviations

Match the following terms with the definitions in the numbered list.

anastomosis	*emetics*	*liver function tests*	*qid*
antacids	*endoscopy*	*lower GI series*	*stat*
bid	*gastroscopy*	*pc, pp*	*stool guaiac*
bilirubin	*intubation*	*ultrasonography*	*stomatoplasty*
choledochoplasty	*laxatives*	*proctosigmoidoscopy*	*upper GI series*

1. _____ after meals

2. _____ breakdown of hemoglobin, normally excreted from the body as bile

3. _____ agents that produce vomiting

4. _____ twice a day

5. _____ surgical reconstruction of a bile duct

6. _____ an enema with a barium solution is administered while a series of radiographs are taken of the large intestine

7. _____ visual examination of the stomach

8. _____ surgical reconstruction of the mouth

9. _____ insertion of a tube into any hollow organ

10. _____ surgical formation of a passage or opening between two hollow viscera or vessels

11. _____ detects presence of blood in the feces; also called Hemoccult

12. _____ visual examination of a cavity or canal using a specialized lighted instrument

13. _____ used to treat constipation

14. _____ neutralize excess acid in the stomach and help to relieve gastritis and ulcer pain

15. _____ procedure in which high-frequency sound waves produce images of internal body structures that are displayed on a monitor

16. _____ measures the levels of certain enzymes, bilirubin, and various proteins

17. _____ four times a day

18. _____ immediately

19. _____ endoscopic procedure for visualization of the rectosigmoid colon

20. _____ barium solution swallowed for a radiographic examination of the esophagus, stomach, and duodenum

✓ Check your answers in Appendix A. Review material that you did not answer correctly.

CORRECT ANSWERS _____ × 5 = _____ **% SCORE**

MEDICAL RECORD ACTIVITIES

The two medical records included in the following activities use common clinical scenarios to show how medical terminology is used to document patient care. Complete the terminology and analysis sections for each activity to help you recognize and understand terms related to the digestive system.

Medical Record Activity 6-1

GI evaluation

Terminology

The terms listed in the chart come from the medical record *GI Evaluation* that follows. Use a medical dictionary such as *Taber's Cyclopedic Medical Dictionary*, the appendices of this book, or other resources to define each term. Then review the pronunciations for each term and practice by reading the medical record aloud.

Term	Definition
appendectomy* ăp-ĕn-DĔK-tō-mē	
cholecystectomy kō-lē-sis-TĔK-tō-mē	
cholecystitis kō-lē-sis-TĪ-tĭs	
cholelithiasis* kō-lē-lĭ-THĪ-ă-sĭs	
crescendo kră-SHĔN-dō	
decrescendo dā-kră-SHĔN-dō	
defecate DĔF-ĕ-kāt	
flatus FLĀ-tŭs	
heme-negative stool hēm-NĔG-ă-tĭv	
hepatomegaly hĕp-ă-tō-MĔG-ă-lē	
intermittent ĭn-tĕr-MĬT-ĕnt	

(Continued)

Term	Definition	(Continued)
nausea NAW-sē-ă		
PMH		
postoperative pōst-ŎP-ĕr-ă-tĭv		
R/O		
splenomegaly splē-nō-MĔG-ă-lē		
tonsillectomy tōn-sĭl-ĔK-tō-mē		

*Refer to Figure 6–5 and Figure 6–8 for a visual illustration of these terms.

GI EVALUATION

HISTORY OF PRESENT ILLNESS: The patient's abdominal pain began 2 years ago when she first had intermittent, sharp epigastric pain. Each episode lasted 2 to 4 hours. Eventually, she was diagnosed as having cholecystitis with cholelithiasis and underwent cholecystectomy. Three to five large calcified stones were found.

Her postoperative course was uneventful until 4 months ago, when she began having continuous deep right-sided pain.

This pain followed a crescendo pattern and peaked several weeks ago, at a time when family stress was also at its climax. Since then, the pain has been following a decrescendo pattern. It does not cause any nausea or vomiting, does not trigger any urge to defecate, and was not alleviated by passage of flatus. Her PMH is significant only for tonsillectomy, appendectomy, and the cholecystectomy. Her PE findings indicate that there was no hepatomegaly or splenomegaly. The rectal examination confirmed normal sphincter tone and heme-negative stool.

IMPRESSION: Abdominal pain. R/O hepatomegaly and splenomegaly.

PLAN: Schedule a complete barium workup for possible obstruction.

Analysis

Review the medical record *GI Evaluation* to answer the following questions.

1. While referring to Figure 6–3, describe the location of the gallbladder in relation to the liver.

_____

2. Why did the patient undergo the cholecystectomy?

_____

3. List the patient's prior surgeries.

_____

4. How does the patient's most recent postoperative episode of discomfort (pain) differ from the initial pain she described?

_____

Medical Record Activity 6-2

Esophagogastroduodenoscopy with biopsy

Terminology

The terms listed in the chart come from the medical record *Esophagogastroduodenoscopy with Biopsy* that follows. Use a medical dictionary such as *Taber's Cyclopedic Medical Dictionary*, the appendices of this book, or other resources to define each term. Then review the pronunciations for each term and practice by reading the medical record aloud.

Term	Definition
Demerol DĔM-ĕr-ŏl	
duodenal bulb dū-ō-DĒ-năl BŬLB	
duodenitis dū-ŏd-ĕ-NĪ-tĭs	
erythema ĕr-ĭ-THĒ-mă	
esophageal varices ē-sŏf-ă-JĒ-ăl VĂR-ĭ-sēz	
esophagogastroduodenoscopy ĕ-SŎF-ă-gō-GĂS-trō-doo-ō-dĕn-ŎS-kō-pē	
etiology ē-tē-ŎL-ō-jē	
friability frī-ă-BĬL-ĭ-tē	
gastric antrum GĂS-trĭk ĂN-trŭm	
gastritis găs-TRĪ-tĭs	
hematemesis hĕm-ăt-ĔM-ĕ-sĭs	
lateral recumbent LĂT-ĕr-ăl rē-KŬM-bĕnt	
oximeter ŏk-SĬM-ĕ-tĕr	
punctate erythema PŬNK-tāt ĕr-ĭ-THĒ-mă	

(Continued)

Term	Definition	(Continued)
tomography tō-MŎG-ră-fē		
Versed VĔR-sĕd		
videoendoscope vĭd-ē-ō-ĔND-ō-skōp		

ESOPHAGOGASTRODUODENOSCOPY WITH BIOPSY

POSTOPERATIVE DIAGNOSIS: Diffuse gastritis and duodenitis.

PROCEDURE: Esophagogastroduodenoscopy with biopsy.

TISSUE TO LABORATORY: Biopsies from gastric antrum and duodenal bulb.

ESTIMATED BLOOD LOSS: Nil.

COMPLICATIONS: None.

TIME UNDER SEDATION: 20 minutes.

INDICATIONS FOR PROCEDURE: This is a patient with hematemesis of unknown etiology.

FINDINGS AND PROCEDURE: After obtaining informed consent regarding the procedure, its risks, and its alternatives, the patient was taken to the GI Laboratory, where she was placed on the examining table in the left lateral recumbent position. She was given nasal oxygen at 3 liters per minute throughout the procedure and monitored with a pulse oximeter throughout the procedure. Through a previously inserted intravenous line, the patient was sedated with a total of 50 mg of Demerol intravenously plus 4 mg of Versed intravenously throughout the procedure.

The Fujinon computed tomography scan videoendoscope was then readily introduced.

Esophagus: The esophageal mucosa appeared normal throughout. No other abnormalities were seen. Specifically, there was prior evidence of esophageal varices.

Stomach: There was diffuse erythema with old blood seen within the stomach. No ulcerations, erosions, or fresh bleeding was seen. A representative biopsy was obtained from the gastric antrum and submitted to the pathology laboratory.

Duodenum: Punctate erythema was noted in the duodenal bulb. There was some friability. No ulcerations, erosions, or active bleeding was seen. A bulbar biopsy was obtained. The second portion of the duodenum appeared normal.

Analysis

Review the medical record *Esophagogastroduodenoscopy with Biopsy* to answer the following questions.

1. What caused the hematemesis?

_____

2. What procedures were carried out to determine the cause of bleeding?

_____

3. How much blood did the patient lose during the procedure?

_____

4. Were there any ulcerations or erosions found during the exploratory procedure that might account for the bleeding?

_____

5. What type of sedation was used during the procedure?

_____

6. What did the doctors find when they examined the stomach and duodenum?

_____

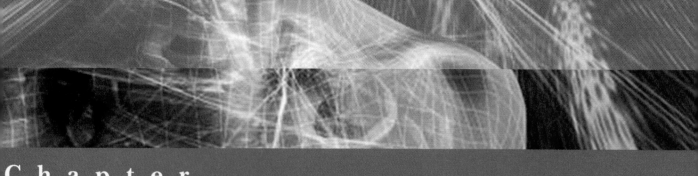

Chapter

7

Respiratory System

CHAPTER OUTLINE

OBJECTIVES

Upon completion of this chapter, you will be able to:

■ Locate and describe the structures of the respiratory system.

■ Recognize, pronounce, spell, and build words related to the respiratory system.

■ Describe pathological conditions, diagnostic and therapeutic procedures, and other terms related to the respiratory system.

■ Explain pharmacology related to the treatment of respiratory disorders.

■ Demonstrate your knowledge of this chapter by completing the learning and medical record activities.

151

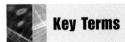

Key Terms

This section introduces important respiratory system terms and their definitions. Word analyses are also provided.

Term	Definition
cytoplasm SĪ-tō-plăzm *cyt/o:* cell *-plasm:* formation, growth	All the material within the cell membrane other than the nucleus
carbon dioxide (CO_2) KĂR-bŏn dī-ŎK-sīd	Tasteless, colorless, odorless gas produced by body cells during the metabolic process *A product of cell respiration, carbon dioxide is carried by the blood to the lungs and exhaled.*
granuloma grăn-ū-LŌ-mă *granul:* granule *-oma:* tumor	Any type of nodular, inflammatory lesion; usually small; may be granular, firm, and persistent and may contain compactly grouped mononuclear phagocytes
mucosa mū-KŌ-să	Moist tissue layer lining hollow organs and cavities of the body that open to the environment; also called *mucous membrane*
mucus MŪ-kŭs	Viscous, slippery secretion of mucous membranes that acts as a lubricant and coats and protects many epithelial surfaces, especially the respiratory and genital tracts
naris NĀ-rĭs	Nostril; opening to the nasal cavity
oxygen (O_2) ŎK-sĭ-jĕn	Tasteless, odorless, colorless gas essential for human respiration
pH	Symbol that indicates the degree of acidity or alkalinity of a substance *Increasing acidity is expressed as a number less than 7; increasing alkalinity as a number greater than 7, with 7 being neutral. Normal blood is slightly alkaline with a pH range from 7.37 to 7.43. When blood pH is less than 7.37 it is called acidosis; greater than 7.43, alkalosis.*
respiratory failure RĔS-pĭ-ră-tō-rē	Inability of the cardiac and pulmonary systems to maintain an adequate exchange of oxygen and carbon dioxide in the lungs
septum SĔP-tŭm	Wall dividing two cavities; for example, the nasal septum that separates the nostrils
sputum SPŪ-tŭm	Secretions produced in the lungs and bronchi that are expelled by coughing and may contain such pathological elements as cellular debris, mucus, blood, pus, caseous material, and microorganisms

Term	Definition
status asthmaticus STĀ-tŭs ăz-MĂ-tĭk-ŭs	Severe, prolonged asthma attack that does not respond to repeated doses of bronchodilators and may lead to respiratory failure and death
surfactant sŭr-FĂK-tănt	Lipoprotein that decreases the surface tension of alveoli and contributes to their elasticity, thereby reducing the work of breathing

Anatomy and Physiology

The organs and structures of the respiratory system are responsible for the exchange of the respiratory gases oxygen and carbon dioxide. Oxygen, essential for life, is delivered to all cells of the body in exchange for carbon dioxide, a waste product. The cardiovascular system assists in this vital function by providing blood vessels, the pathways for transporting these gases. Failure of or deficiency in either system has the same effect on the body: disruption of homeostasis and oxygen starvation in tissues that may result in death.

The lungs and airways bring in fresh, oxygen-enriched air and expel waste carbon dioxide by a process called breathing, or ventilation. Breathing is an important method of regulating the pH of the blood, thereby maintaining homeostasis.

Upper Respiratory Tract

The breathing process begins with inhalation. (See Figure 7–1.) Air is drawn into the (1) **nasal cavity,** a chamber lined with mucous membranes and tiny hairs called *cilia.* Here, air is filtered, heated, and moistened to prepare it for its journey to the lungs. The nasal cavity is divided into a right and left side by a vertical partition of cartilage called the *nasal septum.*

The receptors for the sense of smell are located in the nasal cavity. These receptors, called the *olfactory neurons,* are found among the epithelial cells lining the nasal tract and are covered with a layer of mucus. Because these receptors are located higher in the nasal passage than air normally inhaled during breathing, a person must sniff or inhale deeply to identify weak odors.

Air passes from the nasal cavity to a muscular tube called the *pharynx,* or *throat,* that serves as a passageway for food and air. It consists of three sections: the (2) **nasopharynx,** posterior to the nose; the (3) **oropharynx,** posterior to the mouth; and the (4) **laryngopharynx,** superior to the larynx.

Within the nasopharynx is a collection of lymphatic tissue known as (5) **adenoids,** or *pharyngeal tonsils.* The (6) **palatine tonsils,** more commonly known as *tonsils,* are located in the oropharynx. They protect the opening to the respiratory tract from microscopic organisms that may attempt entry by this route. The (7) **larynx** (voice box) contains the structures that make vocal sounds possible. A leaf-shaped structure on top of the larynx, the (8) **epiglottis,** seals off the air passage to the lungs during swallowing. This function ensures that food or liquids do not obstruct the flow of air to the lungs. The larynx is a short passage that joins the pharynx with the (9) **trachea** (windpipe). The trachea is composed of smooth muscle embedded with C-shaped rings of cartilage, which provide rigidity to keep the air passage open.

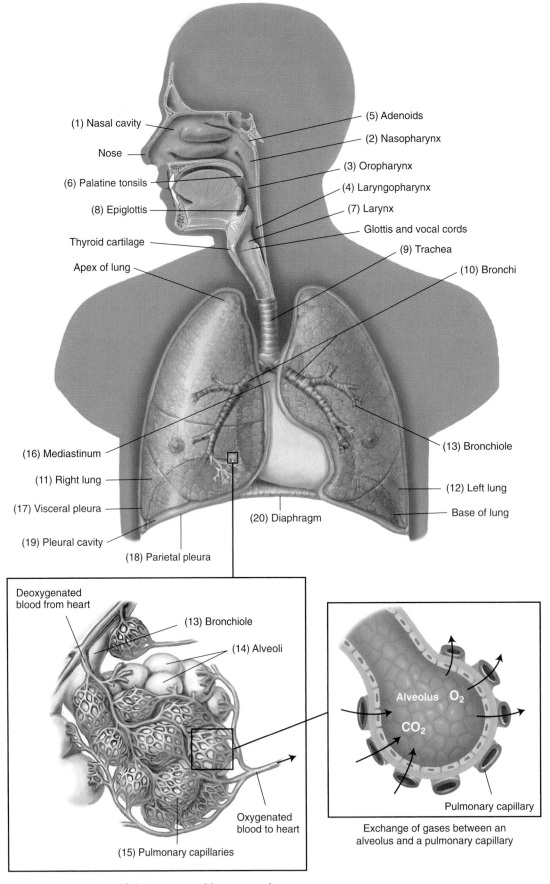

(1) Nasal cavity

Nose

(6) Palatine tonsils

(8) Epiglottis

Thyroid cartilage

Apex of lung

(5) Adenoids

(2) Nasopharynx

(3) Oropharynx

(4) Laryngopharynx

(7) Larynx

Glottis and vocal cords

(9) Trachea

(10) Bronchi

(16) Mediastinum

(11) Right lung

(17) Visceral pleura

(19) Pleural cavity

(18) Parietal pleura

(13) Bronchiole

(12) Left lung

Base of lung

(20) Diaphragm

Deoxygenated
blood from heart

(13) Bronchiole

(14) Alveoli

(15) Pulmonary capillaries

Oxygenated
blood to heart

Alveolus O_2

CO_2

Pulmonary capillary

Exchange of gases between an
alveolus and a pulmonary capillary

Figure 7–1   Anterior view of the upper and lower respiratory tracts.

Lower Respiratory Tract

The trachea divides into two branches called (10) **bronchi** (singular, **bronchus**). One branch leads to the (11) **right lung** and the other to the (12) **left lung.** The inner walls of the trachea and bronchi are composed of a mucous membrane embedded with cilia. This membrane traps incoming particles, and the cilia move the entrapped material upward into the pharynx, where it is coughed out, sneezed out, or swallowed. Like the trachea, bronchi contain C-shaped rings of cartilage.

Each bronchus divides into smaller and smaller branches, eventually forming (13) **bronchioles.** Where bronchioles terminate, tiny air sacs called (14) **alveoli** (singular, **alveolus**) are formed. An alveolus resembles a small balloon because it expands and contracts with inflow and outflow of air. The (15) **pulmonary capillaries** lie adjacent to the thin tissue membranes of the alveoli. Carbon dioxide diffuses from the blood within the pulmonary capillaries and enters the alveolar spaces. Simultaneously, oxygen from the alveoli diffuses into the blood. After the exchange of gases, freshly oxygenated blood returns to the heart. It is now ready for delivery to all body tissues.

The lungs are divided into lobes: three lobes in the right lung and two lobes in the left lung. The space between the right and left lungs, called the (16) **mediastinum,** contains the heart, aorta, esophagus, and bronchi. A serous membrane, the **pleura,** envelops the lobes of the lungs and folds over to line the walls of the thoracic cavity. The innermost membrane lying next to the lung is the (17) **visceral pleura;** the outermost membrane, which lines the thoracic cavity, is the (18) **parietal pleura.** Between these two membranes is the (19) **pleural cavity.** It contains a small amount of lubricating fluid, which permits the visceral pleura to glide smoothly over the parietal pleura during breathing.

Ventilation depends on a pressure differential between the atmosphere and chest cavity. A large muscular partition, the (20) **diaphragm,** lies between the chest and abdominal cavities. The diaphragm assists in changing the volume of the thoracic cavity to produce the needed pressure differential for ventilation. When the diaphragm contracts, it partially descends into the abdominal cavity, thus decreasing the pressure within the chest and drawing air into the lungs. When the diaphragm relaxes, it slowly re-enters the thoracic cavity, thus increasing the pressure within the chest **(inspiration).** As the pressure increases, air leaves the lungs **(expiration).** The **intercostal** muscles assist the diaphragm in changing the volume of the thoracic cavity by elevating and lowering the rib cage. (See Figure 7–2.)

Respiration

Respiration is the overall process by which oxygen is taken from air and transported to body cells for the metabolic process, while carbon dioxide and water, the waste products generated by these cells, are returned to the environment.

Respiration includes four separate processes:

1. ventilation (breathing), the largely involuntary movement of air into (inspiration) and out of (expiration) the lungs in response to changes in oxygen and carbon dioxide levels in the blood and nervous stimulation of the diaphragm and intercostal muscles
2. external respiration, the exchange of oxygen and carbon dioxide between the alveoli and the blood in the pulmonary capillaries
3. transport of respiratory gases through the body by blood in the cardiovascular system
4. internal respiration, the exchange of oxygen and carbon dioxide between tissue cells and the blood in systemic capillaries

 It is time to review respiratory structures by completing Learning Activity 7–1.

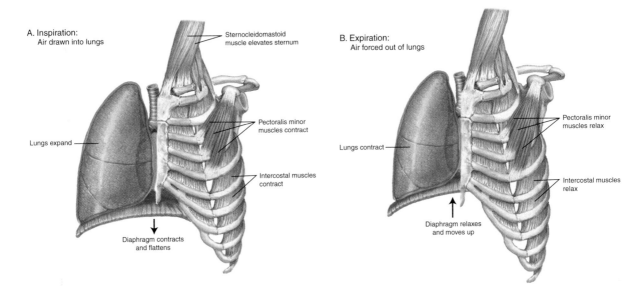

Figure 7–2   Breathing muscles.

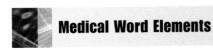
Medical Word Elements

This section introduces combining forms, suffixes, and prefixes related to the integumentary system. Word analyses are also provided.

Element	Meaning	Word Analysis
COMBINING FORMS		
Upper Respiratory Tract		
nas/o	nose	nas/al (NĀ-zl): pertaining to the nose *-al:* pertaining to, relating to
rhin/o		rhin/o/plasty (RĪ-nō-plăs-tē): plastic surgery of the nose to correct a birth defect or breathing problem or for cosmetic purposes *-plasty:* surgical repair
sept/o	septum	sept/o/plasty (sĕp-tō-PLĂS-tē): plastic surgery to correct a deviated septum *-plasty:* surgical repair
sinus/o	sinus, cavity	sinus/o/tomy (sī-nŭs-ŎT-ō-mē): incision of any of the sinuses to improve ventilation or drainage in unresponsive sinusitis *-tomy:* incision

Element	Meaning	Word Analysis
adenoid/o	adenoids	adenoid/ectomy (ăd-ĕ-noyd-ĔK-tō-mē): excision of the adenoids *-ectomy:* excision, removal
tonsill/o	tonsils	peri/tonsill/ar (pĕr-ĭ-TŎN-sĭ-lăr): pertaining to the area surrounding the tonsils *peri-:* around *-ar:* pertaining to, relating to
pharyng/o	pharynx (throat)	pharyng/o/scope (făr-ĬN-gō-skōp): instrument used to examine the pharynx *-scope:* instrument for examining
epiglott/o	epiglottis	epiglott/itis (ĕp-ĭ-glŏt-Ī-tĭs): inflammation of the epiglottis that can lead to severe airway obstruction *-itis:* inflammation
laryng/o	larynx (voice box)	laryng/o/plegia (lă-rĭn-gō-PLĒ-jē-ă): paralysis of the vocal cords and larynx *-plegia:* paralysis
trache/o	trachea (windpipe)	trache/o/stomy (trā-kē-ŎS-tō-mē): opening created through the neck and into the trachea into which a breathing tube may be inserted *-stomy:* forming an opening (mouth) *A tracheostomy is usually performed to bypass an obstructed upper airway; clean and remove secretions from the airway; and deliver oxygen to the lungs.*

Lower Respiratory Tract

Element	Meaning	Word Analysis
bronchi/o	bronchus	bronchi/ectasis (brŏng-kē-ĔK-tă-sĭs): abnormal dilation of one or more bronchi *-ectasis:* dilation, expansion *Bronchiectasis is associated with various lung conditions and is commonly accompanied by chronic infection.*
bronch/o		bronch/o/scope (BRŎNG-kō-skōp): flexible tube that is passed into the lungs through the nose or mouth *-scope:* instrument for examining *A bronchoscope allows inspection of the lungs and collection of tissue biopsies and secretions for analysis.*
bronchiol/o	bronchiole	bronchiol/itis (brŏng-kē-ō-LĪ-tĭs): inflammation of the bronchioles (small passages of the bronchial tree); usually caused by a viral infection *-itis:* inflammation

(Continued)

Element	Meaning	Word Analysis	(Continued)
alveol/o	alveolus	alveol/ar (ăl-VĒ-ō-lăr): pertaining to the alveoli *-ar:* pertaining to, relating to	
pneum/o	air; lung	pneum/ectomy (nūm-ĔK-tō-mē): excision of all or part of a lung *-ectomy:* excision	
pneumon/o		pneumon/ia (nū-MŌ-nē-ă): inflammation of the lungs usually due to bacteria, viruses, or other pathogenic organisms *-ia:* condition	
pulmon/o	lung	pulmon/o/logist (pŭl-mă-NŌL-ă-jĭst): physician specializing in the treatment of lung and respiratory diseases *-logist:* specialist in the study of	
pleur/o	pleura	pleur/o/clysis (ploo-RŎK-lă-sĭs): injection and removal of a fluid into the pleural cavity to wash it out *-clysis:* irrigation, washing	

Other

Element	Meaning	Word Analysis	
anthrac/o	coal, coal dust	anthrac/osis (ăn-thră-KŌ-sĭs): chronic lung disease characterized by the deposit of coal dust in the lungs and the formation of black nodules on the bronchioles *-osis:* abnormal condition; increase (used primarily with blood cells)	
atel/o	incomplete; imperfect	atel/ectasis (ăt-ĕ-LĔK-tă-sĭs): partial or complete collapse of the lung; airless lung *-ectasis:* dilation, expansion	
coni/o	dust	pneum/o/coni/osis (nū-mō-kō-nē-Ō-sĭs): any disease of the lungs caused by chronic inhalation of dust, usually mineral dust of occupational or environmental origin *pneum/o:* air; lung *-osis:* abnormal condition; increase (used primarily with blood cells) *Forms of pneumoconiosis include silicosis, asbestosis, and anthracosis.*	
cyan/o	blue	cyan/osis (sī-ă-NŌ-sĭs): abnormal blueness of the skin and mucous membranes associated with a decrease of oxygen in the blood *-osis:* abnormal condition; increase (used primarily with blood cells) *Cyanosis is associated with cold temperatures, heart failure, lung diseases, and smothering.*	

Element	Meaning	Word Analysis
lob/o	lobe	lob/ectomy (lō-BĔK-tō-mē): surgical removal of a lobe of an organ or gland (such as the lungs, liver, and thyroid gland) *-ectomy:* excision *A lobectomy is performed when a malignancy is confined to a single lobe of the lung.*
orth/o	straight	orth/o/pnea (or-THŎP-nē-ă): condition in which the patient experiences difficulty breathing in any position other than sitting or standing erect *-pnea:* breathing
ox/o	oxygen	hyp/ox/emia (hī-pŏks-Ē-mē-ă): abnormal decrease of oxygen in arterial blood resulting in hypoxia *hyp-:* under, below, deficient *-emia:* blood condition
ox/i		ox/i/meter (ŏk-SĬM-ĕ-tĕr): device used to measure the oxygen saturation of arterial blood *-meter:* instrument for measuring *The oximeter is usually attached to the tip of a finger but may also be placed on a toe or earlobe.*
pector/o	chest	pector/algia (pĕk-tō-RĂL-jē-ă): pain in the chest *-algia:* pain
steth/o		steth/o/scope (STĔTH-ō-skōp): instrument used to evaluate the sounds of the chest and abdomen *-scope:* instrument for examining
thorac/o		thorac/algia (thō-răk-ĂL-jē-ă): pain in the chest wall; also called *thoracodynia* *-algia:* pain
phren/o	diaphragm; mind	phren/o/ptosis (frĕn-ŏp-TŌ-sĭs): abnormal downward displacement of the diaphragm *-ptosis:* prolapse, downward displacement
spir/o	breathe	spir/o/meter (spī-RŎM-ĕt-ĕr): instrument that measures how much air the lungs can hold (vital capacity) as well as how much and how quickly air can be exhaled *-meter:* instrument for measuring
SUFFIXES		
-capnia	carbon dioxide (CO_2)	hyper/capnia (hī-pĕr-KĂP-nē-ă): excess of CO_2 in the blood *hyper-:* excessive, above normal
-osmia	smell	an/osmia (ăn-ŎZ-mē-ă): loss or impairment of the sense of smell *an-:* without, not

(Continued)

Element	Meaning	Word Analysis	(Continued)
-phonia	voice	dys/phonia (dĭs-FŌ-nē-ă): altered or impaired voice quality 　*dys-:* bad; painful; difficult *Dysphonia includes hoarseness, voice fatigue, or decreased projection.*	
-pnea	breathing	a/pnea (ăp-NĒ-ă): temporary loss of breathing 　*a-:* without, not *Types of apnea include sleep apnea, cardiac apnea, and apnea of the newborn.*	
-ptysis	spitting	hem/o/ptysis (hē-MŎP-tĭ-sĭs): coughing up of blood or bloody sputum from the lungs or airway 　*hem/o:* blood	
-thorax	chest	py/o/thorax (pī-ō-THŌ-răks): accumulation of pus in the chest cavity; also called *empyema* 　*py/o:* pus *Pyothorax is usually caused by a penetrating chest wound or spread of infection from another part of the body.*	
PREFIXES			
brady-	slow	brady/pnea (brăd-ĭp-NĒ-ă): abnormally slow respiratory rate 　*-pnea:* breathing	
dys-	bad; painful; difficult	dys/pnea (dĭsp-NĒ-ă): breathing discomfort or significant breathlessness 　*-pnea:* breathing	
eu-	good, normal	eu/pnea (ūp-NĒ-ă): normal, unlabored breathing 　*-pnea:* breathing *The normal range for a resting adult respiratory rate is 12 to 20 breaths/minute.*	
tachy-	rapid	tachy/pnea (tăk-ĭp-NĒ-ă): abnormally rapid respiratory rate 　*-pnea:* breathing	

 It is time to review word elements by completing Learning Activity 7–2.

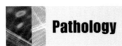 ## Pathology

Common signs and symptoms for many respiratory disorders include cough (dry or productive), chest pain, altered breathing patterns, breathlessness, cyanosis, and fever. Many disorders of the respiratory system, including bronchitis and emphysema, begin as an acute problem but become chronic over time. Chronic respiratory diseases are commonly difficult to treat, and their damaging effects become irreversible.

For diagnosis, treatment, and management of respiratory disorders, the medical services of a specialist may be warranted. **Pulmonology** is the medical specialty concerned with disorders of the respiratory system. The physician who treats these disorders is called a **pulmonologist.**

Chronic Obstructive Pulmonary Disease

Chronic obstructive pulmonary disease (COPD), also called *chronic obstructive lung disease* (*COLD*), includes respiratory disorders characterized by a chronic partial obstruction of the air passages. The patient experiences difficulty breathing **(dyspnea)** on exertion and often exhibits a chronic cough. The three major disorders included in COPD are asthma, chronic bronchitis, and emphysema. (See Figure 7–3.)

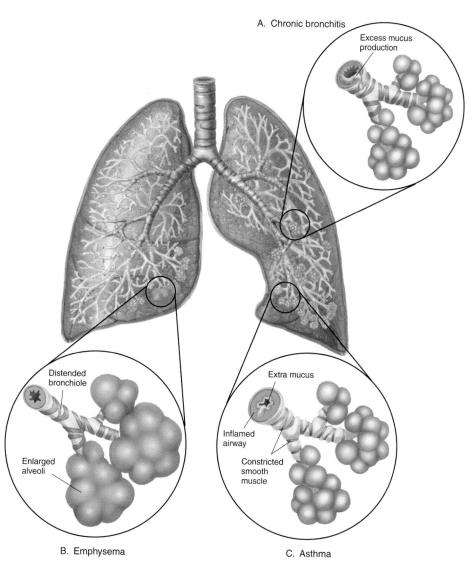

Figure 7–3   COPD. (A) Chronic bronchitis with inflamed airways and excessive mucus. (B) Emphysema with distended bronchioles and alveoli. (C) Asthma with narrowed bronchial tubes and swollen mucous membranes.

Asthma

Asthma produces spasms in the bronchial passages (**bronchospasms**) that are typically sudden and violent (**paroxysmal**), causing dyspnea. Asthma is commonly caused by exposure to allergens or irritants. Other causes include stress, cold, and exercise. During recovery, coughing episodes produce large amounts of mucus (**productive cough**). Over time, the epithelium of the bronchial passages thickens, making breathing difficult. Treatment includes agents that loosen and break down mucus (**mucolytics**) and medications that open up the bronchi (**bronchodilators**) by relaxing their smooth muscles. If bronchospasms are not reversed by usual measures, the patient is said to have **status asthmaticus.**

Chronic Bronchitis

Chronic bronchitis is an inflammation of the bronchi caused primarily by smoking and air pollution. However, other agents, such as viruses and bacteria, may also be responsible for the disorder. Bronchitis is characterized by swelling of the mucosa and a heavy, productive cough commonly accompanied by chest pain. Patients usually seek medical attention when they suffer exercise intolerance, wheezing, and shortness of breath. Bronchodilators and medications that facilitate the removal of mucus (**expectorants**) help to widen air passages. Steroids are commonly needed as the disease progresses.

Emphysema

Emphysema is characterized by decreased elasticity of the alveoli. They expand (**dilate**) but are unable to contract to their original size. Residual air becomes trapped, resulting in a characteristic "barrel-chested" appearance. This disease is often found in combination with another respiratory disorder, such as asthma, tuberculosis, or chronic bronchitis. It is also associated with long-term heavy smoking. Emphysema sufferers often find it easier to breathe when sitting or standing erect (**orthopnea**). As the disease progresses, however, the patient no longer finds relief even in the orthopneic position. Treatment for emphysema is similar to that for chronic bronchitis.

Influenza

Influenza (flu) is an acute infectious respiratory disease caused by viruses. Three major viral types are responsible: type A, type B, and type C. Type A is of primary concern because it is commonly associated with worldwide epidemics (**pandemics**) and is extremely pathogenic (**virulent**). The type A swine flu epidemic of 1918 was responsible for 20 to 40 million deaths worldwide. Influenza type A epidemics occur about every 2 to 3 years. Type B flu is usually limited geographically and tends to be less severe than type A. Both viruses undergo antigenic variations; consequently, new vaccines must continually be developed in anticipation of outbreaks. Type C flu is a mild flu and is not associated with epidemics.

The onset of the flu is usually very rapid. The patient experiences fever, chills, headache, generalized muscle pain (**myalgia**), and loss of appetite. The patient is ill during the acute phase but recovery occurs in about 7 to 10 days. The flu virus rarely causes death. Should death occur, it is usually the result of a secondary pneumonia caused by a lower respiratory invasion by bacteria or viruses. Children should avoid using aspirin for relief of symptoms caused by viruses. An apparent relationship exists between Reye syndrome and the use of aspirin by children 2 to 15 years of age.

Pleural Effusions

Any abnormal fluid in the pleural cavity, the space between the visceral and parietal pleura, is called a *pleural effusion.* The pleural cavity normally contains only a small amount of lubricating fluid but, in many disorders, an abnormal increase in fluid occurs. These disorders include failure of the heart to pump adequate amounts of blood to body tissues **(heart failure),** liver diseases associated with an accumulation of fluid in the abdominal and pleural cavities **(ascites),** infectious lung diseases, and trauma. Different types of pleural effusions include pus in the pleural space **(empyema),** serum in the pleural space **(hydrothorax),** blood in the pleural space **(hemothorax),** air in the pleural space **(pneumothorax),** and a mixture of pus and air in the pleural space **(pyopneumothorax).** (See Figure 7–4.)

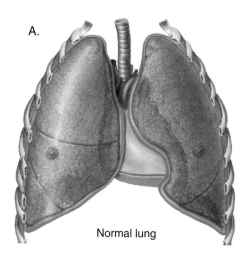

A.

Normal lung

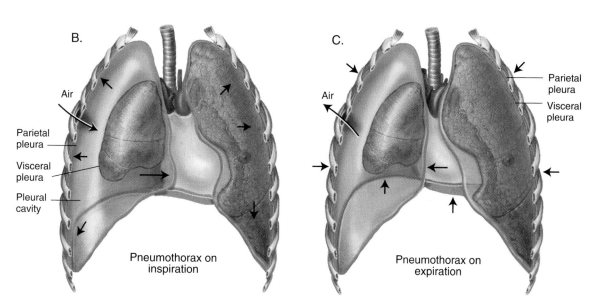

B.

Air

Parietal pleura

Visceral pleura

Pleural cavity

Pneumothorax on inspiration

C.

Air

Parietal pleura

Visceral pleura

Pneumothorax on expiration

Figure 7–4   Pneumothorax. (A) Normal. (B) Open pneumothorax during inspiration. (C) Open pneumothorax during expiration.

Depending on the amount and type of fluid, treatment may include surgical puncture of the chest (**thoracocentesis, thoracentesis**) to remove excess fluid from the pleural cavity using a hollow bore needle. (See Figure 7–5.) Sometimes chest tubes are inserted to facilitate removal of the fluid. Two noninvasive techniques used in the diagnosis of pleural effusion are listening to the sounds of the chest cavity with a stethoscope (**auscultation**) and gently tapping the chest with the fingers to determine the position, size, or consistency of the underlying structures (**percussion**).

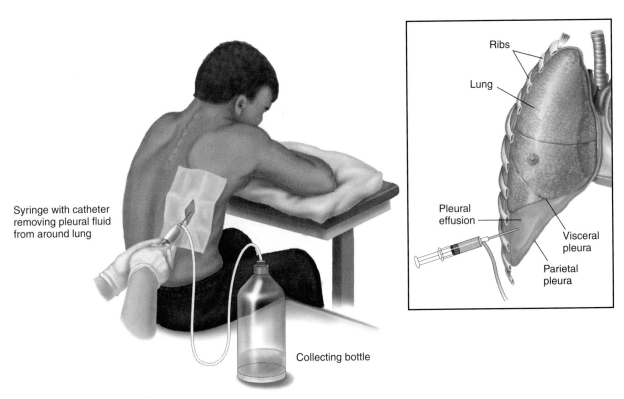

Figure 7–5   Thoracentesis.

Tuberculosis

An alarming increase in tuberculosis occurred in the United States between 1985 and 1992. This increase corresponded with the escalation of drug-resistant TB strains, the number of people with acquired immunodeficiency syndrome (AIDS), and those who were homeless or living in poverty. Since 1992, incidence of the disease has declined primarily because of active surveillance and new treatment methods.

TB is highly communicable and spreads by droplets of respiratory secretions (**aerosol transmission**) or particles of dry sputum containing the TB organism. The waxy coat of the TB organism allows it to remain alive (**viable**) and infectious for 6 to 8 months outside the body.

The first time the TB organism enters the body (**primary tuberculosis**), the disease develops slowly. It eventually produces unique focal **granulomas** called *tubercles*. These granulomas usually remain dormant for years, during which time the patient is asymptomatic. When the immune system becomes impaired (**immunocompromised**) or when the patient is reintroduced to the bacterium, the full-blown disease may develop.

Although primarily a lung disease, TB can infect the bones, genital tract, meninges, and peritoneum. Many of the TB strains that infect AIDS patients are not responsive to standard medications (**drug resistant**), and treatment commonly includes simultaneous use of several antibiotics (**combination therapy**).

Pneumonia

The term *pneumonia* refers to any inflammatory disease of the lungs. Pneumonia may be caused by bacteria, viruses, fungi, chemicals, and other agents. Infectious pneumonias are primarily attributed to bacteria or viruses. A type of pneumonia associated with influenza is sometimes fatal. Other potentially fatal pneumonias may result from food or liquid inhalation (**aspiration pneumonias**). Some pneumonias affect only a lobe of the lung (**lobar pneumonia**), but some are more diffuse (**bronchopneumonia**). Chest pain, mucopurulent sputum, and spitting of blood (**hemoptysis**) are frequent symptoms of the disease. The lungs may undergo solidification (**consolidation**) because of a pathological engorgement.

Pneumocystis carinii pneumonia (PCP) is a type of pneumonia closely associated with AIDS. Recent evidence suggests that it is caused by a fungus that resides in or on most people (**normal flora**) but causes no harm as long as the individual remains healthy. When the immune system becomes compromised, however, this organism becomes infectious (**opportunistic**). Diagnosis relies on examination of biopsied lung tissue or bronchial washings (**lavage**).

Cystic Fibrosis

Cystic fibrosis is a hereditary disorder of the exocrine glands that causes the body to secrete extremely thick (**viscous**) mucus that clogs ducts or tubes of the pancreas, digestive tract, and sweat glands. In the lungs, this mucus blocks airways and impedes natural infection-fighting mechanisms, eventually turning the body's immune system against its own lung tissue. Medication in the form of mists (**aerosols**) along with postural drainage provides relief.

An important diagnostic finding in cystic fibrosis is an increase in the amount of salt excreted in sweat. A laboratory test called a *sweat test* analyzes the amount of chloride in sweat and, when elevated, is indicative of cystic fibrosis. Although the disease is fatal, improved methods of treatment have extended life expectancy, and patient survival is approximately 30 years.

Respiratory Distress Syndrome

Respiratory distress syndrome (RDS) is most commonly caused by absence or impairment in the production of a phospholipid substance of the lungs called **surfactant** that allows the lungs to expand with ease (**compliance**). Without surfactant, the alveoli collapse and inhalation becomes extremely difficult.

When RDS is found in newborn infants, it is called **infant respiratory distress syndrome (IRDS)** or **hyaline membrane disease (HMD)**. IRDS is most commonly seen in premature infants or infants born to diabetic mothers. If the amount of surfactant is inadequate at birth, clinical symptoms include blueness (**cyanosis**) of the extremities, rapid breathing (**tachypnea**), flaring of the nostrils (**nares**), intercostal retraction, and a characteristic grunt audible during exhalation. Radiography shows a membrane that has a ground-glass appearance (**hyaline membrane**). Although severe cases of IRDS result in death, some forms of therapy are effective.

Acute respiratory distress syndrome (ARDS) is caused by an impairment of surfactant production or by exposure to substances that remove surfactant from the lungs. Accidental inhalation of foreign substances, water, smoke, chemical fumes, or vomit is commonly the cause.

Oncology

The most common form of lung cancer is bronchogenic carcinoma, also called *primary pulmonary cancer*. This cancer is most commonly associated with tobacco use. In this type of cancer, the cells at the base of the epithelium (**basal cells**) divide repeatedly until, eventually, the entire epithelium is involved. Within a short time, the epithelium begins to invade the underlying tissues. As masses form, they block air passages and alveoli. Bronchogenic carcinoma spreads (**metastasizes**) rapidly to other areas of the body, commonly to lymph nodes, liver, bones, brain, or kidney. Only about 10% of lung cancers are found in the early stages when the cure rate is high. Treatment of lung cancer includes surgery, radiation, and chemotherapy or a combination of these methods. Nevertheless, lung cancer is difficult to control and survival rates are extremely low.

Diagnostic, Symptomatic, and Related Terms

This section introduces diagnostic, symptomatic, and related terms and their meanings. Word analyses for selected terms are also provided.

Term	Definition
acidosis ăs-ĭ-DŌ-sĭs	Excessive acidity of body fluids, commonly associated with pulmonary insufficiency and the subsequent retention of carbon dioxide
anosmia ăn-ŎZ-mē-ă *an-:* without, not *-osmia:* smell	Absence of or decrease in the sense of smell *Anosmia usually occurs as a temporary condition resulting from an upper respiratory infection or a condition that causes intranasal swelling.*
apnea ăp-NĒ-ă *a-:* without, not *-pnea:* breathing **sleep**	Temporary loss of breathing *There are three types of apnea: obstructive (enlarged tonsils and adenoids), central (failure of the brain to transmit impulses for breathing), and mixed (combination of obstructive and central apnea).* One of several disorders in which breathing during sleep stops for more than 10 seconds and usually more than 20 times/hour, causing measurable blood deoxygenation
asphyxia ăs-FĬK-sē-ă *a-:* without, not *-sphyxia:* pulse	Condition caused by insufficient intake of oxygen *Some common causes of asphyxia are drowning, electrical shock, lodging of a foreign body in the respiratory tract, inhalation of toxic smoke, and poisoning.*
atelectasis ăt-ĕ-LĔK-tă-sĭs *atel-:* incomplete; imperfect *-ectasis:* dilation, expansion	Collapsed or airless state of the lung, which may be acute or chronic and affect all or part of a lung *Atelectasis is a potential complication of some surgical procedures, especially those of the chest because breathing is commonly shallow after surgery to avoid pain from the surgical incision. In fetal atelectasis, the lungs fail to expand normally at birth.*
Cheyne-Stokes respiration CHĀN-STŌKS	Repeated breathing pattern characterized by fluctuation in the depth of respiration, first deeply, then shallow, then not at all *Cheyne-Stokes respiration is usually caused by diseases that affect the respiratory centers of the brain (such as heart failure and brain damage).*

Term	Definition
compliance kŏm-PLĪ-ăns	Ease with which lung tissue can be stretched *Low compliance means lungs are less elastic; therefore, more effort is required to inflate the lungs.*
coryza kŏ-RĪ-ză	Head cold; upper respiratory infection (URI)
croup CROOP	Common childhood condition involving inflammation of the larynx, trachea, bronchial passages and, sometimes, lungs characterized by resonant, barking cough; suffocative and difficult breathing; laryngeal spasm; and, sometimes, the formation of a membrane
deviated nasal septum DĒ-vē-āt-ĕd NĀ-zl SĔP-tŭm	Displacement of cartilage dividing the nostrils
epiglottitis ĕp-i-glŏt-Ī-tĭs *epiglott:* epiglottis *-itis:* inflammation	Severe, life-threatening infection of the epiglottis and supraglottic structures that occurs most commonly in children between 2 and 12 years of age *Symptoms of epiglottitis include fever, dysphagia, inspiratory stridor, and severe respiratory distress. Intubation or tracheostomy may be required to open the obstructed airway.*
epistaxis ĕp-i-STĂK-sĭs	Nosebleed; nasal hemorrhage
finger clubbing KLŬB-ing	Enlargement of the terminal phalanges of the fingers and toes, commonly associated with pulmonary disease
hypoxemia hī-pŏks-Ē-mē-ă *hyp-:* under, below, deficient *ox:* oxygen *-emia:* blood condition	Deficiency of oxygen in the blood; also called *anoxemia* *Hypoxemia is usually a sign of respiratory impairment.*
hypoxia hī-PŎKS-ē-ă *hyp-:* under, below, deficient *-oxia:* oxygen	Absence or deficiency of oxygen in the tissues; also called *anoxia* *Hypoxia is usually a sign of respiratory impairment.*
pertussis pĕr-TŬS-ĭs	Acute infectious disease characterized by a cough that has a "whoop" sound; also called *whooping cough* *Immunization of infants as part of the diphtheria-pertussis-tetanus (DPT) vaccination is very effective in the prevention of this disease.*
pleurisy PLOO-rĭs-ē *pleur:* pleura *-isy:* state of; condition	Inflammation of the pleural membrane characterized by a stabbing pain that is intensified by coughing or deep breathing; also called *pleuritis*

(Continued)

Term	Definition	(Continued)
pneumoconiosis nū-mō-kō-nē-Ō-sĭs *pneum/o:* air; lung *coni:* dust *-osis:* abnormal condition; increase (used primarily with blood cells)	Generally occupational disease caused by inhaling dust particles, including coal dust (anthracosis), stone dust (chalicosis), iron (siderosis), and asbestos (asbestosis)	
pulmonary edema PŬL-mō-nĕ-rē ĕ-DĒ-mă *pulmon:* lung *-ary:* pertaining to, relating to	Accumulation of extravascular fluid in lung tissues and alveoli, caused most commonly by heart failure *The excessive fluid in the lungs induces coughing and dyspnea.*	
pulmonary embolus PŬL-mō-nĕ-rē ĔM-bō-lŭs *pulmon:* lung *-ary:* pertaining to, relating to *embol:* plug *-us:* condition, structure	Mass of undissolved matter (such as a blood clot, tissue, air bubbles, and bacteria) in the pulmonary arteries or its branches	
rale RĂL	Abnormal respiratory sound heard on auscultation, caused by exudates, spasms, hyperplasia, or when air enters moisture-filled alveoli; also called *crackle*	
rhonchus RŎNG-kŭs	Adventitious breath sound that resembles snoring, commonly suggesting secretions in the larger airways	
stridor STRĪ-dor	High-pitched, harsh adventitious breath sound caused by a spasm or swelling of the larynx or an obstruction in the upper airway *The presence of stridor requires immediate intervention.*	
sudden infant death syndrome (SIDS)	Completely unexpected and unexplained death of an apparently normal and healthy infant, usually less than 12 months of age; also called *crib death* *The rate of SIDS has declined more than 30% since parents have been instructed to place their baby on the back for sleeping rather than the stomach.*	
wheeze HWĒZ	Whistling or sighing sound on auscultation that results from narrowing of the lumen of the respiratory passageway *Wheezing is a characteristic of asthma, croup, hay fever, obstructive emphysema, and other obstructive respiratory conditions.*	

 It is time to review pathological, diagnostic, symptomatic, and related terms by completing Learning Activity 7–3.

Diagnostic and Therapeutic Procedures

This section introduces procedures used to diagnose and treat respiratory disorders. Descriptions are provided as well as pronunciations and word analyses for selected terms.

Procedure	Description
DIAGNOSTIC PROCEDURES	
Clinical	
Mantoux test măn-TŪ	Intradermal test to determine tuberculin sensitivity based on a positive reaction where the area around the test site becomes red and swollen *A positive test suggests a past or present exposure to TB or past TB vaccination. However, the Mantoux test does not differentiate between active or inactive infection.*
oximetry ŏk-SĬM-ă-trē *ox/i:* oxygen *-metry:* act of measuring	Noninvasive method of monitoring the percentage of hemoglobin (Hb) saturated with oxygen; also called *pulse oximetry* *In oximetry, a probe is attached to the patient's finger or earlobe and linked to a computer that displays the percentage of hemoglobin saturated with oxygen and, in some units, provides an audible signal for each pulse beat.*
polysomnography pŏl-ē-sŏm-NŎG-ră-fē *poly-:* many, much *somn/o:* sleep *-graphy:* process of recording	Test of sleep cycles and stages using continuous recordings of brain waves (EEGs), electrical activity of muscles, eye movement (electro-oculogram), respiratory rate, blood pressure, blood oxygen saturation, heart rhythm and, sometimes, direct observation of the person during sleep using a video camera
pulmonary function studies *pulmon:* lung *-ary:* pertaining to, relating to	Multiple tests used to evaluate the ability of the lungs to take in and expel air as well as perform gas exchange across the alveolocapillary membrane
spirometry spi-RŎM-ĕ-trē *spir/o:* breathe *-metry:* act of measuring	Measurement of ventilatory ability by assessing lung capacity and flow, including the time necessary for exhaling the total volume of inhaled air *A spirometer produces a graphic record for placement in the patient's chart.*
Endoscopic	
bronchoscopy brŏng-KŎS-kō-pē *bronch/o:* bronchus *-scopy:* visual examination	Visual examination of the bronchi using an endoscope (flexible fiberoptic or rigid) inserted through the mouth and trachea for direct viewing of structures or for projection on a monitor *Bronchoscopy also allows suctioning, biopsy, removal of foreign bodies, and collection of fluid or sputum for examination and diagnosis.*

(Continued)

Procedure	Description	(Continued)
laryngoscopy lăr-in-GŎS-kō-pē *laryng/o:* larynx (voice box) *-scopy:* visual examination	Visual examination of the inside of the larynx to detect tumors, foreign bodies, nerve or structural injury, or other abnormalities	
mediastinoscopy mē-dē-ăs-tǐ-NŎS -kō-pē *mediastin/o:* mediastinum *-scopy:* visual examination	Visual examination of the mediastinal structures including the heart, trachea, esophagus, bronchus, thymus, and lymph nodes *The mediastinoscope is inserted through a very small incision made above the sternum. The attached camera projects images on a monitor. Additional incisions may be made if nodes are removed or other diagnostic or therapeutic procedures are performed.*	

Laboratory

arterial blood gases (ABGs)	Test that measures the partial pressure of oxygen (PaO_2), carbon dioxide ($PaCO_2$), pH (acidity or alkalinity), and bicarbonate level of an arterial blood sample *This test evaluates pulmonary gas exchange and helps to guide treatment of acid-base imbalances.*	
sputum culture SPŪ-tŭm	Microbial test used to identify disease-causing organisms of the lower respiratory tract, especially those that cause pneumonias	
sweat test	Measurement of the amount of salt (sodium chloride) in sweat *This test is used almost exclusively in children to confirm cystic fibrosis.*	
throat culture	Test used to identify pathogens, especially group A streptococci *Untreated streptococcal infections may lead to serious secondary complications, including kidney and heart disease.*	

Radiographic

radiography rā-dē-ŎG-rǎ-fē *radi/o:* radiation, x-ray; radius (lower arm bone on thumb side) *-graphy:* process of recording	Producing images using an x-ray that is passed through the body or area and captured on a film	
chest	Images of the chest taken from anteroposterior (AP), posteroanterior (PA), or lateral projection, or a combination of these projections *Radiography is used to diagnose rib fractures and lung diseases, including atelectasis, masses, pneumonia, and emphysema.*	

Procedure	Description
scan	Term used to describe a computed image by modality (such as CT scan, MRI scan, and nuclear scan) or structure (such as thyroid scan and bone scan)
thoracic (CT) thō-RĂS-ĭk *thorac:* chest *-ic:* pertaining to, relating to	A cross-sectional view of the chest taken with or without an injected contrast medium to visualize injuries, tumors, fluid in the lungs, or other pathologies
lung	Nuclear scanning procedure commonly used to diagnose blood clots and pulmonary emboli

THERAPEUTIC PROCEDURES

Clinical

aerosol therapy ĀR-ō-sŏl	Inhalation of microdrops of medication directly into the respiratory system via a nebulizer (liquid), metered-dose inhaler (gas), or dry-powder inhaler (solid) (See Figure 7–6.) *In aerosol therapy, the medication is deposited directly into the respiratory system, thus allowing lower dosages, providing rapid action, and minimizing side effects and systemic toxicity.*

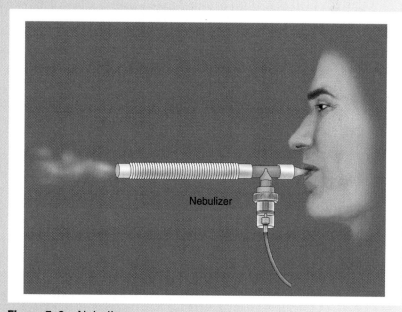

Figure 7–6   Nebulizer.

lavage lă-VĂZH	Irrigating or washing out of an organ, stomach, bladder, bowel, or body cavity with a stream of water or other fluid
antral ĂN-trăl	Irrigation of the paranasal sinuses usually performed to remove mucopurulent material in an immunosuppressed patient or one with known sinusitis that has failed medical management
postural drainage PŎS-tū-răl	Positioning a patient so that gravity aids in the drainage of secretions from the bronchi and lobes of the lungs

(Continued)

Procedure	Description	*(Continued)*

Surgical

rhinoplasty RĪ-nō-plăs-tē *rhin/o:* nose *-plasty:* surgical repair	Reconstructive surgery of the nose to correct deformities or for cosmetic purposes
pleurectomy ploor-ĔK-tō-mē *pleur:* pleura *-ectomy:* excision, removal	Excision of part of the pleura, usually parietal *Pleurectomy is performed to reduce pain caused by a tumor mass or to prevent the recurrence of pleural effusion but is generally ineffective in the treatment of malignancy of the pleura.*
pneumectomy nūm-ĔK-tō-mē *pneum:* air; lung *-ectomy:* excision, removal	Excision of a lung or lobe (lobectomy) of the lung *Other partial types of lung excisions include resection, segmental, and wedge.*
septoplasty sĕp-tō-PLĂS-tē *sept/o:* septum *-plasty:* surgical repair	Surgical repair of a deviated nasal septum usually performed when the septum is encroaching on the breathing passages or nasal structures *Common complications of a deviated septum include interference with breathing and a predisposition to sinus infections.*
thoracentesis thō-ră-sĕn-TĒ-sĭs	Surgical puncture and drainage of the pleural cavity; also called *pleurocentesis* or *thoracocentesis* (See Figure 7–5.) *Thoracentesis is performed as a diagnostic procedure to determine the nature and cause of an effusion or as a therapeutic procedure to relieve the discomfort caused by the effusion. The procedure is usually carried out at the bedside using local anesthetic.*

 Pharmacology

In addition to antibiotics used to treat respiratory infections, there are several classes of drugs that treat pulmonary disorders. (See Table 7–1.) Bronchodilators are especially significant in the treatment of COPD and exercise-induced asthma. They relax smooth muscles of the bronchi, thus increasing airflow. Some bronchodilators are delivered as a fine mist directly to the airways via aerosol delivery devices, including nebulizers and metered-dose inhalers (MDIs). Another method of delivering medications directly to the lungs is dry-powder inhalers (DPIs) that dispense medications in the form of a powder. Steroidal and nonsteroidal anti-inflammatory drugs are important in the control and management of many pulmonary disorders.

Table 7-1   DRUGS USED TO TREAT RESPIRATORY DISORDERS

This table lists common drug classifications used to treat respiratory disorders, their therapeutic actions, and selected generic and trade names.

Classification	Therapeutic Action	Generic and Trade Names
antihistamines	Relieve nasal congestion and seasonal allergic rhinitis symptoms *Antihistamines exert their therapeutic effect by blocking histamine receptors in the nose and throat. They dry up secretions, decrease mucous membrane swelling, and decrease redness and itching.*	**fexofenadine** fĕks-ō-FĔN-ă-dēn *Allegra* **loratadine** lor-ĂH-tă-dēn *Claritin* **diphenhydramine** dī-fĕn-HĪ-dră-mēn *Benadryl*
antitussives	Relieve or suppress coughing *Antitussives are used to alleviate nonproductive dry coughs. Some antitussives contain narcotics, such as codeine and hydrocodone. Other over-the-counter antitussives contain the non-narcotic dextromethorphan or diphenhydramine.*	**hydrocodone** hī-drō-KŌ-dōn *Hycodan* **codeine** KŌ-dēn *no trade names except in combination* **dextromethorphan** dĕk-strō-MĔTH-or-făn *Benylin DM, Sucrets, Vicks Formula 44*
bronchodilators	Relax smooth muscle surrounding the bronchi resulting in increased air flow *Bronchodilators are used to treat chronic symptoms and to prevent acute attacks in respiratory diseases, such as asthma and COPD. The pharmacological agent may be delivered by an inhaler (as in Proventil, Ventolin, and Serevent), orally, or intravenously.*	**albuterol** ăl-BŪ-tĕr-ăl *Proventil, Ventolin* **salmeterol** săl-mē-TĔR-ŏl *Serevent*
corticosteroids	Treat chronic lung disease (including asthma) by suppressing the immune response and decreasing inflammation *Vanceril and Beclovent decrease the frequency and intensity of asthma attacks, thereby preventing pulmonary damage associated with chronic asthma.*	**beclomethasone dipropionate** bĕ-klō-MĔTH-ă-sōn dī-PRŌ-pē-ō-nāt *Vanceril, Beclovent* **triamcinolone** trī-ăm-SĬN-ō-lōn *Azmacort*
decongestants	Decrease mucous membrane swelling to alleviate nasal stuffiness *Decongestants are commonly prescribed for allergies and colds and are usually combined with antihistamines in cold remedies. They can be administered orally or topically as nasal sprays and nasal drops.*	**oxymetazoline** ŏks-ē-mĕt-ĂZ-ō-lēn *Afrin, Dristan, Sinex* **pseudoephedrine** soo-dō-ē-FĔD-rĭn *Drixoral, Sudafed*
expectorants	Reduce the thickness or viscosity of sputum *Reducing the viscosity of secretions aids the patient's ability to cough up sputum. Expectorants are prescribed only for productive coughs.*	**guaifenesin** gwī-FĔN-ĕ-sĭn *Robitussin* **iodinated glycerol** ī-Ō-dĭn-ā-tĭd GLĬS-ĕr-ŏl *Organidin*

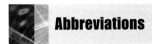

Abbreviations

This section introduces respiratory-related abbreviations and their meanings.

Abbreviation	Meaning
ABGs	arterial blood gases
AFB	acid-fast bacillus (TB organism)
AP	anteroposterior
ARDS	acute respiratory distress syndrome
CO_2	carbon dioxide
COPD	chronic obstructive pulmonary disease
CPR	cardiopulmonary resuscitation
CT scan	computed tomography scan
CXR	chest x-ray, chest radiograph
DPT	diphtheria, pertussis, tetanus
FVC	forced vital capacity
HMD	hyaline membrane disease
IPPB	intermittent positive-pressure breathing
IRDS	infant respiratory distress syndrome
MRI scan	magnetic resonance imaging scan
NMTs	nebulized mist treatments
O_2	oxygen

Abbreviation	Meaning
PA	posteroanterior; pernicious anemia
Pco_2	partial pressure of carbon dioxide
PCP	*Pneumocystis carinii* pneumonia
PFT	pulmonary function tests
pH	symbol for degree of acidity or alkalinity
PND	paroxysmal nocturnal dyspnea
Po_2	partial pressure of oxygen
RD	respiratory distress
RDS	respiratory distress syndrome
Sao_2	arterial oxygen saturation
SIDS	sudden infant death syndrome
SOB	shortness of breath
T & A	tonsillectomy and adenoidectomy
TB	tuberculosis
TPR	temperature, pulse, and respiration
URI	upper respiratory infection
VC	vital capacity

 It is time to review procedures, pharmacology, and abbreviations by completing Learning Activity 7–4.

LEARNING ACTIVITIES

The following activities provide review of the respiratory system terms introduced in this chapter. Complete each activity and review your answers to evaluate your understanding of the chapter.

Learning Activity 7–1

Identifying respiratory structures

Label the illustration on page 177 using the terms listed below.

adenoids	larynx	parietal pleura
alveoli	left lung	pleural cavity
bronchi	mediastinum	pulmonary capillaries
bronchiole	nasal cavity	right lung
diaphragm	nasopharynx	trachea
epiglottis	oropharynx	visceral pleura
laryngopharynx	palatine tonsils	

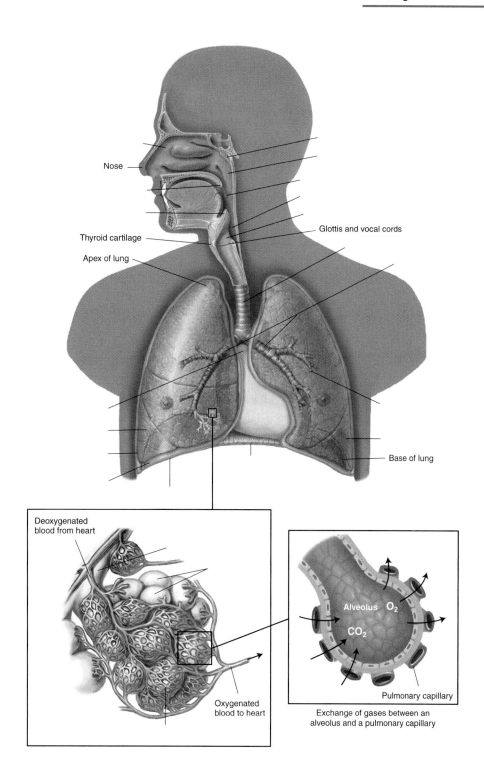

Nose

Thyroid cartilage

Apex of lung

Glottis and vocal cords

Base of lung

Deoxygenated
blood from heart

Oxygenated
blood to heart

Alveolus O₂

CO₂

Pulmonary capillary

Exchange of gases between an
alveolus and a pulmonary capillary

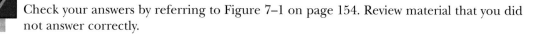

Check your answers by referring to Figure 7–1 on page 154. Review material that you did
not answer correctly.

Learning Activity 7–2

Building medical words

Use **rhin/o** *(nose) to build words that mean:*

1. discharge from the nose _____

2. inflammation of the (mucous membranes of the) nose _____

Use **laryng/o** *(larynx [voice box]) to build words that mean:*

3. visual examination of the larynx _____

4. inflammation of the larynx _____

5. stricture or narrowing of the larynx _____

Use **bronch/o** *or* **bronchi/o** *(bronchus) to build words that mean:*

6. dilation or expansion of the bronchus _____

7. disease of the bronchus _____

8. spasm of the bronchus _____

Use **pneumon/o** *or* **pneum/o** *(air; lung) to build words that mean:*

9. air in the chest (pleural space) _____

10. inflammation of the lungs _____

Use **pulmon/o** *(lung) to build words that mean:*

11. specialist in lung (diseases) _____

12. pertaining to the lung _____

Use **-pnea** *(breathing) to build words that mean:*

13. difficult breathing _____

14. slow breathing _____

15. rapid breathing _____

16. absence of breathing _____

Build surgical words that mean:

17. surgical repair of the nose _____

18. surgical puncture of the chest _____

19. removal of a lung _____

20. forming an opening (mouth) in the trachea _____

Check your answers in Appendix A. Review material that you did not answer correctly.

CORRECT ANSWERS _____ × 5 = _____ **% SCORE**

Learning Activity 7–3

Matching pathological, diagnostic, symptomatic, and related terms

Match the following terms with the definitions in the numbered list.

anosmia	*deviated nasal septum*	*pneumoconiosis*
apnea	*emphysema*	*pulmonary edema*
ascites	*empyema*	*rale, crackle*
atelectasis	*epistaxis*	*stridor*
compliance	*hypoxemia*	*surfactant*
consolidation	*pertussis*	*tubercles*
coryza	*pleurisy*	

1. _____ collapsed or airless lung
2. _____ pus in the pleural cavity
3. _____ phospholipid that allows the lungs to expand with ease
4. _____ solidification of the lungs
5. _____ accumulation of fluid in the abdominal or pleural cavities
6. _____ absence or decrease in the sense of smell
7. _____ deficiency of oxygen in the blood; also called *anoxemia*
8. _____ granulomas associated with tuberculosis
9. _____ temporary loss of breathing
10. _____ disease characterized by decrease in alveolar elasticity
11. _____ ease with which lung tissue can be stretched
12. _____ nosebleed; nasal hemorrhage
13. _____ excessive fluid in the lungs that induces cough and dyspnea
14. _____ abnormal respiratory sound associated with exudates, spasms, or hyperplasia
15. _____ displacement of the cartilage dividing the nostrils
16. _____ head cold; upper respiratory infection
17. _____ condition in which dust particles are found in the lungs
18. _____ inflammation of the pleural membrane
19. _____ abnormal sound caused by spasms or swelling of larynx
20. _____ whooping cough

Check your answers in Appendix A. Review any material that you did not answer correctly.

CORRECT ANSWERS _____ × 5 = _____ **% SCORE**

Learning Activity 7-4

Matching procedures, pharmacology, and abbreviations

Match the following terms with the definitions in the numbered list.

ABGs	*expectorants*	*pulmonary function studies*
aerosol therapy	*laryngoscopy*	*radiography*
AFB	*lung scan*	*rhinoplasty*
antihistamines	*Mantoux test*	*septoplasty*
antitussives	*oximetry*	*sweat test*
antral lavage	*pneumectomy*	*throat culture*
decongestants	*polysomnography*	

1. _____ imaging procedure that uses radionuclide to evaluate blood flow in the lungs

2. _____ test of sleep cycles and stages

3. _____ producing images using an x-ray machine

4. _____ washing or irrigating sinuses

5. _____ relieve nasal congestion and seasonal allergic rhinitis symptoms

6. _____ relieve or suppress coughing

7. _____ test used primarily in children to confirm cystic fibrosis

8. _____ noninvasive test used to monitor percentage of hemoglobin saturated with oxygen

9. _____ TB organism

10. _____ inhalation of medication directly into the respiratory system via a nebulizer

11. _____ decrease mucous membrane swelling to alleviate nasal stuffiness

12. _____ intradermal test to determine presence of TB infections

13. _____ laboratory tests to assess gases and pH of arterial blood

14. _____ reduces the viscosity of sputum to facilitate productive coughing

15. _____ used to identify pathogens, especially group A streptococci

16. _____ multiple tests used to determine the ability of lungs and capillary membranes to exchange oxygen

17. _____ visual examination of the voice box to detect tumors and
other abnormalities

18. _____ surgery to correct a deviated nasal septum

19. _____ excision of the entire lung

20. _____ reconstructive surgery of the nose, commonly for cosmetic
purposes

✓ Check your answers in Appendix A. Review any material that you did not answer correctly.

CORRECT ANSWERS _____ × 5 = _____ **% SCORE**

MEDICAL RECORD ACTIVITIES

The two medical records included in the activities that follow use common clinical scenarios to show how medical terminology is used to document patient care. Complete the terminology and analysis sections for each activity to help you recognize and understand terms related to the respiratory system.

Medical Record Activity 7–1

Respiratory evaluation

Terminology

The terms listed in the chart come from the medical record *Respiratory Evaluation* that follows. Use a medical dictionary such as *Taber's Cyclopedic Medical Dictionary*, the appendices of this book, or other resources to define each term. Then review the pronunciations for each term and practice by reading the medical record aloud.

Term	Definition
anteriorly ăn-TĒR-ē-or-lē	
bilateral bī-LĂT-ĕr-ăl	
COPD	
exacerbation ĕks-ăs-ĕr-BĀ-shŭn	
heart failure hărt FĀL-yĕr	
Hx	
hypertension hī-pĕr-TĔN-shŭn	
interstitial ĭn-tĕr-STĬSH-ăl	
PE	
peripheral vascular disease pĕr-ĬF-ĕr-ăl VĂS-kū-lăr dĭ-ZĒZ	
pleural PLOO-răl	

Term	Definition
posteriorly pŏs-TĒR-ē-or-lē	
rhonchi RŎNG-kī	
SOB	
wheezes HWĒZ-ĕz	

RESPIRATORY EVALUATION

HISTORY OF PRESENT ILLNESS: This 49-year-old man with known history of COPD is admitted because of exacerbation of SOB over the past few days. Patient was a heavy smoker and states that he quit smoking for a short while but now smokes three to four cigarettes a day. He has a Hx of difficult breathing, high blood pressure, COPD, and peripheral vascular disease. He underwent triple bypass surgery in 19xx. PE indicates scattered bilateral wheezes and rhonchi heard anteriorly and posteriorly.

Compared with a portable chest film from 4/17/xx, deterioration since the previous study is noted that most likely indicates interstitial vascular congestion. Some superimposed inflammatory change cannot be excluded. There may also be some pleural reactive change.

DIAGNOSIS:

1. Acute exacerbation of chronic pulmonary disease
2. Heart failure
3. Peripheral vascular disease

Analysis

Review the medical record *Respiratory Evaluation* to answer the following questions.

1. What symptom caused the patient to seek medical help?

   _____

2. What was the patient's previous history?

   _____

3. What were the findings of the physical examination?

   _____

4. What changes were noted from the previous film?

   _____

5. What is the present Dx?

   _____

6. What new diagnosis was made that did not appear in the previous medical history?

   _____

Medical Record Activity 7–2

Chronic interstitial lung disease

Terminology

The terms listed in the chart come from the medical record *Chronic Interstitial Lung Disease* that follows. Use a medical dictionary such as *Taber's Cyclopedic Medical Dictionary*, the appendices of this book, or other resources to define each term. Then review the pronunciations for each term and practice by reading the medical record aloud.

Term	Definition
ABGs	
adenopathy ăd-ĕ-NŎP-ă-thē	
basilar crackles BĂS-ĭ-lăr KRĂK-ĕlz	
cardiomyopathy kăr-dē-ō-mi-ŎP-ă-thē	
chronic KRŎN-ĭk	
diuresis di-ū-RĒ-sĭs	
dyspnea dĭsp-NĒ-ă	
fibrosis fī-BRŌ-sĭs	
interstitial ĭn-tĕr-STĬSH-ăl	
kyphosis ki-FŌ-sĭs	
Lasix LĀ-sĭks	
neuropathy nū-RŎP-ă-thē	
Pco$_2$	
pedal edema PĔD-l ĕ-DĒ-mă	

Term	Definition
pH	
Po$_2$	
pulmonary fibrosis PŬL-mō-ně-rē fĭ-BRŌ-sĭs	
renal insufficiency RĒ-năl ĭn-sŭ-FĬSH-ěn-sē	
rhonchi RŎNG-kī	
silicosis sĭl-ĭ-KŌ-sĭs	
thyromegaly thī-rō-MĔG-ă-lē	

Chronic Interstitial Lung Disease

CHIEF COMPLAINT: Dyspnea with activity; pedal edema

HISTORY OF PRESENT ILLNESS: The patient is an 84-year-old male who carries the diagnosis of cardiomyopathy, renal insufficiency, COPD, and pulmonary fibrosis. He also has peripheral neuropathy, which has improved with Elavil therapy.

ASSESSMENT: BP: 140/70. Pulse: 76. Neck is supple without thyromegaly or adenopathy. Mild kyphosis without scoliosis is present. Chest reveals basilar crackles without wheezing or rhonchi. Cardiac examination shows trace edema without clubbing or murmur. Abdomen is soft and nontender. ABGs on room air demonstrate a Po$_2$ of 55, Pco$_2$ of 45, and pH of 7.42.

IMPRESSION: Chronic interstitial lung disease, likely a combination of pulmonary fibrosis and heart failure. We do believe he would benefit from further diuresis, which was implemented by Dr. Lu. Should there continue to be concerns about his volume status or lack of response to Lasix therapy, then he might benefit from right heart catheterization.

PLAN: Supplemental oxygen will be continued. We plan no change in his pulmonary medication at this time and will see him in return visit in 4 months. He has been told to contact us should he worsen in the interim.

Analysis

Review the medical record *Chronic Interstitial Lung Disease* to answer the following questions.

1. When did the patient notice SOB?

_____

2. Other than the respiratory system, what other body systems are identified in the history of present illness?

_____

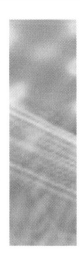

3. What were the findings regarding the neck?

_____

4. What was the finding regarding the spine?

_____

5. What appears to be the likely cause of the chronic interstitial lung disease?

_____

6. Define the following abbreviations: ABGs, P_{O_2}, P_{CO_2}, and pH.

_____

7. What is the therapeutic action of Lasix?

_____

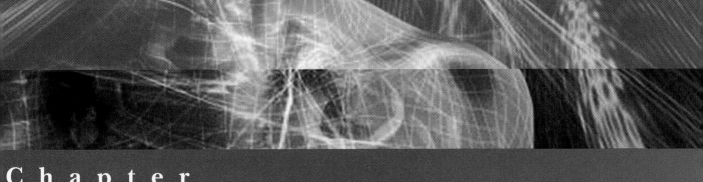

Chapter

8

Cardiovascular System

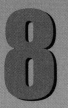

OBJECTIVES

Upon completion of this chapter, you will be able to:

- Locate and describe the structures of the cardiovascular system.
- Recognize, pronounce, spell, and build words related to the cardiovascular system.
- Describe pathological conditions, diagnostic and therapeutic procedures, and other terms related to the cardiovascular system.
- Explain pharmacology related to the treatment of cardiovascular disorders.
- Demonstrate your knowledge of this chapter by completing the learning and medical record activities.

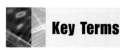

Key Terms

This section introduces important cardiovascular system terms and their definitions. Word analyses are also provided.

Term	Definition
diaphoresis dī-ă-fō-RĒ-sĭs *dia-:* through, across *-phoresis:* carrying, transmission	Profuse sweating
incompetent ĭn-KŎM-pĕ-tĕnt	Inability to adequately perform a given function or action
leaflet	Thin, flattened structure; term used to describe the leaf-shaped structures that compose a heart valve
lumen LŪ-mĕn	Tubular space or channel within any organ or structure of the body; space within an artery, vein, intestine, or tube
malaise mă-LĀZ	Vague, uneasy feeling of body weakness, distress, or discomfort, commonly marking the onset of and persisting throughout a disease
occlusion ŏ-KLOO-zhŭn	Blockage in a canal, vessel, or passage of the body; the state of being closed
patent PĂT-ĕnt	Open and unblocked, such as a patent artery
prophylaxis prō-fĭ-LĂK-sĭs *pro-:* before, in front of *-phylaxis:* protection	Preventive measure or technique commonly involving the use of a biologic, chemical, or mechanical agent to destroy or prevent the entry of infectious organisms
viscosity vĭs-KŎS-ĭ-tē	State of being sticky or gummy *A solution that has high viscosity is relatively thick and flows slowly.*

Anatomy and Physiology

The cardiovascular system is composed of the heart and blood vessels. The heart is a hollow muscular organ lying in the mediastinum, the center of the thoracic cavity between the lungs. The pumping action of the heart propels blood containing oxygen, nutrients, and other vital products to body cells through a vast network of blood vessels called *arteries*. Blood returns to the heart through blood vessels called *veins* to begin the cycle again. On its return trip to the heart, blood picks up waste products from the body cells to deliver them to the organs of excretion. The trillions of body cells rely on the cardiovascular system for their survival. When this transportation system fails, life at the cellular level is not possible and, ultimately, the organism will die.

Vascular System

Three major types of vessels—(1) **artery,** (2) **capillary,** and (3) **vein**—carry blood throughout the body. (See Figure 8–1.) Each type of vessel differs in structure, depending on its function.

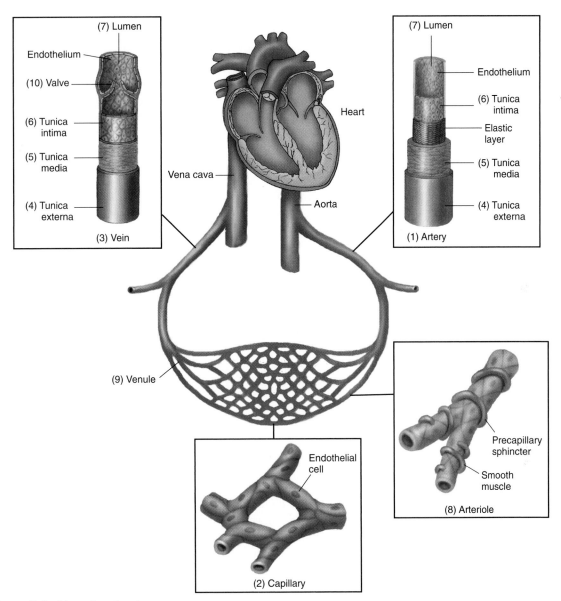

Figure 8–1 Vascular structures.

Arteries

Arteries carry blood from the heart to trillions of body cells that make up an organism. Because blood is propelled thorough the arteries by the pumping action of the heart, the walls of the arteries must be able to withstand the surge of blood that results from each contraction of the heart.

The walls of the large arteries have three layers to provide the necessary strength and flexibility. The (4) **tunica externa** is a tough, outer coat of connective tissue that provides strength. The (5) **tunica media** is a layer of smooth muscular tissue. Depending on the needs of the body, it can cause *vasoconstriction* (reduction of the lumen diameter caused by smooth muscle contraction) or *vasodilation* (widening of the lumen caused by smooth muscle relaxation). The (6) **tunica intima** is a thin, inner lining composed of endothelial cells that provides a smooth surface so blood can flow easily through its (7) **lumen.**

The surge of blood felt in the arteries when blood is pumped from the heart is referred to as a *pulse.* Because of the pressure against arterial walls associated with the pumping action of the heart, a cut or severed artery may lead to profuse bleeding.

Arterial blood (except for that found in the pulmonary artery) contains a high concentration of oxygen. It appears bright red and is said to be *oxygenated.* Oxygenated blood travels to smaller arteries called (8) **arterioles** and finally to the smallest vessels, the capillaries.

Capillaries

Capillaries are microscopic vessels that join the arterial system with the venous system. Although seemingly the most insignificant of the three vessel types because of their microscopic size, they are actually the most important because of their function. At the capillary level, nutrients and oxygen in the blood are exchanged for waste products formed by the surrounding cells. Because capillary walls are composed of a single layer of endothelial cells, they are very thin. This thinness enables the exchange of water, macromolecules, metabolites, and wastes. Because there are vast numbers of capillaries branching from arterioles, blood flows slowly through them, providing sufficient time for exchange of necessary substances.

Blood flow through the highly branched capillary system is regulated by the contraction of smooth muscle precapillary sphincters that lead into the capillary bed. When tissues require more blood, these sphincters open; when less blood is required, they close. Once the exchange of products is complete, blood enters the venous system for its return cycle to the heart.

Veins

Veins return blood to the heart. They are formed from smaller vessels called (9) **venules** that develop from the union of capillaries. Because the extensive network of capillaries absorbs the propelling pressure exerted by the heart, veins use other methods to propel blood to the heart, including:

- skeletal muscle contraction
- gravity
- respiratory activity
- valves

The (10) **valves** are small structures within veins that prevent the backflow of blood. Valves are found predominantly in the extremities and are especially important for returning blood from the legs to the heart because blood must travel a long distance against the force of gravity to reach the heart. Large veins such as those found in the abdomen contain smooth muscle that contract peristaltically to propel blood toward the heart against gravity.

Blood carried in the veins (except for the blood in the pulmonary veins) contains a low concentration of oxygen (**deoxygenated**) with a corresponding high concentration of carbon dioxide. Deoxygenated blood takes on a characteristic purple color. Blood continuously circulates to the lungs so that carbon dioxide can be exchanged for oxygen.

Heart

The heart is contained in a sac called the **pericardium** and has three distinct tissue layers:

1. The **endocardium** is a serous membrane that lines the four chambers of the heart and its valves and is continuous with the endothelium of the arteries and veins.
2. The **myocardium** is the muscular layer of the heart.
3. The **epicardium** is the outermost layer of the heart.

The heart is a four-chambered muscular pump supplied with an electrical conduction system whose function is to propel blood throughout the body through a closed vascular system. (See Figures 8–2A and 8–2B.) The heart is divided into four chambers. The two upper

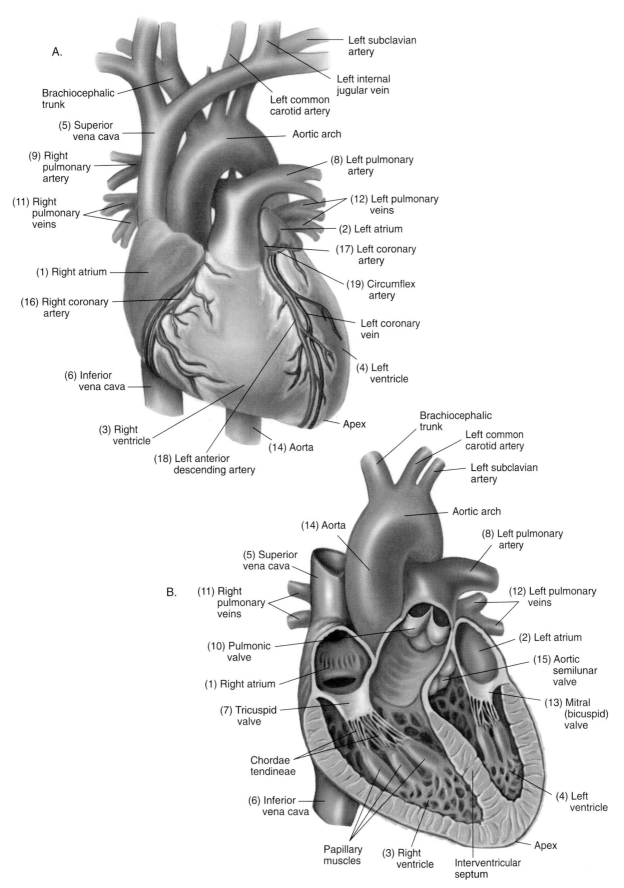

A.

Left subclavian artery

Brachiocephalic trunk

Left internal jugular vein

Left common carotid artery

(5) Superior vena cava

Aortic arch

(9) Right pulmonary artery

(8) Left pulmonary artery

(11) Right pulmonary veins

(12) Left pulmonary veins

(2) Left atrium

(17) Left coronary artery

(1) Right atrium

(19) Circumflex artery

(16) Right coronary artery

Left coronary vein

(6) Inferior vena cava

(4) Left ventricle

(3) Right ventricle

Apex

(18) Left anterior descending artery

(14) Aorta

Brachiocephalic trunk

Left common carotid artery

Left subclavian artery

Aortic arch

(14) Aorta

(8) Left pulmonary artery

(5) Superior vena cava

B. (11) Right pulmonary veins

(12) Left pulmonary veins

(10) Pulmonic valve

(2) Left atrium

(15) Aortic semilunar valve

(1) Right atrium

(13) Mitral (bicuspid) valve

(7) Tricuspid valve

Chordae tendineae

(6) Inferior vena cava

(4) Left ventricle

Apex

Papillary muscles

(3) Right ventricle

Interventricular septum

Figure 8–2 Structures of the heart. (A) Anterior view of the heart. (B) Frontal section of the heart.

chambers, the atria, are composed of the (1) **right atrium** and (2) **left atrium** and collect blood. The two lower chambers, the ventricles, are composed of the (3) **right ventricle** and (4) **left ventricle** and pump blood from the heart. The right side of the heart pumps blood to the lungs (pulmonary circulation) for oxygenation, and the left side of the heart pumps oxygenated blood to all body systems (systemic circulation).

Deoxygenated blood from the body returns to the heart by way of two large veins: the (5) **superior vena cava,** which collects and carries blood from the upper part of the body; and the (6) **inferior vena cava,** which collects and carries blood from the lower part of the body. The superior and inferior venae cavae deposit deoxygenated blood into the upper right chamber of the heart, the right atrium. From the right atrium, blood passes through the (7) **tricuspid valve** to the right ventricle. When the heart contracts, blood leaves the right ventricle by way of the (8) **left pulmonary artery** and (9) **right pulmonary artery** and travels to the lungs. During contraction of the ventricle, the tricuspid valve closes to prevent a backflow of blood to the right atrium. The (10) **pulmonic valve** (or *pulmonary semilunar valve*) prevents a back-flow of blood into the right ventricle. In the lungs, the pulmonary artery branches into millions of capillaries, each lying close to an alveolus. Here, carbon dioxide in the blood is exchanged for oxygen that has been drawn into the lungs during inhalation.

Pulmonary capillaries unite to form four pulmonary veins—two (11) **right pulmonary veins** and two (12) **left pulmonary veins**—which are the vessels that carry oxygenated blood back to the heart. Pulmonary veins deposit blood in the left atrium. From here, blood passes through the (13) **mitral (bicuspid) valve** to the left ventricle. Upon contraction of the ventricles, the oxygenated blood leaves the left ventricle through the largest artery of the body, the (14) **aorta.** The aorta contains the (15) **aortic semilunar valve** (or *aortic valve*) that permits blood to flow in only one direction—from the left ventricle to the aorta. The aorta branches into many smaller arteries that carry blood to all parts of the body. Some arteries derive their names from the organs or areas of the body they vascularize. For example, the splenic artery vascularizes the spleen and the renal arteries vascularize the kidneys.

It is important to understand that oxygen, present in the blood passing through the chambers of the heart, cannot be used by the myocardium as a source of oxygen and nutrients. Instead, an arterial system composed of the coronary arteries branches from the aorta and provides the heart with its own blood supply. These arteries lie over the top of the heart much as a crown fits over a head, hence the name **coronary** (pertaining to a crown). The artery vascularizing the right side of the heart is the (16) **right coronary artery.** The artery vascular-izing the left side of the heart is the (17) **left coronary artery.** The left coronary artery divides into the (18) **left anterior descending artery** and the (19) **circumflex artery.** If blood flow in the coronary arteries is diminished, myocardial damage may result. When severe damage occurs, part of the heart muscle may die.

Conduction System of the Heart

Within the heart, a specialized cardiac tissue known as *conductive tissue* has the sole function of initiating and spreading contraction impulses. (See Figure 8–3.) This tissue consists of four masses of highly specialized cells:

1. **sinoatrial (SA) node**
2. **atrioventricular (AV) node**
3. **bundle of His (AV bundle)**
4. **Purkinje fibers.**

The SA node, located in the upper portion of the right atrium, possesses its own intrin-sic rhythm. Without being stimulated by external nerves, it has the ability to initiate and prop-agate each heartbeat, thereby setting the basic pace for the cardiac rate. For this reason, the SA node is commonly known as the *pacemaker* of the heart. Cardiac rate may be altered by

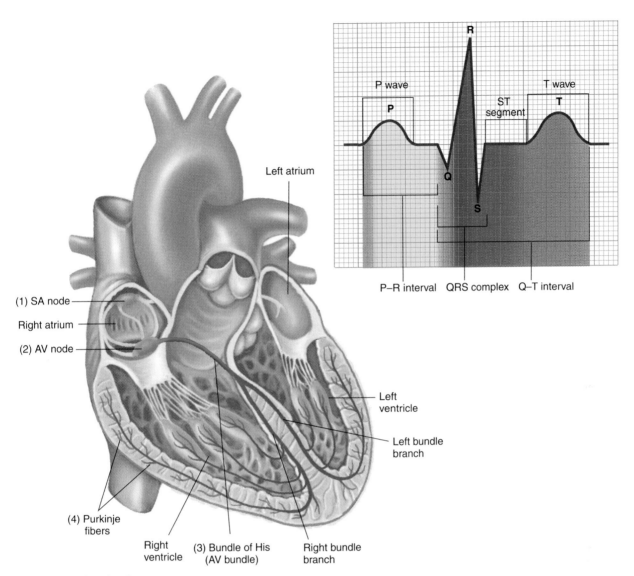

Figure 8–3 Conduction system.

impulses from the autonomic nervous system. Such an arrangement allows outside influences to accelerate or decelerate the heart rate. For example, the heart beats faster during physical exertion and slower during rest.

Each electrical impulse discharged by the SA node is transmitted to the AV node, causing the atria to contract. The AV node is located at the base of the right atrium. From this point, a tract of conduction fibers called the bundle of His, composed of a right and left branch, relays the impulse to the Purkinje fibers. These fibers extend up the ventricle walls. The Purkinje fibers transmit the impulse to both the right and left ventricles, causing them to contract. Blood is now forced from the heart through the pulmonary artery and aorta.

In summary, the sequence of the four structures responsible for conduction of a contraction impulse is as follows:

SA node ——⟶ AV node ——⟶ bundle of His ——⟶ Purkinje fibers

Impulse transmission through the conduction system generates weak electrical currents that can be detected on the surface of the body. These electrical impulses can be recorded on an instrument called an *electrocardiograph*. The needle deflection of the electrocardiograph produces waves or peaks designated by the letters P, Q, R, S, and T, each of which is associated with a specific electrical event:

- The *P wave* is the depolarization (contraction) of the atria.
- The *QRS complex* is the depolarization (contraction) of the ventricles.
- The *T wave*, which appears a short time later, is the repolarization (recovery) of the ventricles.

Blood Pressure

Blood pressure measures the force exerted by blood against the arterial walls during two phases of a heartbeat: the contraction phase, called *systole*, when the blood is forced out of the heart, and the relaxation phase, called *diastole*, when the ventricles are filling with blood. Systole is the maximum force exerted by blood against the arterial walls; diastole, the weakest. These measurements are recorded as two figures separated by a diagonal line; the systolic pressure is given first, followed by the diastolic pressure. For instance, blood pressure may be recorded as 120/80 mm Hg; in this example, 120 is the systolic pressure, 80 the diastolic pressure. A consistently elevated blood pressure is called **hypertension;** decreased blood pressure is called *hypotension*.

Several factors influence blood pressure:

- resistance of blood flow in blood vessels
- pumping action of the heart
- **viscosity,** or thickness, of blood
- elasticity of arteries
- quantity of blood in the vascular system

Fetal Circulation

Blood circulation through a fetus is, by necessity, different from that of a newborn infant. Respiration, the procurement of nutrients, and the elimination of metabolic wastes occur through the maternal blood instead of the organs of the fetus. The capillary exchange between the maternal and fetal circulation occurs within the placenta during pregnancy. This remarkable structure includes part of the mother's uterus and is discharged following delivery.

There are several major structures involved in fetal circulation. (See Figure 8–4.) The (1) **umbilical cord,** containing (2) two **arteries,** carries deoxygenated blood from the fetus to the (3) **placenta.** After oxygenation in the placenta, blood returns to the fetus via the (4) **umbilical vein.** Most of the blood in the umbilical vein enters the (5) **inferior vena cava** through the (6) **ductus venosus,** where it is delivered to the (7) **right atrium.** Some of this blood passes to the (8) **right ventricle;** however, most of it passes to the (9) **left atrium** through a small opening in the atrial septum called the (10) **foramen ovale,** which closes shortly after birth. From the left atrium, blood enters the (11) **left ventricle** and finally exits the heart through the aorta, where it is sent to the head and upper extremities. Because fetal lungs are nonfunctional, most of the blood in the pulmonary arteries is shunted through a connecting vessel called the (12) **ductus arteriosus** to the aorta. Immediately after birth, the ductus arteriosus withers and closes off. As circulation increases in the neonate, the increase of blood flow to the right atrium forces the foramen ovale to close. Normal circulation is now fully established.

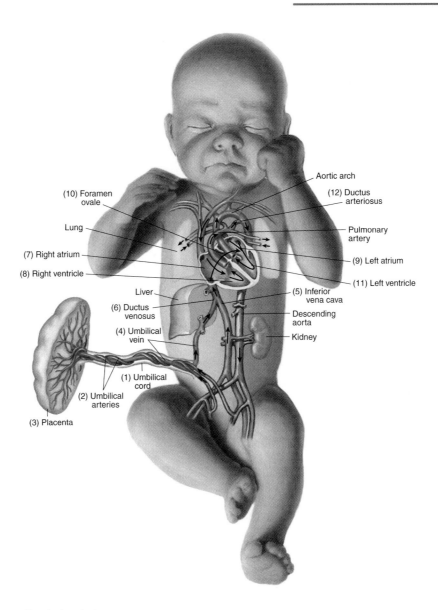

Figure 8–4 Fetal circulation.

 It is time to review cardiovascular structures by completing Learning Activity 8–1.

Medical Word Elements

This section introduces combining forms, suffixes, and prefixes related to the cardiovascular system. Word analyses are also provided.

Element	Meaning	Word Analysis
COMBINING FORMS		
aneurysm/o	a widening, a widened blood vessel	aneurysm/o/rrhaphy (ăn-ū-rĭz-MOR-ă-fē): surgical closure of an aneurysm sac *-rrhaphy:* suture
angi/o	vessel (usually blood or lymph)	angi/o/plasty (ĂN-jē-ō-plăs-tē): any endovascular procedure that reopens narrowed blood vessels and restores blood flow *-plasty:* surgical repair *The blocked vessel is usually opened by balloon dilation.*
vascul/o		vascul/itis (văs-kū-LĪ-tĭs): inflammation of blood vessels *-itis:* inflammation
aort/o	aorta	aort/o/stenosis (ā-or-tō-stĕ-NŌ-sĭs): narrowing of the aorta *-stenosis:* narrowing, stricture
arteri/o	artery	arteri/o/rrhexis (ăr-tē-rē-ō-RĔK-sĭs): rupture of an artery *-rrhexis:* rupture
arteriol/o	arteriole	arteriol/itis (ăr-tēr-ē-ō-LĪ-tĭs): inflammation of the wall of an arteriole *-itis:* inflammation
atri/o	atrium	atri/o/megaly (ā-trē-ō-MĔG-ă-lē): enlargement of the atrium *-megaly:* enlargement
ather/o	fatty plaque	ather/oma (ăth-ĕr-Ō-mă): abnormal condition of fatty-plaque buildup on the inner lining of arterial walls *-oma:* tumor *Atheroma is the most common cause of hardening of the arteries.*
cardi/o	heart	cardi/o/megaly (kăr-dē-ō-MĔG-ă-lē): enlargement of the heart *-megaly:* enlargement
electr/o	electricity	electr/o/cardi/o/gram (ē-lĕk-trō-KĂR-dē-ō-grăm): graphic recording of the electrical impulses of the heart *cardi/o:* heart *-gram:* record, recording *Electrocardiogram is commonly used to diagnose abnormalities of the heart.*

Element	Meaning	Word Analysis
embol/o	plug	embol/ectomy (ĕm-bō-LĚK-tō-mē): removal of an embolus through a surgical procedure or treatment with enzymes *-ectomy:* excision, removal
hemangi/o	blood vessel	hemangi/oma (hē-măn-jē-Ō-mă): benign tumor of dilated blood vessels *-oma:* tumor
my/o	muscle	my/o/cardi/al (mī-ō-KĂR-dē-ăl): pertaining to heart muscle *cardi:* heart *-al:* pertaining to, relating to
phleb/o **ven/o**	vein	phleb/ectasis (flĕ-BĚK-tă-sĭs): dilation of a vein; varicosity *-ectasis:* dilation, expansion ven/o/stasis (vē-nō-STĀ-sĭs): abnormally slow flow of blood in the veins, usually with distension of the vessel; also called *phlebostasis* *-stasis:* standing still
scler/o	hardening; sclera (white of eye)	arteri/o/scler/osis (ăr-tē-rē-ō-sklĕ-RŌ-sĭs): thickening, hardening, and loss of elasticity of arterial walls *arteri/o:* artery *-osis:* abnormal condition; increase (used primarily with blood cells) *Arteriosclerosis results in decreased blood supply that primarily affects the heart, cerebrum, and lower extremities.*
sept/o	septum	sept/o/stomy (sĕp-TŎS-tō-mē): surgical formation of an opening in a septum *-stomy:* forming an opening (mouth) *Septostomy is performed to treat congenital heart defects that affect the aorta and pulmonary arteries.*
sphygm/o	pulse	sphygm/oid (SFĬG-moyd): resembling a pulse *-oid:* resembling
sten/o	narrowing, stricture	sten/o/tic (stĕ-NŎT-ĭk): pertaining to a narrowing or stricture *-tic:* pertaining to, relating to
thromb/o	blood clot	thromb/o/lysis (thrŏm-BŎL-ĭ-sĭs): destruction of a blood clot *-lysis:* separation; destruction; loosening *In thrombolysis, enzymes that destroy the blood clot are infused into the vessel.*
ventricul/o	ventricle (of the heart or brain)	ventricul/ar (vĕn-TRĬK-ū-lăr): pertaining to a ventricle (chamber of the heart or brain) *-ar:* pertaining to, relating to

(Continued)

Element	Meaning	Word Analysis	(Continued)

SUFFIXES

-gram	record, writing	arteri/o/gram (ăr-TĒ-rē-ō-grăm): radiograph of an artery after injection of a radiopaque contrast medium, usually directly into the artery or near its origin *arteri/o:* artery *An arteriogram is used to visualize almost any artery, including those of the heart, head, kidneys, lungs, and other organs.*
-graph	instrument for recording	electr/o/cardi/o/graph (ē-lĕk-trō-KĂR-dē-ō-grăf): device used to record changes in the electrical activity produced by the action of the heart muscles *electr/o:* electricity *cardi/o:* heart
-graphy	process of recording	angi/o/graphy (ăn-jē-ŎG-ră-fē): visualization of the internal anatomy of the heart and blood vessels after introduction of a radiopaque contrast medium *angi/o:* vessel (usually blood or lymph) *Angiography is commonly used to identify atherosclerosis and diagnose heart and peripheral vascular disease.*
-sphyxia	pulse	a/sphyxia (ăs-FĬK-sē-ă): deficiency of oxygen and excess of carbon dioxide in the blood and body tissues; also called *suffocation* *a-:* without, not
-stenosis	narrowing, stricture	aort/o/stenosis (ā-or-tō-stĕ-NŌ-sĭs): narrowing of the aorta *aort/o:* aorta

PREFIXES

brady-	slow	brady/cardia (brăd-ē-KĂR-dē-ă): abnormally slow heart rate *-cardia:* heart condition
endo-	in, within	endo/vascul/ar (ĕn-dō-VĂS-kū-lăr): relating to the inside of a vessel *vascul:* vessel *-ar:* pertaining to, relating to
extra-	outside	extra/vascul/ar (ĕks-tră-VĂS-kū-lăr): relating to the outside of a vessel *vascul:* vessel *-ar:* pertaining to, relating to

Element	Meaning	Word Analysis
peri-	around	peri/cardi/o/tomy (pĕr-ĭ-kăr-dē-ŎT-ō-mē): incision of the pericardium, usually performed to drain a pericardial effusion *cardi/o:* heart *-tomy:* incision
tachy-	rapid	tachy/cardia (tăk-ē-KĂR-dē-ă): abnormally rapid heart rate *-cardia:* heart condition
trans-	across	trans/sept/al (trăns-SĔP-tăl): across the septum *sept:* septum *-al:* pertaining to, relating to

 It is time to review medical word elements by completing Learning Activity 8–2.

Pathology

Many cardiac disorders, especially coronary artery disease, and valvular disorders are associated with a genetic predisposition. Thus, a complete history as well as a physical examination is essential in the diagnosis of cardiovascular disease. Although some of the most serious cardiovascular diseases have few signs and symptoms, when they occur they may include pain, palpitations, dyspnea, and syncope. The pain's location, duration, pattern of radiation, and severity are important qualities in differentiating the various forms of cardiovascular disease and are sometimes characteristic of specific disorders. Because of the general nature of the signs and symptoms of CV disorders, both invasive and noninvasive tests are usually required to confirm or rule out a suspected disease.

For diagnosis, treatment, and management of cardiovascular disorders, the medical services of a specialist may be warranted. *Cardiology* is the medical specialty concerned with disorders of the cardiovascular system. The physician who treats these disorders is called a *cardiologist.*

Arteriosclerosis

Arteriosclerosis is a hardening of arterial walls that causes them to become thickened and brittle. It commonly results from an accumulation of a plaquelike substance composed of cholesterol, lipids, and cellular debris (**atheroma**) that builds up on the innermost lining (**tunica intima**) of the arterial walls. Over time, the plaque hardens (**atherosclerosis**) causing a loss of vascular elasticity. The vascular channel (**lumen**) narrows as the plaque enlarges. Eventually, it becomes difficult for blood to pass through the occluded areas, and tissue distal to the occlusion becomes ischemic. Commonly, blood hemorrhages into the plaque and forms a clot (**thrombus**) that may dislodge. When a thrombus travels though the vascular system it is called an *embolus.* Emboli that travel in venous circulation may cause death. Emboli that travel in arterial circulation frequently lodge in a capillary bed and cause a localized infarct. Plaque sometimes weakens the vessel wall to such an extent that it forms a bulge (**aneurysm**) that may rupture. (See Figure 8–5.)

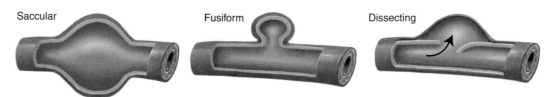

Figure 8–5   Aneurysms.

Arteriosclerosis usually affects large- or medium-sized arteries, including the abdominal aorta, the coronary, cerebral, and renal arteries, and major arteries of the legs **(femoral arteries).** One of the major risk factors for developing arteriosclerosis is an elevated cholesterol level **(hypercholesterolemia).** Other major risk factors include age, family history, smoking, hypertension, and diabetes.

Treatment for arthrosclerosis varies depending on the location and symptoms. In one method, especially in the carotid or femoral arteries, the innermost layer of the artery is surgically removed **(endarterectomy).** Other, less invasive methods include using a catheter with a balloon at its tip and inserting it into the affected area. The balloon is inflated to stretch the narrowed artery **(angioplasty).** After the procedure, the balloon is deflated and removed. A hollow, thin mesh tube **(stent)** is usually placed on the balloon and positioned against the artery wall. It remains in place after the balloon catheter is removed and acts as scaffolding to hold the artery open.

Coronary Artery Disease

Any disease that interferes with the ability of coronary arteries to deliver sufficient blood to the myocardium is referred to as **coronary artery disease (CAD).** The major cause of CAD is arteriosclerosis. About 20% of the total cardiac output is needed to meet the oxygen requirements of the heart muscle. When coronary arteries are unable to deliver sufficient oxygen, localized areas of the heart experience oxygen deprivation **(ischemia)** and, with total lack of oxygen, the affected area of the heart muscle dies **(myocardial infarction [MI]).** (See Figure 8–6.) The clin-

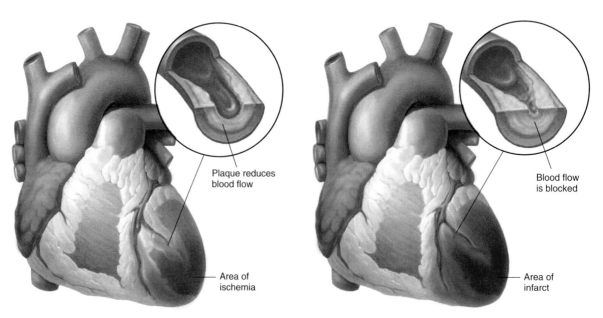

Plaque reduces
blood flow

Area of
ischemia

Blood flow
is blocked

Area of
infarct

Figure 8–6   Occlusions. (A) Partial occlusion. (B) Total occlusion.

ical signs and symptoms of an MI include intense chest pain **(angina)**, diaphoresis, paleness **(pallor)**, and dyspnea. An arrhythmic heartbeat with tachycardia or bradycardia may also accompany MI.

As the heart muscle undergoes necrotic changes, several highly specific cardiac enzymes, including troponin T, troponin I, and creatinine kinase (CK-MB), are released. The rapid elevation of these enzymes at predictable times following MI helps differentiate MI from pericarditis, aortic aneurysm, and acute pulmonary embolism.

When angina cannot be controlled with medication, surgical repair of the vessel **(angioplasty)** may be necessary. In one method of treatment, a deflated balloon is passed through a small incision in the skin and into the diseased blood vessel **(percutaneous transluminal coronary angioplasty [PTCA])**. When it is inflated, the balloon presses the occluding material against the lumen walls to increase their diameter. (See Figure 8–7.) A more invasive procedure involves rerouting blood around the occluded area using a small graft of a vein to bypass the obstruction **(coronary artery bypass graft [CABG])**. One end of the graft vessel is sutured to the aorta and the other end is sutured to the coronary artery below the blocked area. This re-establishes blood flow to the heart muscle. (See Figure 8–8.)

Endocarditis

Endocarditis is an inflammation of the inner lining of the heart and its valves. It may be noninfective in nature, caused by thrombi formation, or infective, caused by various microorganisms. Although the infecting organism can be viral or fungal, the usual culprit is a bacterium.

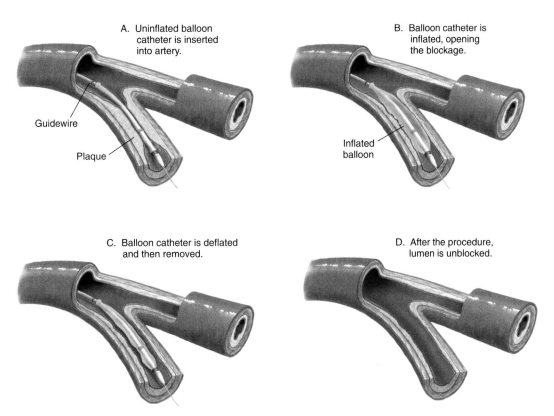

A. Uninflated balloon catheter is inserted into artery.

Guidewire

Plaque

B. Balloon catheter is inflated, opening the blockage.

Inflated balloon

C. Balloon catheter is deflated and then removed.

D. After the procedure, lumen is unblocked.

Figure 8–7   Balloon angioplasty.

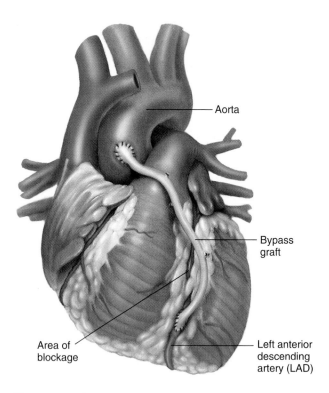

Figure 8–8   Coronary artery bypass graft.

Congenital valvular defects, scarlet fever, rheumatic fever, bicuspid or calcific aortic valves, mitral valve prolapse, and prosthetic valves are predisposing factors. Bacteria, traveling in the bloodstream **(bacteremia),** lodge in the weakened heart tissue and form small masses called *vegetations* composed of fibrin and platelets. Vegetations frequently collect on the leaflets of the valves and their cords, causing a backflow of blood **(regurgitation).** With valve scarring, there may be a narrowing of the valves **(stenosis)** or an inability of the valves to close properly **(insufficiency).** Some may dislodge and travel as emboli to the brain, lungs, kidneys, or spleen. Although medications may prove helpful, if heart failure develops as a result of damaged heart valves, surgery may be the only recourse. Whenever possible, the original valve is repaired. When the damage is extensive, a mechanical or bioprosthetic valve may be used.

Patients who are susceptible to endocarditis are given antibiotic treatment to protect against infection prior to invasive procedures **(prophylactic treatment).** Because many of the bacteria that are normally found in the mouth are also responsible for endocarditis, prophylactic treatment is warranted for tooth removal, root canal procedures, and even routine cleaning.

Varicose Veins

Varicose veins are enlarged, twisted, superficial veins. They develop when the valves of the veins do not function properly **(incompetent)** and fail to prevent the backflow of blood in the vein. Blood accumulates and the vein appears engorged and distended. Excess fluid eventually seeps from the vein, causing swelling in surrounding tissues **(edema).** Varicose veins may develop in almost any part of the body, but occur most commonly in the lower legs, involving the greater and lesser saphenous veins. Types of varicose veins include reticular veins, which appear as small blue veins seen through the skin, and "spider" veins, which look like short, fine lines, starburst clusters, or a weblike maze.

Varicose veins of the legs are not typically painful but may be unsightly in appearance. However, if open lesions or pain is present, treatment includes laser ablation, microphlebectomies, ligation, stripping, and sclerotherapy. The same methods are used as an elective procedure to enhance the appearance of the legs. Treatment of mild cases of varicose veins includes use of elastic stockings and rest periods during which the legs are elevated.

Oncology

Although rare, the most common primary tumor of the heart is composed of mucous connective tissue (**myxoma**); however, these tumors tend to be benign. Although some myxomas originate in the endocardium of the heart chambers, most arise in the left atrium. Occasionally, they interfere with mitral valve function and cause a decrease in exercise tolerance, dyspnea, fluid in the lungs (**pulmonary edema**), and systemic disturbances, including joint pain (**arthralgia**), **malaise,** and anemia. These tumors are usually identified and located by two-dimensional echocardiography. The tumor should be excised surgically.

Most malignant tumors of the heart are the result of a malignancy originating in another area of the body (**primary tumor**) that has spread (**metastasized**) to the heart. The type usually found originates as a darkly pigmented mole or tumor (**malignant melanoma**) of the skin. Other primary sites of malignancy that metastasize to the heart are bone marrow and lymphatic tissue. Treatment of the metastatic tumor of the heart involves treating the primary tumor.

Diagnostic, Symptomatic, and Related Terms

This section introduces diagnostic, symptomatic, and related terms and their meanings. Word analyses for selected terms are also provided.

Term	Definition
aneurysm ĂN-ū-rĭzm	Localized abnormal dilation of a vessel, usually an artery (See Figure 8–5.)
arrest ă-RĔST	Condition of being stopped or bringing to a stop

cardiac
   KĂR-dē-ăk
 	
    cardi: heart
    -ac: pertaining to, relating to
	Loss of effective cardiac function, which results in cessation of circulation
	Cardiac arrest may be due to ventricular fibrillation or asystole in which there is no observable myocardial activity.

circulatory SĔR-kū-lă-tor-ē	Cessation of the circulation of blood due to ventricular standstill or fibrillation

(Continued)

Term	Definition	(Continued)
arrhythmia ă-RĬTH-mē-ă	Inability of the heart to maintain a steady rhythm, possibly including a rapid or slow beat or "skipping" a beat	
bruit brwē	Soft blowing sound heard on auscultation, possibly due to vibrations associated with the movement of blood, valvular action, or both; also called *murmur*	
cardiomyopathy kăr-dē-ō-mi-ŎP-ă-thē *cardi/o:* heart *my/o:* muscle *-pathy:* disease	Any disease of heart muscle that diminishes cardiac function *Cardiomyopathy may be caused by viral infections, metabolic disorders, or general systemic disease.*	
catheter KĂTH-ĕ-tĕr	Thin, flexible, hollow plastic tube that is small enough to be threaded through a vein, artery, or tubular structure	
coarctation kō-ărk-TĀ-shŭn	Narrowing of a vessel, especially the aorta	
heart failure hărt FĀL-yĕr	Failure of the heart to supply an adequate amount of blood to tissues and organs *Heart failure is commonly caused by impaired coronary blood flow, cardiomyopathies, and heart valve disease. The term* heart failure *is currently replacing the term* congestive heart failure (CHF).	
embolus ĔM-bō-lŭs *embol:* plug *-us:* condition, structure	Mass of undissolved matter (foreign object, air, gas, tissue, thrombus) circulating in blood or lymphatic channels until it becomes lodged in a vessel	
fibrillation fĭ-brĭl-Ā-shŭn	Quivering or spontaneous muscle contractions, especially of the heart, causing ineffectual contractions *Fibrillation is commonly corrected with a* defibrillator.	
hemostasis hē-mō-STĀ-sĭs *hem/o:* blood *-stasis:* standing still	Arrest of bleeding or circulation	
hyperlipidemia hi-pĕr-lĭp-ĭ-DĒ-mē-ă *hyper-:* excessive, above normal *lipid:* fat *-emia:* blood condition	Excessive amounts of lipids (cholesterol, phospholipids, and triglycerides) in the blood	

Term	Definition
hypertension hī-pĕr-TĔN-shŭn *hyper-:* excessive, above normal *-tension:* to stretch	Common disorder characterized by elevated blood pressure persistently exceeding 140 mm Hg systolic or 90 mm Hg diastolic
primary	Hypertension in which there is no identifiable cause; also called *essential hypertension* *Primary hypertension is the most common form of hypertension and is associated with obesity, a high serum sodium level, hypercholesterolemia, or family history.*
secondary	Hypertension that results from an underlying, identifiable, commonly correctable cause
hypertensive heart disease hī-pĕr-TĔN-sĭv	Any heart disorder caused by prolonged hypertension, including left ventricular hypertrophy, coronary artery disease, cardiac arrhythmias, and heart failure
implantable cardioverter-defibrillator (ICD) ĭm-PLĂN-tă-băl KĂR-dē-ō-vĕr-tĕr-dē-FĬB-rĭ-lā-tor	Implantable battery-powered device that monitors and, if necessary, corrects an irregular heart rhythm by sending impulses to the heart *ICD is a therapeutic device that automatically terminates ventricular arrhythmias.*
infarct ĭn-FĂRCT	Area of tissue that undergoes necrosis following cessation of blood supply
ischemia ĭs-KĒ-mē-ă	Local and temporary deficiency of blood supply due to circulatory obstruction
mitral valve prolapse (MVP) MĪ-trăl, PRŌ-lăps	Common and occasionally serious condition in which the leaflets of the mitral valve prolapse into the left atrium during systole causing a characteristic murmur heard on auscultation *Common signs and symptoms of MVP include palpitations of the heart and, occasionally, panic attacks with pounding heartbeat. Because of the possibility of valve infection, prophylactic treatment with antibiotics is suggested before undergoing invasive procedures such as dental work.*
radioisotope rā-dē-ō-Ī-sō-tōp	Chemical radioactive substance used as a tracer to follow a substance through the body or a structure
palpitation păl-pĭ-TĀ-shŭn	Sensation that the heart is not beating normally, possibly including "thumping," "fluttering," "skipped beats," or a pounding feeling in the chest *Although most palpitations are harmless, those caused by arrhythmias may be serious. Medical attention should be sought if palpitations are accompanied by pain, dizziness, overall weakness, or shortness of breath.*
patent ductus arteriosus PĂT-ĕnt DŬK-tŭs ăr-tē-rē-O-sŭs	Failure of the ductus arteriosus to close after birth, allowing blood to flow from the aorta into the pulmonary (lung) artery
perfusion pĕr-FŪ-zhŭn	Circulation of blood through tissues or the passage of fluids through vessels of an organ

(Continued)

Term	Definition	(Continued)
tetralogy of Fallot tĕ-TRĂL-ō-jē, făl-Ō	Congenital anomaly consisting of four elements: (1) pulmonary artery stenosis; (2) interventricular septal defect; (3) transposition of the aorta, so that both ventricles empty into the aorta; (4) right ventricular hypertrophy caused by increased workload of the right ventricle	
stent STĔNT	Slender or threadlike device used to hold open vessels, tubes, or an obstructed artery *Stents are used to support tubular structures that are being anastomosed or to induce or maintain patency within these tubular structures.*	
Stokes-Adams syndrome stōks-ĂD-ăms SĬN-drōm	Altered state of consciousness or fainting due to decreased blood flow to the brain caused by prolonged asystole (absence of muscular contraction of the heart)	
thrombus THRŎM-bŭs *thromb:* blood clot *-us:* condition; structure	Blood clot that obstructs a vessel	

 It is time to review pathological, diagnostic, symptomatic, and related terms by completing Learning Activity 8–3.

 ## Diagnostic and Therapeutic Procedures

This section introduces procedures used to diagnose and treat cardiovascular disorders. Descriptions are provided as well as pronunciations and word analyses for selected terms.

Procedure	Description
DIAGNOSTIC PROCEDURES	
Clinical	
cardiac catheterization KĂR-dē-ăk kăth-ĕ-tĕr-ĭ-ZĀ-shŭn *cardi:* heart *-ac:* pertaining to, relating to	Passage of a catheter into the heart through a vein or artery to provide a comprehensive evaluation of the heart *Cardiac catheterization gathers information about the heart, such as blood supply through the coronary arteries and blood flow and pressure in the chambers of the heart as well as enabling blood sample collection and x-rays of the heart.*

Procedure	Description
electrocardiogram (ECG, EKG) ē-lĕk-trō-KĂR-dē-ō-grăm *electr/o:* electricity *cardi/o:* heart *-gram:* record, writing	Graphic line recording that shows the spread of electrical excitation to different parts of the heart using small metal electrodes applied to the chest, arms, and legs *ECGs help diagnose abnormal heart rhythms and myocardial damage.*
Holter monitor test HŎL-tĕr MŎN-ĭ-tor	Electrocardiogram (ECG) taken with a small portable recording system capable of storing up to 24 hours of ECG tracings *Holter monitoring is particularly useful in obtaining a cardiac arrhythmia record that would be missed during an ECG of only a few minutes' duration.*
stress test	ECG taken under controlled exercise stress conditions *A stress test may show abnormal ECG tracings that do not appear during an ECG taken when the patient is resting*
nuclear	Utilizes a radioisotope to evaluate coronary blood flow *In a nuclear stress test, the radioisotope is injected at the height of exercise. The area not receiving sufficient oxygen is visualized by decreased uptake of the isotope.*
Laboratory	
cardiac enzyme studies KĂR-dē-ăk ĔN-zīm	Blood test that measures troponin T, troponin I, and creatinine kinase (CK-MB) *Cardiac enzymes are most specific to cardiac injury and are released into the bloodstream from damaged heart muscle. Along with other less specific enzymes, these enzymes are used as a diagnostic marker for myocardial injury.*
lipid panel LĬP-ĭd	Series of tests (total cholesterol, high density lipoprotein, low density lipoprotein, and triglycerides) used to assess risk factors of ischemic heart disease
Radiographic	
aortography ā-or-TŎG-ră-fē *aort/o:* aorta *-graphy:* process of recording	Radiological examination of the aorta and its branches following the injection of a contrast medium via a catheter
coronary angiography KOR-ō-nă-rē ăn-jē-ŎG-ră-fē *angi/o:* vessel (usually blood or lymph) *-graphy:* process of recording	Radiological examination of the blood vessels of and around the heart

(Continued)

Procedure	Description	(Continued)

echocardiography
ĕk-ō-kăr-dē-
ŎG-ră-fē

  echo-: a repeated sound
  cardi/o: heart
  -graphy: process of recording

Noninvasive diagnostic method that uses ultrasound to visualize internal cardiac structures and produce images of the heart

A transducer is placed on the chest to direct ultra-high-frequency sound waves toward cardiac structures. Reflected echoes are then converted to electrical impulses and displayed on a screen.

  Doppler ultrasound
  DŎP-lĕr

Noninvasive adaptation of ultrasound technology in which blood flow velocity is assessed in different areas of the heart

Sound waves strike moving red blood cells and are reflected back to a recording device that graphically records blood flow.

magnetic resonance imaging (MRI)
māg-NĔT-ĭc RĔZ-ĕn-ăns

Noninvasive imaging technique that uses radiowaves and a strong magnetic field rather than an x-ray beam to produce multiplanar cross-sectional images

magnetic resonance angiography (MRA)
māg-NĔT-ĭc RĔZ-ĕn-ăns ăn-jē-ŎG-ră-fē

  angi/o: vessel (usually blood or lymph)
  -graphy: process of recording

Magnetic resonance imaging technique used to visualize vascular structures

MRA is used to diagnose such vascular disorders as aneurysms, occlusions, atherosclerotic plaque, vascular rupture, and stenosis.

phonocardiography
fō-nō-kăr-dē-
ŎG-ră-fē

  phon/o: voice, sound
  cardi/o: heart
  -graphy: process of recording

Imaging technique that provides a graphic display of heart sounds and murmurs during the cardiac cycle

In phonocardiography, a transducer sends ultrasonic pulses through the chest wall and the echoes are converted into images on a monitor to assess overall cardiac performance. An electrocardiograph is simultaneously displayed to provide a reference point for each of the sounds and their duration.

subtraction angiography
sŭb-TRĂK-shĕn
ăn-jē-ŎG-ră-fē

  angi/o: vessel (usually blood or lymph)
  -graphy: process of recording

Imaging technique used to display soft tissue structures such as blood vessels without the confusing overlay of bone images

In subtraction angiography, two images are obtained—the first before a contrast medium is administered and the second, after the contrast. A computer "subtracts" the first image from the second image, leaving only the contrasted image with all other structures removed.

scintigraphy
sĭn-TĬG-ră-fē

Injection and subsequent detection of radioactive isotopes to create images of body parts and identify body functions and diseases

In scintigraphy, abnormal uptake of the radioactive isotope indicates abnormality.

thallium study (resting)
THĂL-ē-ŭm

Scintigraphy procedure that identifies infarcted or scarred areas of the heart that show up as "cold spots" (areas of reduced radioactivity), taken when the patient is at rest

In a thallium study, radioactive thallium is injected and the uptake of the isotope is recorded by a gamma camera to produce the image. A stress thallium study is commonly performed at the same time as a resting study, and the two images are compared to further identify abnormalities.

Procedure	Description
venography vē-NOG-ră-fē *ven/o:* vein *-graphy:* process of recording	Radiography of a vein after injection of a contrast medium; incomplete filling of a vein indicates obstruction

THERAPEUTIC PROCEDURES

Clinical

cardioversion KĂR-dē-ō-vĕr-zhŭn *cardi/o:* heart *-version:* turning	Process of restoring the normal rhythm of the heart by applying a controlled electrical shock to the exterior of the chest
embolization ĕm-bō-lĭ-ZĀ-shŭn *embol:* plug *-izaton:* process (of)	Technique used to block blood flow to a site by passing a catheter to the area and injecting a synthetic material or medication specially designed to occlude the blood vessel *Embolization may serve to eliminate an abnormal communication between an artery and a vein, stop bleeding, or close vessels that are supporting tumor growth.*

Surgical

angioplasty ĂN-jē-ō-plăs-tē *angi/o:* vessel (usually blood or lymph) *-plasty:* surgical repair	Procedure that alters a vessel through surgery or dilation of the vessel using a balloon catheter
coronary artery bypass graft (CABG) KOR-ō-nă-rē ĂR-tĕr-ē	Surgical procedure that uses a vessel graft from another part of the body to bypass the blocked part of a coronary artery and restore blood supply to the heart muscle
percutaneous transluminal coronary angioplasty (PTCA) pĕr-kū-TĀ-nē-ŭs trăns-LŪ-mĭ-năl KOR-ō-nă-rē *per-:* through *cutane:* skin *-ous:* pertaining to, relating to	Dilation of an occluded vessel using a balloon catheter under fluoroscopic guidance *In PTCA, the catheter is inserted transcutaneously and the balloon is inflated, thereby dilating the narrowed vessel. A stent is commonly positioned to hold the vessel open.*
atherectomy ăth-ĕr-ĒK-tō-mē *ather:* fatty plaque *-ectomy:* excision, removal	Removal of material from an occluded vessel using a specially designed catheter fitted with a cutting or grinding device
biopsy BĪ-ŏp-sē	Removal and examination of a small piece of tissue for diagnostic purposes
arterial ăr-TĒ-rē-ăl *arteri:* artery *-al:* pertaining to, relating to	Removal and examination of a segment of an arterial vessel wall to confirm inflammation of the wall or arteritis, a type of vasculitis

(Continued)

Procedure	Description	(Continued)
catheter ablation KĂTH-ĕ-tĕr ăb-LĀ-shŭn	Destruction of conductive tissue of the heart to interrupt abnormal contractions, thus allowing normal heart rhythm to resume *Catheter ablation is usually performed under fluoroscopic guidance.*	
commissurotomy kŏm-ĭ-shūr-ŎT-ō-mē	Surgical separation of the leaflets of the mitral valve, which have fused together at their "commissures" (points of touching) *Many candidates for commissurotomy are now treated with balloon mitral valvuloplasty.*	
laser ablation	Procedure used to remove or treat varicose veins *In laser ablation, the laser's heat coagulates blood inside the vessel, causing it to collapse and seal. Later, the vessels dissolve within the body, becoming less visible, or disappear altogether.*	
ligation and stripping lĭ-GĀ-shŭn, STRĬP-ĭng	Tying a varicose vein (ligation) followed by removal (stripping) of the affected segment *Ligation and stripping are being replaced by laser ablation, in combination with microphlebectomies and sclerotherapy.*	
open heart surgery	Surgical procedure performed on or within the exposed heart, usually with the assistance of a heart-lung machine *During the operation, the heart-lung machine takes over circulation to allow surgery on the resting (nonbeating) heart. After the heart has been restarted and is beating, the patient is disconnected from the heart-lung machine. Types of open heart surgery include coronary artery bypass graft, valve replacement, and heart transplant.*	
pericardiocentesis pĕr-ĭ-kăr-dē-ō- sĕn-TĒ-sĭs *peri-:* around *cardi/o:* heart *-centesis:* surgical puncture	Puncturing of the pericardium to remove fluid to test for protein, sugar, and enzymes or determine the causative organism of pericarditis	
phlebotomy flē-BŎT-ō-mē *phleb/o:* vein *-tomy:* incision	Incision or puncture of a vein to remove blood or introduce fluids or medications	
thrombolysis thrŏm-BŎL-ĭ-sĭs *thromb/o:* blood clot *-lysis:* separation; destruction; loosening	Destruction of a blood clot using anticlotting agents called "clot-busters" such as tissue plasminogen activator *Prompt thrombolysis can restore blood flow to tissue before serious irreversible damage occurs. However, many thrombolytic agents also pose the risk of hemorrhage.*	
intravascular ĭn-tră-VĂS-kū-lăr *intra-:* in, within *vascul/o:* vessel *-ar:* pertaining to, relating to	Infusion of a thrombolytic agent into a vessel to dissolve a blood clot	

Procedure	Description

valvotomy
văl-VŎT-ō-mē
 	
   valv/o: valve
   -tomy: incision
	Incision of a valve to increase the size of the opening; used in treating mitral stenosis

venipuncture VĔN-ĭ-pŭnk-chŭr	Puncture of a vein by a needle attached to a syringe or catheter to withdraw a specimen of blood, perform a phlebotomy, instill a medication, start an intravenous infusion, or inject a radiopaque substance for radiological examination

 Pharmacology

A healthy, functional cardiovascular system is needed to ensure adequate blood circulation and efficient delivery of oxygen and nutrients to all parts of the body. When any part of the cardiovascular system malfunctions or becomes diseased, drug therapy plays an integral role in establishing and maintaining perfusion and homeostasis.

Medications are used to treat a variety of cardiovascular conditions, including angina pectoris, myocardial infarction, heart failure (HF), arrhythmias, hypertension, hyperlipidemia, and vascular disorders. (See Table 8–1.) Many of the cardiovascular drugs treat multiple problems simultaneously.

Table 8-1   DRUGS USED TO TREAT CARDIOVASCULAR DISORDERS

This table lists common drug classifications used to treat cardiovascular disorders, their therapeutic actions, and selected generic and trade names.

Classification	Therapeutic Action	Generic and Trade Names
angiotensin converting enzyme (ACE) inhibitors	Decrease blood pressure *ACE inhibitors lower blood pressure by dilating arterial blood vessels and inhibiting the conversion of angiotensin I (an inactive enzyme) to angiotensin II (a potent vasoconstrictor).*	**benazepril** bĕn-Ā-ză-prĭl *Lotensin* **captopril** KĂP-tō-prĭl *Capoten* **quinapril** KWĬN-ă-prĭl *Accupril*
antiarrhythmics	Help establish a regular heartbeat *Most antiarrhythmic drugs exert a therapeutic effect by stabilizing the electrical cycle of the heart. These drugs are used to treat atrial and ventricular arrhythmias.*	**flecainide** flă-KĀ-nĭd *Tambocor* **ibutilide** ī-BŪ-tĭ-lĭd *Corvert*

(Continued)

Table 8-1   DRUGS USED TO TREAT CARDIOVASCULAR DISORDERS *(Continued)*

Classification	Therapeutic Action	Generic and Trade Names

beta blockers	Treat and manage angina, hypertension, and ventricular arrhythmias
	
	Beta blockers control heart rate to prevent tachycardia, which helps control hypertension and arrhythmias. They also dilate coronary blood vessels to increase blood flow to the myocardium and, thus, may relieve angina.
		atenolol
		ă-TĔN-ō-lŏl
		  Tenormin
		metoprolol
		mĕ-TŌ-prō-lŏl
		  Lopressor, Toprol
		propranolol
		prō-PRĂN-ō-lŏl
		  Inderal

calcium channel blockers	Treat and manage angina, hypertension, and arrhythmias
	
	Calcium channel blockers block the movement of calcium in and out of the SA node and cause the heart to beat less forcefully and less frequently. They also dilate the coronary arteries and prevent coronary artery spasm, which can trigger angina.
		amlodipine
		ăm-LŌ-dĭ-pēn
		  Norvasc
		diltiazem
		dĭl-TĪ-ă-zĕm
		  Cardizem
		nifedipine
		nī-FĔD-ĭ-pēn
		  Adalat, Procardia

diuretics	Manage edema associated with heart failure and treat hypertension *Diuretics increase the excretion of water and sodium by the kidneys to reduce peripheral edema, a common symptom of heart failure. They also reduce total blood volume to treat certain types of hypertension.*	**furosemide** fū-RŌ-sĕ-mĭd *Lasix*

statins	Reduce low density lipoprotein (LDL) cholesterol in blood and possibly slightly increase high density lipoprotein (HDL) cholesterol
	
	LDL has been implicated in cardiovascular disease; HDL appears to have a beneficial cardiovascular effect.
		atorvastatin
		ăh-tŏr-vă-STĂ-tĭn
		  Lipitor
		simvastatin
		SĬM-vă-stă-tĭn
		  Zocor

nitrates	Treat angina pectoris *Nitrates act as vasodilators to increase the amount of oxygen delivered to the myocardium. Nitrates can be administered in several ways: sublingually as a spray or tablet, orally as a tablet, transdermally as a patch, topically as an ointment, or intravenously in an emergency setting.*	**nitroglycerin** nī-trō-GLĬS-ĕr-ĭn *Nitro-Dur, Nitrolingual, Nitrogard, Nitrostat*

peripheral vasodilators	Increase peripheral blood flow to treat peripheral vascular diseases, diabetic peripheral vascular insufficiency, and Raynaud disease
	
	Peripheral vasodilators selectively act to dilate arteries in skeletal muscles, thus improving peripheral blood flow.
		cyclandelate
		sī-KLĂN-dĕ-lāt
		  Cyclan
		isoxsuprine
		ī-SŎK-sū-prēn
		  Vasodilan

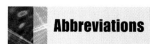

Abbreviations

This section introduces cardiovascular-related abbreviations and their meanings.

Abbreviation	Meaning
AAA	abdominal aortic aneurysm
AF	atrial fibrillation
AS	aortic stenosis
ASD	atrial septal defect
ASHD	arteriosclerotic heart disease
AST	angiotensin sensitivity test; aspartate aminotransferase (cardiac enzyme, formerly called *SGOT*)
AV	atrioventricular, arteriovenous
BBB	bundle branch block
BP	blood pressure
CA	cancer; chronological age; cardiac arrest
CABG	coronary artery bypass graft
CAD	coronary artery disease
CC	cardiac catheterization
CCU	coronary care unit
CHD	coronary heart disease
Chol	cholesterol
CK	creatine kinase (cardiac enzyme)
CPR	cardiopulmonary resuscitation
CV	cardiovascular
DOE	dyspnea on exertion
DSA	digital subtraction angiography
DVT	deep vein thrombosis
ECG, EKG	electrocardiogram

(Continued)

Abbreviation	Meaning	(Continued)
ECHO	echocardiogram; echoencephalogram	
HDL	high-density lipoprotein	
HF	heart failure	
I.V., IV	intravenous	
LD	lactate dehydrogenase; lactic acid dehydrogenase (cardiac enzyme)	
LDL	low-density lipoprotein	
MI	myocardial infarction	
MS	musculoskeletal; multiple sclerosis; mental status; mitral stenosis	
MVP	mitral valve prolapse	
PAC	premature atrial contraction	
PAT	paroxysmal atrial tachycardia	
PTCA	percutaneous transluminal coronary angioplasty	
PVC	premature ventricular contraction	
RV	residual volume; right ventricle	
SA	sinoatrial	
VSD	ventricular septal defect	
VT	ventricular tachycardia	

It is time to review procedures, pharmacology, and abbreviations by completing Learning Activity 8–4.

LEARNING ACTIVITIES

The following activities provide review of the cardiovascular system terms introduced in this chapter. Complete each activity and review your answers to evaluate your understanding of the chapter.

Learning Activity 8–1

Identifying cardiovascular structures

Label the following illustration using the terms listed below.

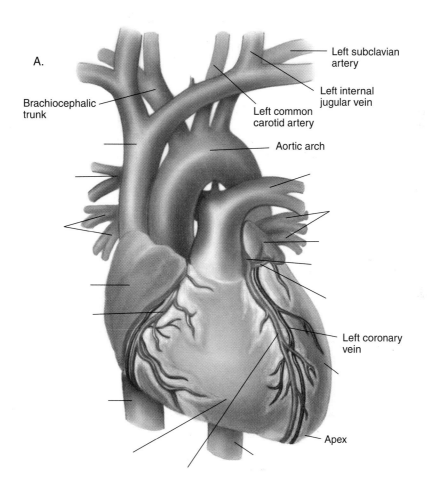

A.

Brachiocephalic trunk

Left subclavian artery

Left internal jugular vein

Left common carotid artery

Aortic arch

Left coronary vein

Apex

aorta	*left coronary artery*	*right coronary artery*
circumflex artery	*left pulmonary artery*	*right pulmonary artery*
inferior vena cava	*left pulmonary veins*	*right pulmonary veins*
left anterior descending artery	*left ventricle*	*right ventricle*
left atrium	*right atrium*	*superior vena cava*

Label the following illustration using the terms listed below.

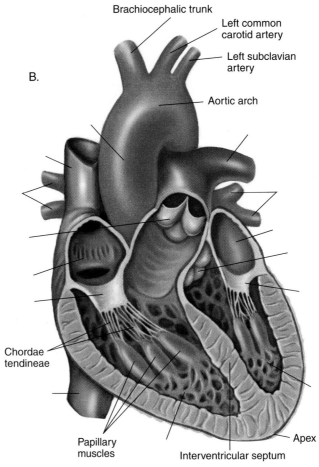

B.

Brachiocephalic trunk

Left common carotid artery

Left subclavian artery

Aortic arch

Chordae tendineae

Papillary muscles

Interventricular septum

Apex

aorta	left pulmonary veins	right pulmonary veins
aortic semilunar valve	left ventricle	right ventricle
inferior vena cava	mitral (bicuspid) valve	superior vena cava
left atrium	pulmonic valve	tricuspid valve
left pulmonary artery	right atrium	

✓ Check your answers by referring to Figures 8–2A and 8–2B on page 191. Review material that you did not answer correctly.

Learning Activity 8-2

Building medical words

*Use **ather/o** (fatty plaque) to build words that mean:*

1. tumor of fatty plaque _____
2. hardening of fatty plaque _____

*Use **phleb/o** (vein) to build words that mean:*

3. inflammation of a vein (wall) _____
4. abnormal condition of a blood clot in a vein _____

*Use **ven/o** (vein) to build words that mean:*

5. pertaining to or relating to a vein _____
6. spasm of a vein _____

*Use **cardi/o** (heart) to build words that mean:*

7. specialist in the study of the heart _____
8. rupture of the heart _____
9. poisonous to the heart _____
10. enlargement of the heart _____

*Use **angi/o** (vessel) to build words that mean:*

11. softening of a vessel (wall) _____
12. tumor of a vessel _____

*Use **thromb/o** (blood clot) to build words that mean:*

13. beginning or formation of a blood clot _____
14. abnormal condition of a blood clot _____

*Use **aort/o** (heart) to build words that mean:*

15. abnormal condition of narrowing or stricture of the aorta _____
16. process of recording the aorta _____

Build surgical words that mean:

17. puncture of the heart _____
18. suture of an artery _____
19. removal of an embolus _____
20. separation, destruction, or loosening of a blood clot _____

Check your answers in Appendix A. Review material that you did not answer correctly.

CORRECT ANSWERS _____ × 5 = _____ **% SCORE**

Learning Activity 8–3

Matching pathological, diagnostic, symptomatic, and related terms

Match the following terms with the definitions in the numbered list.

aneurysm	*catheter*	*infarct*	*secondary*
angina	*embolus*	*lumen*	*stent*
arrest	*hyperlipidemia*	*palpitation*	*thrombolysis*
arrhythmia	*hypertension*	*perfusion*	*varices*
bruit	*incompetent*	*primary*	*vegetations*

1. _____ area of tissue that undergoes necrosis

2. _____ chest pain

3. _____ inability of a valve to close completely

4. _____ small masses of inflammatory material found on the leaflets of valves

5. _____ varicose veins of the esophagus

6. _____ soft, blowing sound heard on auscultation; murmur

7. _____ thin, flexible, hollow tube that can be inserted into a vessel or cavity (vein or artery) of the body

8. _____ sensation of the heart not beating normally

9. _____ vascular channel

10. _____ localized abnormal dilation of a vessel

11. _____ mass of undissolved matter circulating in blood or lymph channels

12. _____ inability of the heart to maintain a steady beat

13. _____ condition of being stopped or bringing to a stop

14. _____ destruction of a blood clot using anticlotting agents

15. _____ slender or threadlike device used to support tubular structures or hold arteries open during and after angioplasty

16. _____ common disorder characterized by persistent elevated blood pressure

17. _____ excessive amounts of lipids in the blood

18. _____ hypertension without an identifiable cause

19. _____ hypertension due to an underlying, identifiable cause

20. _____ circulation of blood through tissues

✓ Check your answers in Appendix A. Review any material that you did not answer correctly.

CORRECT ANSWERS _____ × 5 = _____ % SCORE

Learning Activity 8–4

Matching procedures, pharmacology, and abbreviations

Match the following terms with the definitions in the numbered list.

angioplasty	catheter ablation	embolization	scintigraphy
arterial biopsy	commissurotomy	Holter monitor test	statins
atherectomy	coronary angiography	ligation and stripping	stress test
CABG	diuretics	nitrates	thrombolysis
cardiac enzyme studies	echocardiography	PTCA	venipuncture

1. _____ 24-hour ECG tracing taken with a small, portable recording system

2. _____ noninvasive ultrasound diagnostic test used to visualize internal cardiac structures

3. _____ radiological examination of the blood vessels of and around the heart

4. _____ agents used to treat angina pectoris

5. _____ drugs that have powerful lipid-lowering properties

6. _____ management of edema associated with heart failure and hypertension

7. _____ includes troponin T, troponin I, and creatinine kinase

8. _____ injection and detection of radioactive isotopes to create images and identify function and disease

9. _____ ECG taken under controlled exercise stress conditions

10. _____ tying of a varicose vein and subsequent removal

11. _____ surgical separation of the leaflets of the mitral valve

12. _____ removal of a small segment of an artery for diagnostic purposes

13. _____ destruction of conductive tissue of the heart to interrupt abnormal contractions

14. _____ technique used to block flow to a site by injecting an occluding agent

15. _____ procedure that alters a vessel through surgery or dilation

16. _____ dilation of an occluded vessel using a balloon catheter

17. _____ surgery that creates a bypass around a blocked segment of a coronary artery

18. _____ removal of occluding material using a cutting or grinding device

19. _____ incision or puncture of a vein to remove blood or introduce fluids

20. _____ destruction of a blood clot

Check your answers in Appendix A. Review any material that you did not answer correctly.

CORRECT ANSWERS _____ × 5 = _____ **% SCORE**

MEDICAL RECORD ACTIVITIES

The two medical records included in the activities that follow use common clinical scenarios to show how medical terminology is used to document patient care. Complete the terminology and analysis sections for each activity to help you recognize and understand terms related to the cardiovascular system.

Medical Record Activity 8–1

Acute myocardial infarction

Terminology

The terms listed in the chart come from the medical record *Acute Myocardial Infarction* that follows. Use a medical dictionary such as *Taber's Cyclopedic Medical Dictionary*, the appendices of this book, or other resources to define each term. Then review the pronunciations for each term and practice by reading the medical record aloud.

Term	Definition
acute ă-KŪT	
cardiac enzymes KĂR-dē-ăk ĔN-zīmz	
CCU	
ECG	
heparin HĔP-ă-rĭn	
infarction ĭn-FĂRK-shŭn	
inferior ĭn-FĒ-rē-or	
ischemia ĭs-KĒ-mē-ă	
lateral LĂT-ĕr-ăl	
MI	
myocardial mī-ō-KĂR-dē-ăl	

Term	Definition
partial thromboplastin time thrŏm-bō-PLĂS-tĭn	
streptokinase strĕp-tō-KĪ-nās	
substernal sŭb-STĔR-năl	

ACUTE MYOCARDIAL INFARCTION

HISTORY OF PRESENT ILLNESS: The patient is a 68-year-old woman hospitalized for acute anterior myocardial infarction. She has a history of sudden onset of chest pain. Approximately 2 hours before hospitalization, she had severe substernal pain with radiation to the back. ECG showed evidence of abnormalities. She was given streptokinase and treated with heparin at 800 units/hr. She will be evaluated with a partial thromboplastin time and cardiac enzymes in the morning.

The patient had been seen in 20xx, with a history of an inferior MI in approximately 19xx or 19xx, but she was stable and underwent a treadmill test, the results of which showed no ischemia and she had no chest pain. Her records confirmed an MI with enzyme elevation and evidence of a previous inferior MI.

At this time the patient is stable, is in the CCU, and will be given appropriate follow-up and supportive care.

IMPRESSION: Acute lateral anterior MI and old, healed inferior MI

Analysis

Review the medical record *Acute Myocardial Infarction* to answer the following questions.

1. How long had the patient experienced chest pain before she was seen in the hospital?

   _____

2. Did the patient have a previous history of chest pain?

   _____

3. What are the cardiac enzymes that are tested to confirm the diagnosis of MI?

   _____

4. Initially, what medications were administered to stabilize the patient?

   _____

5. During the current admission, what part of the heart was damaged?

   _____

6. Was the location of damage to the heart for this admission the same as for the initial MI?

   _____

Medical Record Activity 8–2

Operative report: Rule out temporal arteritis

Terminology

The terms listed in the chart come from the medical record *Operative Report: Rule Out Temporal Arteritis* that follows. Use a medical dictionary such as *Taber's Cyclopedic Medical Dictionary*, the appendices of this book, or other resources to define each term. Then review the pronunciations for each term and practice by reading the medical record aloud.

Term	Definition
arteritis ăr-tĕ-RĪ-tĭs	
Betadine BĀ-tă-dīn	
biopsy BĪ-ŏp-sē	
dissected dī-SĔKT-ĕd	
distally DĬS-tă-lē	
incised ĭn-SĪZD	
IV	
ligated LĪ-gā-tĕd	
palpable PĂL-pă-b'l	
preauricular prē-aw-RĬK-ū-lăr	
proximally PRŎK-sĭ-mă-lē	
superficial fascia soo-pĕr-FĬSH-ăl FĂSH-ē-ă	
supine sū-PĪN	
temporal TĔM-por-ăl	
Xylocaine ZĪ-lō-kān	

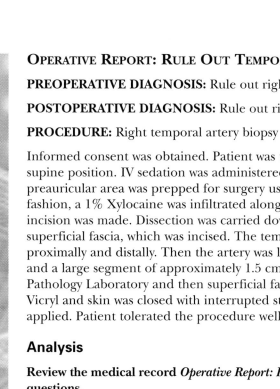

OPERATIVE REPORT: RULE OUT TEMPORAL ARTERITIS

PREOPERATIVE DIAGNOSIS: Rule out right temporal arteritis

POSTOPERATIVE DIAGNOSIS: Rule out right temporal arteritis

PROCEDURE: Right temporal artery biopsy

Informed consent was obtained. Patient was taken to the surgical suite and placed in the supine position. IV sedation was administered. Patient was turned to her left side and the preauricular area was prepped for surgery using Betadine. Having been draped in sterile fashion, a 1% Xylocaine was infiltrated along the palpable temporal artery and a vertical incision was made. Dissection was carried down through the subcutaneous tissue and superficial fascia, which was incised. The temporal artery was located and dissected proximally and distally. Then the artery was ligated with 6–0 Vicryl proximally and distally and a large segment of approximately 1.5 cm was removed. The specimen was sent to Pathology Laboratory and then superficial fascia was closed with interrupted stitches of 6–0 Vicryl and skin was closed with interrupted stitches of 6–0 Prolene. A sterile dressing was applied. Patient tolerated the procedure well. There were no apparent complications.

Analysis

Review the medical record *Operative Report: Rule Out Temporal Arteritis* to answer the following questions.

1. Why was the right temporal artery biopsied?

2. In what position was the patient placed?

3. What was the incision area?

4. How was the temporal artery described in the report?

5. How was the dissection carried out?

6. What was the size of the specimen?

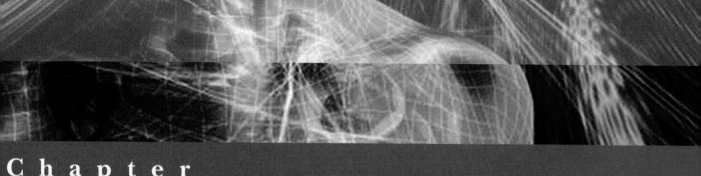

Chapter

9

Blood, Lymph, and Immune Systems

OBJECTIVES

Upon completion of this chapter, you will be able to:

- Identify and describe the components of blood.
- Locate and identify the structures associated with the lymphatic system.
- Identify the cells associated with the acquired immune response and describe their function.

- Recognize, pronounce, spell, and build words related to the blood, lymph, and immune systems.
- Describe pathological conditions, diagnostic and therapeutic procedures, and other terms related to the blood, lymph, and immune systems.
- Explain pharmacology related to the treatment of blood, lymph, and immune disorders.
- Demonstrate your knowledge of this chapter by completing the learning and medical record activities.

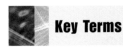 **Key Terms**

This section introduces important blood, lymph, and immune system terms and their definitions. Word analyses are also provided.

Term	Definition
anaphylaxis ăn-ă-fĭ-LĂK-sĭs *ana-:* against; up; back *-phylaxis:* protection	Exaggerated, life-threatening hypersensitivity reaction to a previously encountered antigen
antibody ĂN-tĭ-bŏd-ē	Protective protein produced by B lymphocytes in response to the presence of a foreign substance called an *antigen,* which the immune system regards as harmful to the host
antigen ĂN-tĭ-jĕn	Substance that is recognized as harmful to the host and stimulates the formation of antibodies in an immunocompetent individual
cellular immunity SĔL-ū-lăr ĭ-MŪ-nĭ-tē	Acquired specific resistance, mediated by T cells, that produces reactive substances or directly exerts a cytotoxic effect on a cell that is identified as harmful
host	Organism in or on which another, usually parasitic, organism is nourished and harbored
humoral immunity HŪ-mor-ăl ĭ-MŪ-nĭ-tē	Acquired specific resistance, mediated by B cells, that produces antibodies that bind to and dispose of antigens
immunocompetent ĭm-ū-nō-KŎM-pĕ-tĕnt	Able to develop an immune response; able to recognize antigens and respond to them
immunopathology ĭm-ū-nō-pă-THŎL-ō-jē *immun/o:* immune, immunity, safe *path/o:* disease *-logy:* study of	Study of disease states associated with overreactivity or underreactivity of the immune response

Term	Definition
opportunistic infection ŏp-or-too-NĬS-tĭk	Infection occurring in a person with a weakened immune system and caused by a microorganism that, under normal conditions, would not bring about disease
palliative treatment PĂL-ē-ā-tĭv	Treatment that provides relief, but not a cure
serum SĒ-rŭm	Liquid portion of blood that remains after the removal of fibrinogen *Blood collected without an anticoagulant yields a serum sample. Blood collected with an anticoagulant yields a plasma sample.*

 ## Anatomy and Physiology

The blood, lymph, and immune systems share common cells, structures, and functions. Blood is the source of certain immune cells that locate, identify, and destroy disease-causing agents. These immune cells either actively engage in the destruction of the invading agent or produce proteins that seek out and tag it for destruction. Immune cells rely on lymph vessels and blood vessels to deliver their protective benefits to the entire body. Furthermore, immune cells use lymph structures (the spleen and nodes) to provide permanent or temporary lodging sites where they monitor the extracellular fluid of the body. When disease-causing agents are identified, the immune cells destroy them before irreparable damage occurs in the **host.** The lymph system operates in close association with blood, returning lymph and immune substances back to the circulatory system for redelivery to the entire body. Although these three systems are discussed separately, they commonly function as a single entity to keep the body healthy.

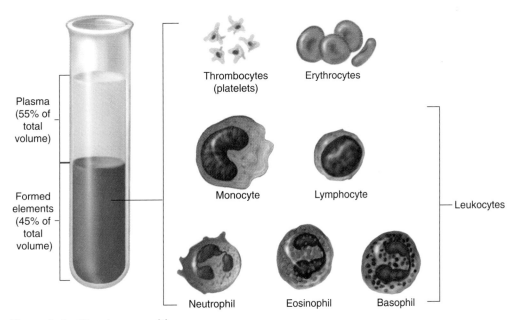

Figure 9–1 Blood composition.

Blood

Blood is connective tissue composed of a liquid medium called *plasma* in which solid components are suspended. These solid components are *erythrocytes* **(red blood cells),** *leukocytes* **(white blood cells),** and cell fragments called *thrombocytes* **(platelets).** (See Figure 9–1.) In adults, blood cells are formed in the bone marrow (myelogenic) tissue of the skull, ribs, sternum, vertebrae, and pelvis as well as at the ends of the long bones of the arms and legs. Blood cells develop from an undifferentiated cell called a *stem cell.* The development and maturation of blood cells is called *hematopoiesis* or *hemopoiesis.* (See Figure 9–2.) Red blood cell (RBC) development is called *erythropoiesis;* white blood cell development, *leukopoiesis;* and platelet development, *thrombopoiesis.* When blood cells are mature, they enter the circulatory system.

Red blood cells transport oxygen and carbon dioxide; white blood cells provide defenses against invasion by foreign substances and aid in tissue repair; and platelets provide mechanisms for blood coagulation, in case the blood vessels become severed. Although it makes up only about 8% of all body tissues, blood is essential to life.

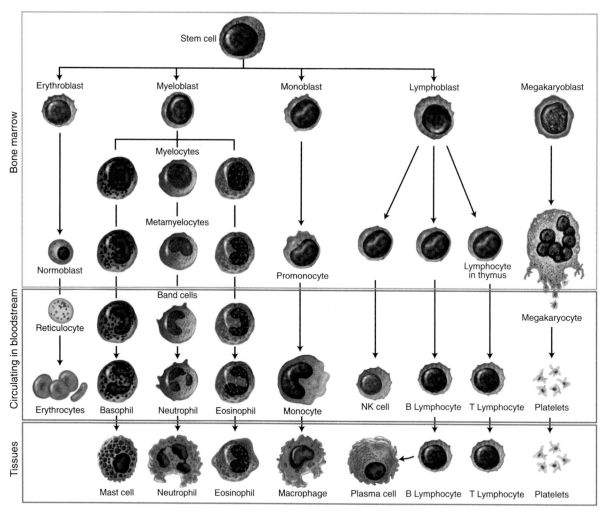

Figure 9–2 Hematopoiesis.

Erythrocytes

Erythrocytes, or RBCs, are the most numerous of the circulating blood cells. In their mature form, they resemble a biconcave disk. During erythropoiesis, erythrocytes develop a specialized iron-containing compound called *hemoglobin* that gives them their red color. Hemoglobin carries oxygen to body tissues, and exchanges it for carbon dioxide. The millions of hemoglobin molecules in each of the billions of RBCs attest to the magnitude of the job they perform. During development, RBCs decrease in size and, just before maturity, the nucleus is extruded from the cell, leaving behind a small fragment of nuclear material that resembles a fine, lacy net, giving this cell its name, *reticulocyte*. Although a few reticulocytes are found in circulation, most erythrocytes lose their nuclear material prior to entering the circulatory system.

Red blood cells live about 120 days and then rupture, releasing hemoglobin and cell fragments. Hemoglobin breaks down into *hemosiderin* (an iron compound) and several bile pigments. Most hemosiderin returns to the bone marrow and is reused to manufacture new blood cells. The liver eventually excretes the bile pigments.

Leukocytes

The chief functions of leukocytes (WBCs) include protecting the body against invasion by bacteria and foreign substances, removing debris from injured tissue, and aiding in the healing process. Whereas RBCs remain in the bloodstream, WBCs are able to migrate through the endothelial walls of capillaries and venules and enter tissue spaces through a process called *diapedesis*. (See Figure 9–3.) There they can initiate inflammatory or immune responses at sites of injury or infection. Leukocytes are divided into two groups: **granulocytes** and **agranulocytes**.

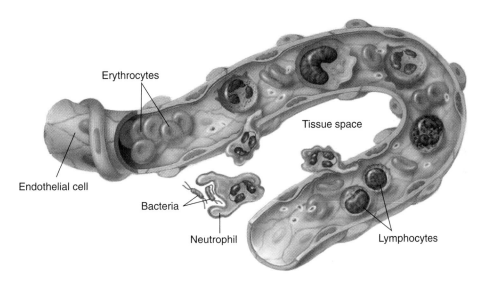

Figure 9–3   Diapedesis.

Granulocytes. **Granulocytes** are the most abundant type of leukocyte. They contain granules in their cytoplasm and, in their mature form, exhibit a multilobed nucleus (**polymorphonuclear**). The three types of granulocytes are **neutrophils,** *eosinophils,* and *basophils*. These names are derived from the type of dye that stains their cytoplasmic granules when a blood smear is stained in the laboratory.

- *Neutrophils* are the most numerous circulating type of leukocyte. They are very motile and highly phagocytic, permitting them to ingest and devour bacteria and other particulate matter. They are the first cell to appear at a site of injury or infection to begin the work of phagocytizing foreign material. (See Figure 9–4.) Their importance in body protection cannot be underestimated. Someone with a serious deficiency of this blood cell type will die, despite protective attempts by other body defenses.

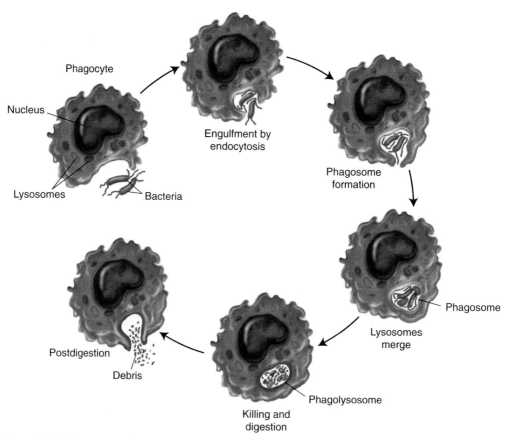

Figure 9–4   Phagocytosis.

- *Eosinophils* protect the body by releasing many substances capable of neutralizing toxic compounds, especially of a chemical nature. Eosinophils increase in number during allergic reactions and animal parasite infestations.
- *Basophils* release histamines and heparin when tissue is damaged. Histamines initiate inflammation, leading to increased blood flow. This brings additional blood cells to injured areas to help in damage containment and tissue repair. Heparin acts to prevent blood from clotting.

Agranulocytes. *Agranulocytes* arise in the bone marrow from stem cells. Because their nuclei do not form lobes, they are frequently called *mononuclear leukocytes.* Agranulocytes include mono-cytes and lymphocytes:

- *Monocytes* are mildly phagocytic when found within blood vessels. However, they remain there only a short time. When they exit the vascular system, they transform into **macrophages,** voracious phagocytes capable of ingesting pathogens, dead cells, and debris found at sites of inflammation. Macrophages play a chief role in many activities associated with specific immunity.
- *Lymphocytes* include B cells, T cells, and natural killer cells. B cells and T cells provide a specialized type of defense called the **specific immune response.** This mode of

protection is custom-made and aimed at a specific antigen. Its dual response includes **humoral immunity** and **cellular immunity.** Natural killer cells are highly effective against cancer cells and other infected cells. They release potent chemicals that destroy these aberrant cells. (See Table 9–1.)

Table 9–1   PROTECTIVE ACTIONS OF WHITE BLOOD CELLS

This chart lists the two main categories of white blood cells: granulocytes and agranulocytes along with their subcategories and the protective actions of each.

Cell Type	Protective Action
Granulocytes	
Neutrophils	Phagocytosis
Eosinophils	Allergy, animal parasites
Basophils	Inflammation mediators, immediate allergic reactions
Agranulocytes	
Monocytes	Phagocytosis

Lymphocytes
  B cells
  T cells
  Natural killer
	
	Humoral immunity
	Cellular immunity
	Destruction without specificity

Platelets

The smallest formed elements found in blood are platelets. Although they are sometimes called *thrombocytes,* they are not true cells, as this term erroneously suggests, but merely fragments of cells. Platelets initiate blood clotting (**hemostasis**) when injury occurs.

Blood clotting is not a single reaction but, rather, a chain of interlinked reactions that can be summarized as follows:

- Thromboplastin is released by traumatized tissue or ruptured platelets.
- Thromboplastin and other blood clotting factors combine with calcium ions to form prothrombin activator.
- Prothrombin activator reacts with prothrombin and calcium ions to form thrombin.
- Thrombin converts the soluble blood protein, fibrinogen, to fibrin, an insoluble protein that forms a "protein net" entangling blood cells and platelets. This jellylike mass of fibrin, blood cells, and platelets is known as a blood clot.

Plasma

Plasma is the liquid portion of the blood in which blood cells are suspended. When blood cells are absent, plasma is a thin, almost colorless fluid. It is composed of about 92% water and contains proteins (albumins, globulins, and fibrinogen), gases, nutrients, salts, hormones, and excretory products. Plasma makes possible the chemical communication between all body cells by transporting these products to all parts of the body.

Blood **serum** is a product of blood plasma. It differs from plasma in that the clotting elements have been removed. When a blood sample is placed in a test tube and permitted to clot, the resulting clear fluid that remains after the clot is removed is serum, because fibrinogen and other clotting elements are used to form the clot.

Blood Groups

Human blood is divided into four groups based on the presence or absence of specific antigens on the surface of RBCs. (See Table 9–2.) Four blood groups, A, B, AB, and O, are identified by the presence or absence of these antigens. In each of these four blood groups, the plasma does not contain the antibody against the antigen that is present on the RBCs. Rather, the plasma contains the opposite antibodies. These antibodies occur naturally; that is, they are present or develop shortly after birth even though there has been no previous exposure to the antigen.

In addition to antigens to the four blood groups, there are numerous other antigens that may be present on RBCs. One such antigen group includes the Rh blood factor. This particular factor is implicated in hemolytic disease of the newborn (HDN) caused by an incompatibility between maternal and fetal blood.

Blood groups are medically important in transfusions, transplants, and maternal-fetal incompatibilities. Although hematologists have identified more than 300 different blood antigens, most of these are not of medical concern.

Table 9–2	ABO SYSTEM

The table below lists the four blood types along with their respective antigens and antibodies and the percentage of the population that have each type.

Blood Type	Antigen (RBC)	Antibody (plasma)	% Population
A	A	anti-B	41
B	B	anti-A	10
AB	A and B	none	4
O	none	anti-A and anti-B	45

Lymph System

The lymph system consists of a fluid called lymph (in which lymphocytes and monocytes are suspended), a network of transporting vessels called *lymph vessels,* and a multiplicity of other structures, including nodes, spleen, thymus, and tonsils. Lymph vessels are a one-way transport system that begin as capillaries within tissues, which gradually increase in size as they transport lymph to the bloodstream. Along the journey, lymph passes through lymph nodes and other lymphoid tissue. Functions of the lymph system include:

- maintaining the fluid balance of the body by draining extracellular fluid from tissue spaces and returning it to the blood
- transporting lipids away from the digestive organs for use by body tissues
- filtering and removing unwanted or infectious products in lymph nodes.

Lymph vessels begin as closed-ended capillaries in tissue spaces and terminate at the right lymphatic duct and the thoracic duct in the chest cavity. (See Figure 9–5.) As whole blood circulates, a small amount of plasma seeps out of (1) **blood capillaries.** This fluid, now called *extracellular* fluid **(interstitial or tissue fluid),** resembles plasma but contains slightly less protein. Extracellular fluid carries needed products to tissue cells while removing their wastes. As extracellular fluid moves through tissues, it also collects cellular debris, bacteria, and particulate matter. Eventually, extracellular fluid returns to blood capillaries or enters (2) **lymph capillaries.** If it enters a lymph capillary, it is called **lymph.** Lymph passes into larger and larger vessels on its return trip to the bloodstream. Before it reaches its destination, it first enters (3) **lymph nodes.** These nodes serve as depositories for cellular debris. In the node, macrophages phagocytize bacteria and other harmful material while T cells and B cells exert their protective influence. When a local infection exists, the number of bacteria entering a node is so great and their destruction so powerful that the node frequently enlarges and becomes tender.

Lymph vessels from the right chest and arm join the (4) **right lymphatic duct.** This duct drains into the (5) **right subclavian vein,** a major vessel in the cardiovascular system. Lymph from all other parts of the body enters the (6) **thoracic duct** and drains into the (7) **left subclavian vein.** Lymph is redeposited into the circulating blood and becomes plasma. This cycle continually repeats itself.

The three organs associated with the lymphatic system are the (8) **spleen,** (9) **thymus,** and (10) **tonsils:**

- Like lymph nodes, the *spleen* acts as a filter. Phagocytic cells within the spleen lining remove cellular debris, bacteria, parasites, and other infectious agents. The spleen also destroys old RBCs and serves as a repository for healthy blood cells that are placed into circulation when needed.
- The *thymus* gland is located in the upper part of the chest **(mediastinum).** It partially controls the immune system by transforming lymphocytes into T cells, the cell responsible for cellular immunity.
- *Tonsils* are masses of lymphatic tissue located in the pharynx. They act as a filter to protect the upper respiratory structures from invasion by pathogens.

Immune System

Although exposed to a vast number of harmful substances, most people suffer relatively few diseases throughout their lives. Numerous body defenses called resistance work together to protect against disease. Resistance includes physical barriers (skin, mucous membranes), and chemical and cellular barriers (tears, saliva, gastric juices, and neutrophils). These barriers are present at birth. Another form of resistance called *acquired immune response* develops after birth. This form of resistance is, by far, the most complex in both structure and function. It develops throughout life as a result of exposure to one disease after another. With each exposure, the immune system identifies the invader (antigen), musters a unique response to destroy it, and then retreats with a memory of both the invader and the method of destruction. In the event of a second encounter by the same invader, the immune system is armed and ready to destroy it before it can cause disease. The WBCs responsible for the specific immune response include monocytes and lymphocytes.

Monocytes

After a brief stay in the vascular system, monocytes enter tissue spaces and become highly phagocytic *macrophages*. In this form, they consume large numbers of bacteria and other antigens. They process these substances and place their antigenic property on their cell surface, thus becoming antigen-presenting cells **(APCs).** The APC awaits an encounter with an immunocompetent lymphocyte (one capable of responding to that specific antigen) to initiate the specific immune response.

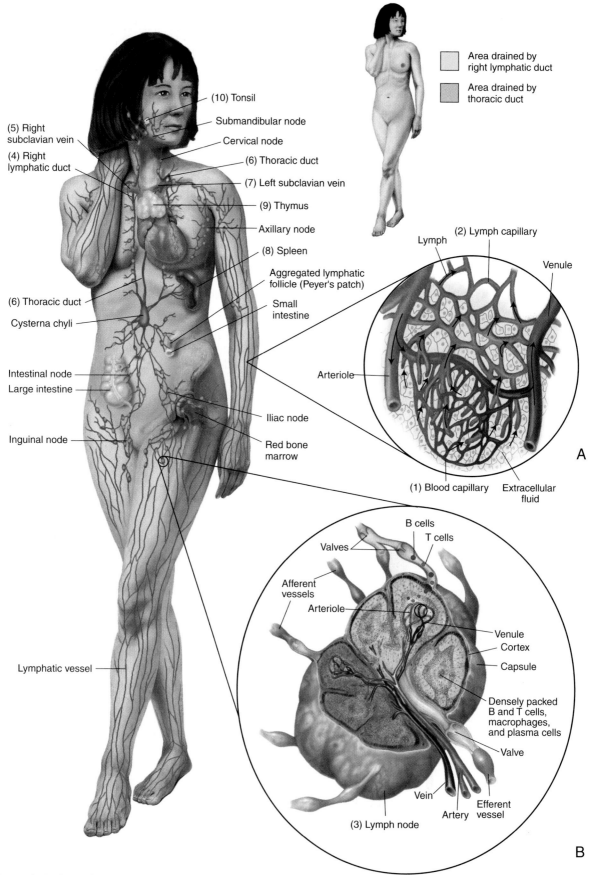

(10) Tonsil
Submandibular node
(5) Right subclavian vein
Cervical node
(4) Right lymphatic duct
(6) Thoracic duct
(7) Left subclavian vein
(9) Thymus
Axillary node
(8) Spleen
Aggregated lymphatic follicle (Peyer's patch)
(6) Thoracic duct
Small intestine
Cysterna chyli
Intestinal node
Large intestine
Iliac node
Inguinal node
Red bone marrow
Lymphatic vessel

Area drained by right lymphatic duct
Area drained by thoracic duct

(2) Lymph capillary
Lymph
Venule
Arteriole
(1) Blood capillary
Extracellular fluid

A

B cells
T cells
Valves
Afferent vessels
Arteriole
Venule
Cortex
Capsule
Densely packed B and T cells, macrophages, and plasma cells
Valve
Vein
Artery
Efferent vessel
(3) Lymph node

B

Figure 9–5 Lymph system. (A) Capillary. (B) Lymph node.

Lymphocytes

Two types of lymphocytes, T cells and B cells, are the active cells in the acquired immune response. Each cell type mediates a specific response: humoral or cellular immunity.

- **Humoral immunity** protects primarily against extracellular antigens, such as bacteria and viruses, that have not yet entered a cell. It is mediated by B cells, which originate and mature in the bone marrow. During maturation, these B cells develop receptors for a specific antigen. Upon an encounter with their specific antigen, B cells produce a clone of cells called *plasma cells*. Plasma cells produce proteins called **antibodies.** Antibodies enter the circulatory system and travel throughout the body in plasma, tissue fluid, and lymph. When antibodies encounter their specific antigen, they form an antigen-antibody complex that inactivates, neutralizes, or tags the antigen for destruction. All such reactions are highly specific; that is, the antibody reacts only against the specific antigen that caused its formation, a characteristic called *specificity*. After the encounter, B memory cells migrate to lymph tissue and are available for immediate recall, should the antigen be encountered again.

- **Cellular immunity** protects primarily against intracellular antigens such as viruses and also has the ability to destroy cancer cells. It is mediated by T cells, which originate in the bone marrow but migrate and mature in thymus. Four types of T cells include the cytotoxic T cell (T_C), helper T cell (T_H), suppressor T cell (T_S), and memory T cell (T_M). T_C is the cell that actually destroys the invading antigen. It determines its specific weakness and uses this weakness as a point of attack to destroy the antigen. The T_H is essential to the proper functioning of both humoral and cellular immunity. It activates other cells of the immune system using chemical messengers called *cytokines*. If the T_H cell is unavailable, the immune system essentially shuts down and the patient becomes a victim of even the most harmless organisms and eventually dies. The T_S monitors the progression of the infection. When the infection is resolved, the T_S suppresses, or "shuts down," the immune system until the next encounter with an antigen. Finally, like the humoral response, the cellular response also produces memory cells. These T_M cells find their way to the lymph system and remain there long after the encounter with the antigen. (See Table 9–3.)

Table 9–3   LYMPHOCYTES AND IMMUNE RESPONSE

The chart below lists the lymphocytes involved in humoral and cellular immunity along with their specific functions and their sites of origin and maturation in the blood and lymph systems.

Lymphocyte	Function	Origin	Maturation
Humoral immunity			
B lymphocytes		Bone	Bone marrow
• Plasma cells	• Antibody formation for destruction of extracellular antigens		
• Memory cells	• Provides active immunity		
Cellular immunity			
T lymphocytes		Bone marrow	Thymus
• Cytotoxic T cell (T_C)	• Destruction of infected cells and cancer cells		
• Helper T cell (T_H)	• Assistance for B cells and cytotoxic T cells (T_C)		
• Suppressor T cell (T_S)	• Suppression (shutting down) of humoral and cellular response when infection resolves		
• Memory T cell (T_M)	• Provides active immunity		

The memory component is unique to the acquired immune system. These memory cells are able to "recall" how the B cells and T cells previously disposed of the antigen and are able to repeat the process. The repeat performance is immediate, powerful, and sustained. Disposing of the antigen during the second and all subsequent exposures is extremely rapid and much more effective than it was during the first exposure.

Finally, a unique type of lymphocyte called the *natural killer (NK) cell*, works independently of the specific immune response. It will attack any cell that appears abnormal, and does not require the specificity needed by T cells and B cells. Although NK cells have the ability to kill over and over again, they do not have a memory component like B cells and T cells.

 It is time to review lymph structures by completing Learning Activity 9–1.

 ## Medical Word Elements

This section introduces combining forms, suffixes, and prefixes related to the blood, lymph, and immune systems. Word analyses are also provided.

Element	Meaning	Word Analysis
COMBINING FORMS		
aden/o	gland	aden/oid (ĂD-ĕ-noyd): having the appearance or resembling a gland *-oid:* resembling
agglutin/o	clumping, gluing	agglutin/ation (ă-gloo-tĭ-NĀ-shŭn): process of clumping *-ation:* process (of)
bas/o	base (alkaline, opposite of acid)	bas/o/phil (BĀ-sō-fĭl): granulocytic white blood cell whose granules have an attraction for alkaline dyes *-phil:* attraction for *The granules of the basophil appear dark blue when stained with methylene blue, an alkaline dye used in hematology.*
blast/o	embryonic cell	erythr/o/blast/osis (ĕ-rĭth-rō-blăs-TŌ-sĭs): abnormal condition marked by embryonic red cells in circulating blood *erythr/o:* red (cell) *-osis:* abnormal condition; increase (used primarily with blood cells)
chrom/o	color	hypo/chrom/ic (hī-pō-KRŌM-ĭk): refers to red blood cells with less color (paler) than normal and, therefore, containing less hemoglobin than normal *hypo-:* under, below *-ic:* pertaining to, relating to *Hypochromic cells are commonly associated with iron-deficiency anemia.*

Element	Meaning	Word Analysis
eosin/o	dawn (rose-colored)	eosin/o/phil (ē-ō-SĬN-ō-fĭl): granulocytic leukocyte whose granules have an attraction for eosin -phil: attraction for *The granules of an eosinophil appear red when stained with eosin, a dye used in hematology.*
erythr/o	red	erythr/o/cyte (ĕ-RĬTH-rō-sīt): red blood cell -cyte: cell
granul/o	granule	granul/o/cyte (GRĂN-ū-lō-sīt): group of leukocytes that have cytoplasmic granules -cyte: cell *The three types of granulocytes include neutrophils, basophils, and eosinophils.*
hem/o hemat/o	blood	hem/o/phobia (hē-mō-FŌ-bē-ă): an aversion to seeing blood -phobia: fear hemat/oma (hē-mă-TŌ-mă): mass of extravasated, usually clotted blood; caused by a break or leak in a blood vessel -oma: tumor *A hematoma may be found in organs, tissues, or spaces within the body.*
immun/o	immune, immunity, safe	immun/o/logy (ĭm-ū-NŎL-ō-jē): study of the components and function of the immune system -logy: study of
kary/o nucle/o	nucleus	kary/o/lysis (kăr-ē-ŎL-ĭ-sĭs): destruction of the nucleus of a cell resulting in cell death -lysis: separation; destruction; loosening mono/nucle/ar (mŏn-ō-NŪ-klē-ăr): pertaining to cells that have a single nucleus mono-: one -ar: pertaining to, relating to *The two mononuclear leukocytes are monocytes and lymphocytes.*
leuk/o	white	leuk/emia (loo-KĒ-mē-ă): any of several types of malignancy that affect white blood cells -emia: blood condition *Leukemia involves a profoundly elevated white blood cell count and a very low red blood cell count.*

(Continued)

Element	Meaning	Word Analysis	(Continued)
lymphaden/o	lymph gland (node)	lymphaden/o/pathy (lĭm-făd-ĕ-NŎP-ă-thē): any disease of lymph nodes *-pathy:* disease *Lymphadenopathy is characterized by changes in size, consistency, or number of lymph nodes.*	
lymph/o	lymph	lymph/oid (LĬM-foyd): resembling lymph or lymph tissue *-oid:* resembling	
lymphangi/o	lymph vessel	lymphangi/oma (lĭm-făn-jē-Ō-mă): benign tumor composed of a mass of dilated lymph vessels *-oma:* tumor	
morph/o	form, shape, structure	morph/o/logy (mor-FŎL-ō-jē): study of form, shape, and structure *-logy:* study of	
myel/o	bone marrow, spinal cord	myel/o/gen/ic (mī-ĕ-lō-JĔN-ĭk): relating to or having origin in bone marrow *gen:* forming, producing, origin *-ic:* pertaining to, relating to *All blood cells are formed in the bone marrow and are thus considered myelogenic.*	
neutr/o	neutral, neither	neutr/o/phil/ic (nū-trō-FĬL-ĭk): pertaining to a neutrophil, a granular leukocyte that stains easily with neutral dyes *-phil:* attraction for *-ic:* pertaining to, relating to	
phag/o	swallowing, eating	phag/o/cyte (FĂG-ō-sīt): cell that surrounds, engulfs, and digests microorganisms and cellular debris *-cyte:* cell	
plas/o	formation, growth	a/plas/tic (ā-PLĂS-tĭk): failure of a tissue or organ to develop or grow normally *a-:* without, not *-tic:* pertaining to, relating to	
poikil/o	varied, irregular	poikil/o/cyt/osis (poy-kĭl-ō-si-TŌ-sĭs): abnormal increase in red blood cells that are irregular in shape *cyt:* cell *-osis:* abnormal condition; increase (used primarily with blood cells)	
reticul/o	net, mesh	reticul/o/cyte (rĕ-TĬK-ū-lō-sīt): immature erythrocyte characterized by a meshlike pattern of threads and particles at the former site of the nucleus *-cyte:* cell	

Element	Meaning	Word Analysis
sider/o	iron	sider/o/penia (sĭd-ĕr-ō-PĒ-nē-ă): deficiency of iron in the blood *-penia:* decrease, deficiency
ser/o	serum	ser/o/logy (sē-RŎL-ō-jē): study of the serum components of blood, especially antigens and antibodies *-logy:* study of *Serology also includes the study of antigens and antibodies from sources other than serum.*
splen/o	spleen	splen/o/rrhagia (splē-nō-RĀ-jē-ă): hemorrhaging from a ruptured spleen *-rrhagia:* bursting forth
thromb/o	blood clot	thromb/o/cyt/osis (thrŏm-bō-sī-TŌ-sĭs): abnormal increase in the number of platelets in the blood *cyt:* cell *-osis:* abnormal condition; increase (used primarily with blood cells)
thym/o	thymus gland	thym/o/pathy (thī-MŎP-ă-thē): any disease of the thymus gland *-pathy:* disease
xen/o	foreign, strange	xen/o/graft (ZĔN-ō-grăft): transplantation of tissues from one species to another; also called *heterograft* *-graft:* transplantation *Xenograft is used as a temporary measure when there is insufficient tissue available from the patient or other human donors.*

SUFFIXES

Element	Meaning	Word Analysis
-blast	embryonic cell	erythr/o/blast (ĕ-RĬTH-rō-blăst): embryonic red blood cell *erythr/o:* red
-emia	blood condition	an/emia (ă-NĒ-mē-ă): blood condition characterized by a reduction in the number of red blood cells or a deficiency in their hemoglobin *an-:* without, not
-globin	protein	hem/o/globin (HĒ-mō-glō-bĭn): blood protein found in erythrocytes *hem/o:* blood *Hemoglobin contains iron, gives blood its red color, and transports oxygen.*

(Continued)

Element	Meaning	Word Analysis	(Continued)
-graft	transplantation	auto/graft (AW-tō-grăft): surgical transplantation of tissue from one part of the body to another location in the same individual *auto-:* self, own	
-osis	abnormal condition; increase (used primarily with blood cells)	leuk/o/cyt/osis (loo-kō-si-TŌ-sĭs): abnormal increase in white blood cells *leuk/o:* white *cyt/o:* cell	
-penia	decrease, deficiency	erythr/o/penia (ĕ-rith-rō-PĒ-nē-ă): abnormal decrease in red blood cells *erythr/o:* red	
-phil	attraction for	neutr/o/phil (NŪ-trō-fĭl): leukocyte whose granules have an attraction for a neutral dye *neutr/o:* neutral, neither *Neutrophils are the most numerous type of leukocyte. They provide phagocytic protection for the body.*	
-phoresis	carrying, transmission	electr/o/phoresis (ē-lĕk-trō-fō-RĒ-sĭs): laboratory technique that uses an electric current to separate various plasma proteins *electr/o:* electricity	
-phylaxis	protection	ana/phylaxis (ăn-ă-fĭ-LĂK-sĭs): exaggerated, life-threatening hypersensitivity reaction to a previously encountered antigen *ana-:* against	
-poiesis	formation, production	hem/o/poiesis (hē-mō-poy-Ē-sĭs): production of blood cells, normally within the bone marrow *hem/o:* blood	
-stasis	standing still	hem/o/stasis (hē-mō-STĀ-sĭs): termination of bleeding by mechanical or chemical means or by coagulation *hem/o:* blood	
PREFIXES			
a-	without, not	a/morph/ic (ā-MOR-fĭk): lacking a definite form *morph:* form, shape, structure *ic:* pertaining to, relating to	
allo-	other, differing from the normal	allo/graft (ĂL-ō-grăft): graft transplanted between genetically nonidentical individuals of the same species; also called *homograft* *-graft:* transplantation *An allograft is a transplant between two individuals who are not identical twins.*	

Element	Meaning	Word Analysis
aniso-	unequal, dissimilar	aniso/cyt/osis (ăn-ĭ-sō-sĭ-TŌ-sĭs): condition of the blood characterized by red blood cells of variable and abnormal size *cyt:* cell *-osis:* abnormal condition; increase (used primarily with blood cells)
iso-	same, equal	iso/chrom/ic (ī-sō-KRŌM-ĭk): having the same color *chrom:* color *ic:* pertaining to, relating to
macro-	large	macro/cyte (MĂK-rō-sīt): abnormally large erythrocyte *-cyte:* cell
micro-	small	micro/cyte (MĪ-krō-sīt): abnormally small erythrocyte *-cyte:* cell
mono-	one	mono/nucle/osis (mŏn-ō-nū-klē-Ō-sĭs): presence of an abnormally high number of mononuclear leukocytes in the blood *nucle:* nucleus *-osis:* abnormal condition; increase (used primarily with blood cells)
poly-	many, much	poly/morph/ic (pŏl-ē-MOR-fĭk): occurring in more than one form *morph:* form, shape, structure *ic:* pertaining to, relating to

It is time to review medical word elements by completing Learning Activity 9–2.

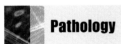

Pathology

Pathology associated with blood includes anemias, leukemias, and coagulation disorders. These three disorders typically share common signs and symptoms that generally include paleness, weakness, shortness of breath, and heart palpitations.

Lymphatic disorders are commonly associated with edema and lymphadenopathy. In these disorders, tissues are swollen with enlarged, tender nodes.

Immunopathies include either abnormally heightened immune responses to antigens (allergies, hypersensitivities, and autoimmune disorders) or abnormally depressed responses (immunodeficiencies and cancers). Many immunologic disorders are manifested in other body systems. For example, asthma and hay fever are immunologic disorders that affect the respiratory system; atopic dermatitis and eczema are immunologic disorders that affect the integumentary system. Some of the most devastating diseases, such as rheumatoid arthritis, cancer, and AIDS, are caused by disordered immunity.

For diagnosis, treatment, and management of diseases that affect blood and blood-forming organs, the medical services of a specialist may be warranted. *Hematology* is the branch of medicine that studies blood cells, blood-clotting mechanisms, bone marrow, and lymph nodes. The physician who specializes in this branch of medicine is called a *hematologist*. *Allergy and immunology* is the branch of medicine involving disorders of the immune system, including asthma and anaphylaxis, adverse reactions to drugs, autoimmune diseases, organ transplantations, and malignancies of the immune system. The physician who specializes in this combined branch of medicine is called an *allergist and immunologist*.

Anemias

Anemia is any condition in which the oxygen-carrying capacity of blood is less than that required by the body. It is not a disease but rather a symptom of various diseases. Some of the causes of anemias include excessive blood loss, excessive blood-cell destruction, decreased blood formation, and faulty hemoglobin production. It results from a decrease in the number of circulating RBCs (erythropenia), amount of hemoglobin (hypochromasia) within them, or volume of packed erythrocytes (hematocrit).

Anemia commonly causes changes in the appearance of RBCs when observed microscopically. In healthy individuals, RBCs fall within a normal range for size **(normocytic)** and amount of hemoglobin **(normochromic).** Variations in these normal values include RBCs that are excessively large **(macrocytic),** are excessively small **(microcytic),** or have decreased amounts of hemoglobin **(hypochromic).** The signs and symptoms associated with most anemias include difficulty breathing **(dyspnea),** weakness, rapid heartbeat **(tachycardia),** paleness **(pallor),** low blood pressure **(hypotension)** and, commonly, a slight fever. (See Table 9–4.)

Table 9–4   COMMON ANEMIAS

This chart lists various types of anemia along with descriptions and causes for each.

Type of Anemia	Description	Causes
Aplastic (hypoplastic)	• Associated with bone marrow failure • Diminished numbers of white blood cells and platelets due to bone marrow suppression • Serious form of anemia that may be fatal	Commonly caused by exposure to cytotoxic agents, radiation, hepatitis virus, and certain medications
Folic-acid deficiency anemia	• Normal levels achieved by increasing folic acid in the diet or eliminating contributing causes	Caused by insufficient folic acid intake, due to poor diet, impaired absorption, prolonged drug therapy, or increased requirements (pregnancy or rapid growth as seen in children)
Hemolytic	• Associated with premature destruction of red blood cells • Usually accompanied by jaundice	Caused by the excessive destruction of red blood cells or such disorders as erythroblastosis and sickle cell anemia
Hemorrhagic	• Associated with loss of blood volume • Normal levels achieved with correction of underlying disorder	Commonly caused by acute blood loss (as in trauma), childbirth, or chronic blood loss (as in bleeding ulcers)

Table 9-4	COMMON ANEMIAS	
Type of Anemia	**Description**	**Causes**
Iron-deficiency anemia	• Most common type of anemia worldwide	Caused by a greater demand on stored iron than can be supplied, commonly as a result of inadequate dietary iron intake or malabsorption of iron
Pernicious anemia	• Chronic, progressive disorder found mostly in people older than age 50 • Treated with B_{12} injections	Caused by low levels of vitamin B_{12} in peripheral red blood cells that may be the result of a lack of "intrinsic factor" in the stomach, which then inhibits absorption of vitamin B_{12}
Sickle cell anemia	• Most common genetic disorder in people of African descent • Characterized by red blood cells that change from their normal shape to crescents and other irregular shapes that cannot enter capillaries when oxygen levels are low, resulting in severe pain and internal bleeding • Manifest only in patients with both genes for the trait, not those with only one gene for the trait, who are merely carriers of the disease	Caused by a defect in the gene responsible for hemoglobin synthesis

Acquired Immunodeficiency Syndrome (AIDS)

AIDS is a transmissible infectious disease caused by the human immunodeficiency virus (HIV), which slowly destroys the immune system. Eventually the immune system becomes so weak **(immunocompromised)** that, in the final stage of the disease, the patient falls victim to infections that usually do not affect healthy individuals **(opportunistic infections).** Gradually, the patient begins to display the symptoms of AIDS: swollen lymph glands **(lymphadenopathy),** malaise, fever, night sweats, and weight loss. Kaposi sarcoma, a neoplastic disorder, and *Pneumocystic carinii* pneumonia (PCP) are two diseases closely associated with AIDS.

Transmission of HIV occurs primarily through body fluids—mostly blood, semen, and vaginal secretions. The virus attacks the most important cell in the immune system, the T_H cell. Once infected by HIV, the T_H cell becomes a "mini-factory" for the replication of the virus. More importantly, the virus destroys the T_H, which is essential to both the humoral and cellular arms of the immune system. Without this cell, the entire acquired immune system completely closes down and the patient ultimately dies.

Although there is no cure for HIV, there are highly effective treatments available that can significantly slow the progression of both the virus and the disease. However, many of the medications have serious adverse effects, and once the decision for medical management is made, the patient should not discontinue treatment, as this causes the virus to become resistant.

Allergy

An allergy is an acquired abnormal immune response. It requires initial exposure to an allergen **(antigen)** that causes an allergic response **(sensitization).** Subsequent exposures to the allergen produce increasing allergic reactions that cause a broad range of inflammatory changes. One common manifestation is hives **(urticaria).** Other manifestations include eczema, allergic rhinitis, coryza, asthma and, in the extreme, anaphylactic shock, a life-threatening condition.

The offending allergens are identified by allergy sensitivity tests. Usually small scratches are made on the patient's back and a liquid suspension of the allergen is introduced into the scratch. If antibodies to the allergen are present in the patient, the scratch becomes red, swollen, and hardened **(indurated).**

Desensitization involves repeated injections of a dilute solution containing the allergen. The initial concentration of the solution is too weak to cause symptoms. Additional exposure to higher concentrations promotes tolerance of the allergen.

Autoimmune Disease

Failure of the body to distinguish accurately between "self" and "nonself" leads to a phenomenon called autoimmunity. In this abnormal response, the immune system attacks the antigens found on its own cells to such an extent that tissue injury results. Types of autoimmune disorders range from those that affect only a single organ to those that affect many organs and tissues **(multisystemic).**

Myasthenia gravis is an autoimmune disorder that affects the neuromuscular junction. Muscles of the limbs and eyes and those affecting speech and swallowing are usually involved. Other autoimmune diseases include rheumatoid arthritis, idiopathic thrombocytopenic purpura (ITP), vasculitis, and systemic lupus erythematosus (SLE).

Treatment consists of attempting to reach a balance between suppressing the immune response to avoid tissue damage while still maintaining the immune mechanism sufficiently to protect against disease. Most autoimmune diseases have periods of flare-up **(exacerbations)** and latency **(remissions).** Autoimmune diseases are commonly chronic, requiring lifelong care and monitoring, even when the person may look or feel well. Currently, few autoimmune diseases can be cured; however, with treatment, those afflicted can live relatively normal lives.

Edema

Edema is an abnormal accumulation of fluids in the intercellular spaces of the body. One of the major conditions that cause edema is a decrease in the blood protein level **(hypoproteinemia),** especially albumin, which controls the amount of plasma leaving the vascular system. Other causes of edema include poor lymph drainage, high sodium intake, increased capillary permeability, and heart failure.

Edema limited to a specific area **(localized)** may be relieved by elevation of that body part and application of cold packs. Systemic edema may be treated with medications that promote urination **(diuretics).**

Closely associated with edema is a condition called *ascites,* in which fluid collects within the peritoneal or pleural cavity. The chief causes of ascites are interference in venous return during cardiac disease, obstruction of lymphatic flow, disturbances in electrolyte balance, and liver disease.

Hemophilia

Hemophilia is a hereditary disorder in which the blood clotting mechanism is impaired. There are two types of hemophilia: hemophilia A, a deficiency in clotting factor VIII, and hemophilia B, a deficiency in clotting factor IX. The degree of deficiency varies from mild to severe. The disease is sex-linked and found most commonly in men. Women are the carriers of the trait but generally do not have symptoms of the disease.

Mild symptoms include nosebleeds, easy bruising, and bleeding from the gums. Severe symptoms produce areas of blood seepage **(hematomas)** deep within muscles. If blood enters joints **(hemarthrosis),** it is associated with pain and, possibly, permanent deformity. Uncontrolled bleeding anyplace in the body may lead to shock and death. Treatment involves a simple I.V. injection of the deficient factor directly into the individual's vein. The amount of factor replaced varies for a minor and major bleed.

Infectious Mononucleosis

One of the acute infections caused by the Epstein-Barr virus (EBV) is infectious mononucleosis. It is found mostly in young adults and appears in greater frequency in early spring and early fall. Saliva and respiratory secretions have been implicated as significant infectious agents, hence the name "kissing disease." Sore throat, fever, and enlarged cervical lymph nodes characterize this disease. Other signs and symptoms include gum infection **(gingivitis),** headache, tiredness, loss of appetite **(anorexia),** and general malaise. In most cases, the disease resolves spontaneously and without complications. In some cases, however, the liver and spleen enlarge **(hepatomegaly** and **splenomegaly**). Less common clinical findings include hemolytic anemia with jaundice and thrombocytopenia. Recovery usually ensures a lasting immunity.

Oncology

Oncological disorders associated with the blood, lymph, and immune systems include leukemia, Hodgkin disease, and Kaposi sarcoma.

Leukemia

Leukemia is an oncological disorder of the blood-forming organs characterized by an overgrowth **(proliferation)** of blood cells. With this condition, malignant cells replace healthy bone marrow cells. The disease is generally categorized by the type of leukocyte population affected: granulocytic **(myelogenous)** or lymphocytic.

The various types of leukemia may be further classified as either chronic or acute. In acute form, the cells are highly embryonic **(blastic)** and lack mature forms resulting in severe anemia, infections, and bleeding disorders. This situation is commonly life threatening. Although there is a proliferation of blastic cells in the chronic forms of leukemia, there are usually a sufficient number of mature cells to carry on the functions of the various cells types.

Although the specific causes of leukemia are unknown, viruses, environmental conditions, high-dose radiation, and genetic factors have been implicated. Bone marrow aspiration and bone marrow biopsy are used to diagnose leukemia. Treatment methods include one or more of the following: chemotherapy with one or more of the anticancer drugs, radiation, biologic therapy, and bone marrow transplant. Left untreated, leukemias are fatal.

Hodgkin Disease

Hodgkin disease (Hodgkin lymphoma) is a malignant disease that affects the lymphatic system, primarily the lymph nodes. Although it usually remains only in neighboring nodes, it may spread to the spleen, GI tract, liver, or bone marrow.

Hodgkin disease usually begins with a painless enlargement of lymph nodes, typically on one side of the neck, chest, or underarm. Other symptoms include extreme itching **(pruritus),** weight loss, progressive anemia, and fever. If nodes in the neck become excessively large, they may press on the trachea, causing difficulty in breathing **(dyspnea),** or on the esophagus, causing difficulty in swallowing **(dysphagia).**

Radiation and chemotherapy are important methods of controlling the disease. Newer methods of treatment include bone marrow transplants. Treatment is highly effective.

Kaposi Sarcoma

Kaposi sarcoma is a malignancy of connective tissue including bone, fat, muscle, and fibrous tissue. It is closely associated with AIDS and is commonly fatal because the tumors readily metastasize to various organs. Its close association with HIV has resulted in this disorder being classified as one of several "AIDS-defining conditions." The lesions emerge as purplish-brown macules and develop into plaques and nodules. The lesions initially appear over the lower extremities and tend to spread symmetrically over the upper body, particularly the face and oral mucosa. Treatment for AIDS-related Kaposi sarcoma is usually palliative, relieving the pain and discomfort that accompany the lesions, but there is little evidence that it prolongs life.

Diagnostic, Symptomatic, and Related Terms

This section introduces diagnostic, symptomatic, and related terms and their meanings. Word analyses for selected terms are also provided.

Term	Definition
anisocytosis ăn-ī-sō-sī-TŌ-sĭs *an-:* without, not *iso-:* same, equal *cyt:* cell *-osis:* abnormal condition, increase (used primarily with blood cells)	Condition of marked variation in the size of erythrocytes, when observed on a blood smear *With anisocytosis, the blood smear will show macrocytes (large RBCs) and microcytes (small RBCs) as well as normocytes (RBCs that are normal in size).*
ascites ă-SĪ-tēz	Accumulation of serous fluid in the peritoneal or pleural cavity
bacteremia băk-tĕr-Ē-mē-ă *bacter:* bacteria *-emia:* blood condition	Presence of viable bacteria circulating in the bloodstream, and considered as "travelers" rather than a blood infection
graft rejection GRĂFT	Recipient's immune system attacks a transplanted organ or tissue resulting in its distruction
graft-versus-host reaction (GVHR) GRĂFT	Condition that occurs following bone marrow transplants where the immune cells in the transplanted marrow produce antibodies against the host's tissues *Bone marrow graft-vs.-host disease can be acute or chronic. The acute form appears within 2 months of the transplant; the chronic form usually appears within 3 months. The symptoms are similar to an autoimmune disease called scleroderma.*
hematoma hēm-ă-TŌ-mă *hemat:* blood *-oma:* tumor	Localized accumulation of blood, usually clotted, in an organ, space, or tissue due to a break in or severing of a blood vessel

Term	Definition
hemoglobinopathy hē-mō-glō- bĭ-NŎP-ă-thē *hem/o:* blood *globin/o:* protein *-pathy:* disease	Any disorder caused by abnormalities in the hemoglobin molecule *One of the most common hemoglobinopathies is sickle cell anemia.*
hemolysis hē-MŎL-ĭ-sĭs *hem/o:* blood *-lysis:* separation; destruction; loosening	Destruction of RBCs with a release of hemoglobin that diffuses into the surrounding fluid
hemostasis hē-mō-STĀ-sĭs *hem/o:* blood *-stasis:* standing still	Arrest of bleeding or circulation
immunity ĭ-MŪ-nĭ-tē	State of being protected against infectious diseases
active	Immunity developed as a consequence of exposure to an antigen and the subsequent development of antibodies *Active immunity is generally long-lived because memory cells are formed. Two forms of active immunity include* natural immunity *and* artificial immunity. *In the natural active immunity, the individual acquires a disease and subsequently recovers from it. In artificial active immunity, the individual receives a vaccination or immunizing injection.*
passive	Immunity in which antibodies or other immune substances formed in one individual are transferred to another individual to provide immediate, temporary immunity *Passive immunity is short-lived because memory cells are not transferred to the recipient. Two forms of passive immunity include* natural passive immunity *and* artificial passive immunity. *In the natural form, medical intervention is not required (infant receiving antibodies through breast milk). In the artificial form, antibodies, antitoxins, or toxoids (generally produced in sheep or horses) are transfused or injected into the individual to provide immediate protection.*
lymphadenopathy lĭm-făd-ĕ-NŎP-ă-thē *lymph:* lymph *aden/o:* gland *-pathy:* disease	Any disease of the lymph nodes *In lymphadenopathy, the number, consistency, or size of the lymph nodes varies from the normal. In localized lymphadenopathy, only one area of the body is affected. In systemic lymphadenopathy, two or more noncontiguous areas are affected.*
lymphosarcoma lĭm-fō-săr-KŌ-mă *lymph/o:* lymph *sarc:* flesh (connective tissue) *-oma:* tumor	Malignant neoplastic disorder of lymphatic tissue (not related to Hodgkin disease)

(Continued)

Term	Definition	(Continued)
septicemia sĕp-tĭ-SĒ-mē-ă	Systemic disease associated with the presence and persistence of pathogenic microorganisms or their toxins in the blood; also called *blood infection* *Septicemia is characterized by chills and fever, purpuric pustules, and abscesses. If left untreated, it may lead to shock and death.*	
serology sē-RŎL-ō-jē *ser/o:* serum *-logy:* study of	Blood test to detect the presence of antibodies, antigens, or immune substances	
titer TĪ-tĕr	Blood test that measures the amount of antibodies in blood; commonly used as an indicator of immune status	

It is time to review pathological, diagnostic, symptomatic, and related terms by completing Learning Activity 9–3.

Diagnostic and Therapeutic Procedures

This section introduces procedures used to diagnose and treat blood, lymph, and immune disorders. Descriptions are provided as well as pronunciations and word analyses for selected terms.

Procedure	Description
DIAGNOSTIC	
Laboratory	
activated partial thromboplastin time (APTT) thrŏm-bō-PLĂS-tĭn	Test that screens for deficiencies of some clotting factors; valuable for preoperative screening for bleeding tendencies
blood culture	Test to determine the presence of pathogens in the bloodstream
complete blood count (CBC)	Series of tests that includes hemoglobin; hematocrit; red blood cell (RBC), white blood cell (WBC), and platelet counts; differential WBC count; RBC indices; and RBC and WBC morphology
differential count dĭf-ĕr-ĔN-shăl	Test that enumerates the distribution of WBCs in a stained blood smear by counting the different kinds of WBCs and reporting each as a percentage of the total examined *Because differential values change considerably in pathology, this test is commonly used as a first step in diagnosing a disease.*

Procedure	Description
erythrocyte sedimentation rate (ESR; sed rate) ĕ-RĬTH-rō-sīt sĕd-ĭ-mĕn-TĀ-shŭn *erythr/o:* red *-cyte:* cell	Measurement of the distance RBCs settle in 1 hour when whole blood is placed in a narrow tube *The sedimentation rate increases in inflammatory diseases, cancer, and pregnancy and decreases in liver disease.*
hemoglobin (Hgb, Hb) HĒ-mō-glō-bĭn *hem/o:* blood *-globin:* protein	Measurement of the amount of hemoglobin found in a whole blood sample *Hemoglobin values decrease in anemia and increase in dehydration, polycythemia vera, and thrombocytopenia purpura.*
hematocrit (Hct) hē-MĂT-ō-krĭt	Measurement of the percentage of packed RBCs in a whole blood sample; also called *crit*
Monospot	Serological test performed on a blood sample to detect the presence of a nonspecific antibody called the *heterophile antibody* that is present in the serum of patients with infectious mononucleosis
prothrombin time (PT) prō-THRŎM-bĭn	Test used to evaluate portions of the coagulation system and indirectly measure prothrombin; also called *pro time* *Prothrombin time is commonly used to manage patients undergoing anticoagulant therapy.*
RBC indices	Mathematical calculation of the size, volume, and concentration of hemoglobin for an average red blood cell
Schilling test	Test used to assess the absorption of radioactive vitamin B_{12} by the GI system *Schilling test is the definitive test for diagnosing pernicious anemia because vitamin B_{12} is not absorbed in this disorder and passes from the body by way of stool.*
Radiographic	
lymphadenography lĭm-făd-ĕ-NŎG-ră-fē *lymph:* lymph *aden/o:* gland *-graphy:* process of recording	Radiographic examination of lymph nodes after injection of a contrast medium
lymphangiography lĭm-făn-jē-ŎG-ră-fē *lymph:* lymph *angi/o:* vessel *-graphy:* process of recording	Radiographic examination of lymph nodes or tissues after injection of contrast medium in lymph vessels

(Continued)

Procedure	Description	(Continued)

Surgical

aspiration
ăs-pĭ-RĀ-shŭn

Draw in or out using suction

    bone marrow

Procedure using a syringe with a thin aspirating needle that is inserted (usually in the sternum or pelvic bone) to withdraw a small sample of bone marrow fluid for microscopic evaluation. (See Figure 9–6.)

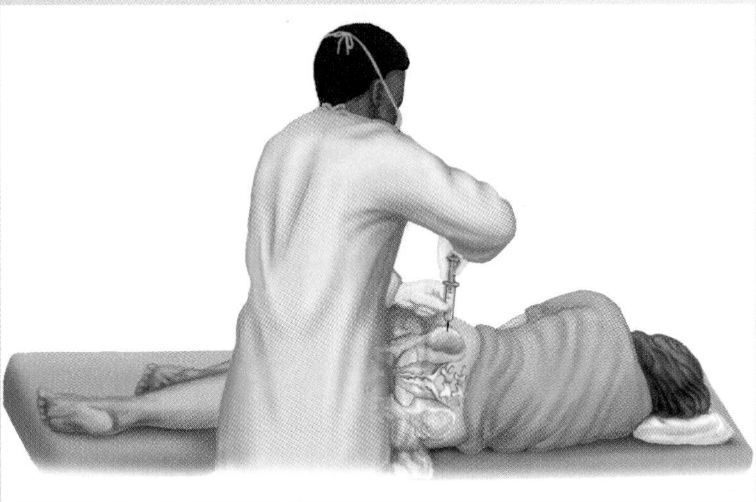

Figure 9–6 Bone marrow aspiration.

biopsy
BĪ-ŏp-sē

Representative tissue sample removed from a body site for microscopic examination, usually to establish a diagnosis

    bone marrow

Removal of a small core sample of tissue from bone marrow for examination under a microscope and, possibly, for analysis using other tests

    sentinel node
    SĔNT-nĕl NŌD

Removal of the first lymph node (also called the sentinel node) that receives drainage from cancer-containing areas and the one most likely to contain malignant cells

If the sentinel node does not contain malignant cells, there may be no need to remove additional lymph nodes.

THERAPEUTIC

Surgical

lymphangiectomy
lĭm-făn-jē-ĔK-tō-mē

lymph: lymph
angi: vessel
-ectomy: excision

Removal of a lymph vessel

Procedure	Description
transfusion trăns-FŪ-zhŭn	Injecting of blood or blood components into the bloodstream
autologous aw-TŎL-ō-gŭs	Transfusion prepared from the recipient's own blood
homologous hō-MŎL-ō-gŭs	Transfusion prepared from another individual whose blood is compatible with that of the recipient
transplantation	Grafting of living tissue from its normal position to another site or from one person to another
autologous bone marrow aw-TŎL-ō-gŭs	Harvesting, freezing (cryopreserving), and reinfusing the patient's own bone marrow; used to treat bone marrow hypoplasia following cancer therapy
homologous bone marrow hō-MŎL-ō-gŭs	Transplantation of bone marrow from one individual to another; used for treating aplastic anemia and immunodeficiency disorders

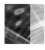

Pharmacology

Various drugs are prescribed to treat blood, lymph, and immune systems disorders. (See Table 9–5.) These drugs act directly on individual components of each system. For example, anticoagulants are used to prevent clot formation but are ineffective in destroying formed clots. Instead, thrombolytics are used to dissolve clots that obstruct coronary, cerebral, or pulmonary arteries, and, conversely, hemostatics are used to prevent or control hemorrhage. In addition, chemotherapy and radiation are commonly used to treat diseases of the immune system. For example, antineoplastics prevent cellular replication to halt the spread of cancer in the body; antivirals prevent viral replication within cells and have been effective in slowing the progression of HIV and AIDS.

Table 9–5   DRUGS USED TO TREAT BLOOD, LYMPH, AND IMMUNE DISORDERS

This table lists common drug classifications used to treat blood, lymph, and immune disorders, their therapeutic actions, and selected generic and trade names.

Classification	Therapeutic Action	Generic and Trade Names
anticoagulants	Prevent blood clot formation by inhibiting one or more clotting factors *Anticoagulants are used to prevent deep venous thrombosis (DVT), prevent postoperative clot formation, and decrease the risk of stroke.*	**enoxaparin** ē-nŏk-să-PĂR-ĭn *Lovenox* **heparin** HĔP-ă-rĭn *Hep-Lock, Hep-Lock U/P* **warfarin** WOR-făr-ĭn *Coumadin*

(Continued)

| Table 9–5 | DRUGS USED TO TREAT BLOOD, LYMPH, AND IMMUNE DISORDERS (Continued) |

Classification	Therapeutic Action	Generic and Trade Names

antineoplastics	Kill or damage rapidly metabolizing cells
	
	Antineoplastics are commonly used in combination with other treatment modalities and have been successful in the treatment of various cancers.
		doxorubicin hydrochloride
		dŏk-sō-RŪ-bĭ-sĭn
		  Adriamycin PFS, Adriamycin RDF, Rubex
		bleomycin
		blē-ō-MĪ-sĭn
		  Blenoxane

antiprotozoals, antibiotics, and sulfa drugs (to treat PCP)	Treat Pneumocystis carinii pneumonia (PCP)
	
	Neutrexin is an antibiotic; Bactrim and Septra are sulfonamides, and NebuPent and Pentam-300 are antiprotozoals. Pneumocystis carinii shares characteristics of protozoa and fungi. It seldom causes symptoms in healthy individuals.
		trimetrexate glucuronate
		trĭ-mĕ-TRĔK-sāt gloo-KŪ-rō-nāt
		  Neutrexin
		trimethoprim, sulfamethoxazole
		trĭ-MĔTH-ō-prĭm, sŭl-fă-mĕth-ŎK-să-zōl
		  Bactrim, Septra
		pentamidine
		pĕn-TĂM-ĭ-dēn
		  NebuPent, Pentam-300

antivirals (to treat HIV-AIDS)	Prevent the replication of viruses within host cells
	
	Combinations of antivirals are commonly given for treatment and management of HIV infection and AIDS.
		nelfinavir
		nĕl-FĬN-ă-vēr
		  Viracept
		lamivudine/zidovudine
		lă-MĬV-ŭ-dēn/zĭ-DŌ-vŭ-dēn
		  Combivir
		zidovudine
		zĭ-DŌ-vŭ-dēn
		  AZT, Retrovir

fat-soluble vitamins	Prevent and treat bleeding disorders resulting from a lack of prothrombin, which is commonly caused by vitamin K deficiency	**phytonadione** fī-tō-nă-DĪ-ōn Vitamin K_1 Mephyton
hemostatics	Prevent or control bleeding Hemostatics are used to treat certain bleeding problems associated with surgery, blood disorders, and liver disease.	**aminocaproic acid** ă-mē-nō-kă-PRŌ-ĭk ĂS-ĭd Amicar

thrombolytics	Dissolve blood clots by destroying the fibrin strands that make up the clot
	
	Thrombolytics are used to break apart or lyse thrombi, especially those that obstruct coronary, pulmonary, and cerebral arteries.
		alteplase
		ĂL-tĕ-plās
		  Activase, t-PA
		streptokinase
		strĕp-tō-KĪ-nās
		  Streptase
		urokinase
		ū-rō-KĪ-nās
		  Abbokinase, Abbokinase Open-Cath

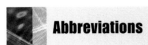

Abbreviations

This section introduces blood, lymph, and immune system abbreviations and their meanings.

Abbreviation	Meaning
AB, ab	abortion, antibodies
ABO	blood groups A, AB, B, and O
AIDS	acquired immunodeficiency syndrome
ALL	acute lymphocytic leukemia
AML	acute myelogenous leukemia
APTT	activated partial thromboplastin time
baso	basophil (type of white blood cell)
CBC	complete blood count
CLL	chronic lymphocytic leukemia
CML	chronic myelogenous leukemia
diff	differential count (white blood cells)
EBV	Epstein-Barr virus
eos	eosinophil (type of white blood cell)
ESR, sed rate	erythrocyte sedimentation rate; sedimentation rate
Hb, Hgb	hemoglobin
HCT, Hct	hematocrit
HDN	hemolytic disease of the newborn
HIV	human immunodeficiency virus
Igs	immunoglobulins
ITP	idiopathic thrombocytopenia purpura
I.V., IV	intravenous
lymphos	lymphocytes

(Continued)

Abbreviation	Meaning	(Continued)
MCH	mean corpuscular hemoglobin; mean cell hemoglobin (average amount of hemoglobin per cell)	
MCHC	mean cell hemoglobin concentration (average concentration of hemoglobin in a single red cell)	
MCV	mean cell volume (average volume or size of a single red blood cell; high MCV = macrocytic cells; low MCV = microcytic cells)	
mL, ml	milliliters	
PA	posteroanterior; pernicious anemia	
PCV	packed cell volume	
poly, PMN, PMNL	polymorphonuclear leukocyte	
PT	prothrombin time, physical therapy	
PTT	partial thromboplastin time	
RBC, rbc	red blood cell, red blood count	
segs	segmented neutrophils	
SLE	systemic lupus erythematosus	
WBC, wbc	white blood cell, white blood count	

It is time to review procedures, pharmacology, and abbreviations by completing Learning Activity 9–4.

LEARNING ACTIVITIES

The following activities provide review of the blood, lymph, and immune system terms introduced in this chapter. Complete each activity and review your answers to evaluate your understanding of the chapter.

Learning Activity 9–1

Identifying lymph structures

Label the following illustration using the terms listed below.

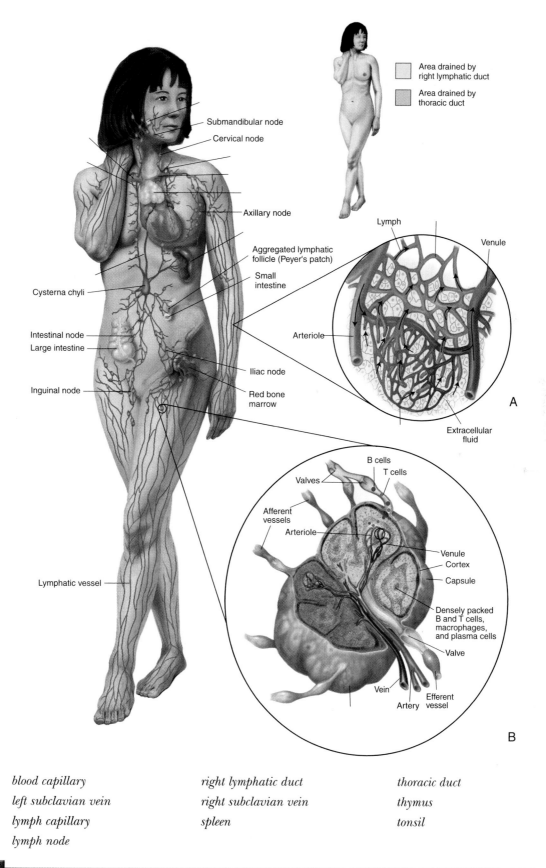

Submandibular node
Cervical node
Axillary node
Aggregated lymphatic follicle (Peyer's patch)
Small intestine
Cysterna chyli
Intestinal node
Large intestine
Inguinal node
Iliac node
Red bone marrow
Lymphatic vessel

Area drained by right lymphatic duct
Area drained by thoracic duct

Lymph
Venule
Arteriole
Extracellular fluid
A

B cells
T cells
Valves
Afferent vessels
Arteriole
Venule
Cortex
Capsule
Densely packed B and T cells, macrophages, and plasma cells
Valve
Vein
Artery
Efferent vessel
B

blood capillary

left subclavian vein

lymph capillary

lymph node

right lymphatic duct

right subclavian vein

spleen

thoracic duct

thymus

tonsil

Check your answers by referring to Figure 9–5 on page 234. Review material that you did not answer correctly.

Learning Activity 9–2

Building medical words

Use -osis (abnormal condition, increase) to build words that mean:

1. abnormal increase in RBCs _____
2. abnormal increase in WBCs _____
3. abnormal increase in lymphocytes _____
4. abnormal increase in reticulocytes _____

Use -penia (deficiency, decrease) to build words that mean:

5. decrease in RBCs _____
6. decrease in WBCs _____
7. decrease in platelets _____
8. decrease in lymphocytes _____

Use -poiesis (formation, production) to build words that mean:

9. production of blood _____
10. production of white cells _____
11. production of platelets _____

Use immun/o (immune, immunity, safe) to build words that mean:

12. specialist in the study of immunity _____
13. study of immunity _____

Use splen/o (spleen) to build words that mean:

14. herniation of the spleen _____
15. destruction of the spleen _____

Build surgical words that mean:

16. excision of the spleen _____
17. removal of the thymus _____
18. destruction of the thymus _____
19. incision of the spleen _____
20. fixation of (a displaced) spleen _____

Learning Activity 9–3

Matching pathological, diagnostic, symptomatic, and related terms

Match the following terms with the definitions in the numbered list.

active	*hemoglobinopathy*	*lymphadenopathy*
anisocytosis	*hemolysis*	*myelogenous*
artificial	*hemophilia*	*normocytic*
bacteremia	*hemostasis*	*passive*
exacerbations	*immunocompromised*	*septicemia*
graft rejection	*infectious mononucleosis*	*titer*
hematoma	*Kaposi sarcoma*	

1. _____ periods of flare-up
2. _____ any disorder due to abnormalities in the hemoglobin molecule
3. _____ presence of bacteria in blood, more as travelers, rather than a blood infection
4. _____ arrest of bleeding or circulation
5. _____ type of immunity where memory cells are formed
6. _____ malignancy of connective tissue commonly associated with HIV
7. _____ used to denote an erythrocyte that is normal in size
8. _____ swollen or diseased lymph glands
9. _____ term that denotes a weakened immune system
10. _____ blood clotting disorder
11. _____ common viral disorder caused by the Epstein-Barr virus
12. _____ leukemia that affects granulocytes
13. _____ type of immunity where memory cells are not transferred to the recipient
14. _____ immunity where medical intervention is required
15. _____ destruction of erythrocytes with the release of hemoglobin
16. _____ localized accumulation of blood in tissue; blood clot
17. _____ destruction of a transplanted organ or tissue by the recipient's immune system
18. _____ condition of marked variation in the size of erythrocytes
19. _____ blood test that measures the amount of antibodies in blood
20. _____ blood infection

Check your answers in Appendix A. Review any material that you did not answer correctly.

CORRECT ANSWERS _____ × 5 = _____ **% SCORE**

Learning Activity 9–4

Matching procedures, pharmacology, and abbreviations

Match the following terms with the definitions in the numbered list.

anticoagulants	*hemostatics*	*RBC*
aspiration	*homologous*	*RBC indices*
autologous	*lymphadenography*	*Shilling*
differential	*lymphangiectomy*	*thrombolytics*
hematocrit	*Monospot*	*WBC*

1. _____ drawing in or out by suction

2. _____ measurement of packed erythrocytes in a whole blood sample

3. _____ serologic test for infectious mononucleosis

4. _____ used to prevent blood clot formation

5. _____ leukocyte

6. _____ term used to describe a transplantation from another individual

7. _____ removal of a lymph vessel

8. _____ mathematical calculation of the size, volume, and concentration of hemoglobin for an average RBC

9. _____ definitive test for pernicious anemia

10. _____ radiographic examination of lymph nodes

11. _____ term used to describe a transfusion from the recipient's own blood

12. _____ used to prevent or control bleeding

13. _____ erythrocyte

14. _____ used to dissolve blood clots

15. _____ test to enumerate the distribution of WBCs in a stained blood smear

✔ Check your answers in Appendix A. Review any material that you did not answer correctly.

CORRECT ANSWERS _____ × 6.67 = _____ **% SCORE**

MEDICAL RECORD ACTIVITIES

The two medical records included in the activities that follow use common clinical scenarios to show how medical terminology is used to document patient care. Complete the terminology and analysis sections for each activity to help you recognize and understand terms related to the integumentary system.

Medical Record Activity 9–1

Discharge summary: Sickle cell crisis

Terminology

The terms listed in the chart come from the medical record *Discharge Summary: Sickle Cell Crisis* that follows. Use a medical dictionary such as *Taber's Cyclopedic Medical Dictionary,* the appendices of this book, or other resources to define each term. Then review the pronunciations for each term and practice by reading the medical record aloud.

Term	Definition
ambulating ĂM-bū-lāt-ĭng	
analgesia ăn-ăl-JĒ-zē-ă	
anemia ă-NĒ-mē-ă	
crisis KRĪ-sĭs	
CT scan	
hemoglobin HĒ-mō-glō-bĭn	
ileus ĬL-ē-ŭs	
infarction ĭn-FĂRK-shŭn	
morphine MOR-fēn	

(Continued)

Term	Definition	(Continued)
sickle cell SĬK-ăl SĔL		
splenectomy splē-NĔK-tō-mē		
Vicodin VĪ-kō-dĭn		

DISCHARGE SUMMARY: SICKLE CELL CRISIS

ADMITTING AND DISCHARGE DIAGNOSES:

(1) Sickle cell crisis

(2) Abdominal pain

PROCEDURES: Two units of packed red blood cells and CT scan of the abdomen

REASON FOR ADMISSION: This is a 46-year-old African-American man who reports a history of sickle cell anemia, which results in abdominal cramping when he is in crisis. His hemoglobin was 6 upon admission. He says his baseline runs 7 to 8. The patient states that he has not had a splenectomy. He describes the pain as midabdominal and cramplike. He denied any chills, fevers, or sweats.

HOSPITAL COURSE BY PROBLEM: (1) Sickle cell crisis. The patient was admitted to a Medical/Surgical bed, and placed on oxygen and IV fluids. He received morphine for analgesia, as well as Vicodin. At discharge his abdominal pain had resolved; however, he reported weakness. He was kept for an additional day for observation.

(2) A CT scan was performed on the belly and showed evidence of ileus in the small bowel with somewhat dilated small bowel loops and also an abnormal enhancement pattern in the kidney. The patient has had no nausea or vomiting. He is moving his bowels without any difficulty. He is ambulating. He even goes outside to smoke cigarettes, which he has been advised not to do. Certainly, we should obtain some information on his renal function and have his regular doctor assess this problem.

DISCHARGE INSTRUCTIONS: The patient has been advised to stop smoking and to see his regular doctor for follow-up on renal function.

Analysis

Review the medical record *Discharge Summary: Sickle Cell Crisis* to answer the following questions.

1. What blood product was administered to the patient?

_____

2. Why was this blood product given to the patient?

_____

3. Why was a CT scan performed on the patient?

_____

4. What were the three findings of the CT scan?

_____

5. Why should the patient see his regular doctor?

_____

Medical Record Activity 9–2

Discharge summary: PCP and HIV

Terminology

The terms listed in the chart come from the medical record *Discharge Summary: PCP and HIV* that follows. Use a medical dictionary such as *Taber's Cyclopedic Medical Dictionary*, the appendices of this book, or other resources to define each term. Then review the pronunciations for each term and practice by reading the medical record aloud.

Term	Definition
alveolar lavage ăl-VĒ-ō-lăr lă-VĂZH	
Bactrim BĂK-trĭm	
bronchoscopy brŏng-KŎS-kō-pē	
diffuse dĭ-FŪS	
HIV	
human immunodeficiency virus ĭm-ū-nō-dē-FĬSH-ĕn-sē	
infiltrate ĬN-fĭl-trāt	
Kaposi sarcoma KĂP-ō-sē săr-KŌ-mă	
leukoencephalopathy loo-kō-ĕn-sĕf-ă-LŎP-ă-thē	
multifocal mŭl-tĭ-FŌ-kăl	
PCP	
PMN	

(Continued)

Term	Definition	(Continued)
Pneumocystis carinii pneumonia nū-mō-SĬS-tĭs kă-RĪ-nē-ĭ nū-MŌ-nē-ă		
thrush THRŬSH		
vaginal candidiasis VĂJ-ĭn-ăl kăn-dĭ-DĪ-ă-sĭs		

Discharge Summary: PCP and HIV

FINAL DIAGNOSES:

(1) _Pneumocystis carinii_ pneumonia

(2) Human immunodeficiency virus infection

(3) Wasting

SOCIAL HISTORY: The patient's husband is deceased from AIDS 1 year ago with progressive multifocal leukoencephalopathy (PMN) and Kaposi sarcoma. She denies any history of intravenous drug use, transfusion, and identifies three lifetime sexual partners.

PAST MEDICAL HISTORY: The patient's past medical history is significant for HIV and several episodes of diarrhea, sinusitis, thrush, and vaginal candidiasis. She gave a history of a 10-pound weight loss. The chest x-ray showed diffuse lower lobe infiltrates, and she was diagnosed with presumptive _Pneumocystis carinii_ pneumonia and placed on Bactrim. She was admitted for a bronchoscopy with alveolar lavage to confirm the diagnosis. The antiretroviral treatment was reinitiated, and she was counseled as to the need to strictly adhere to her therapeutic regimen.

DISCHARGE INSTRUCTIONS: Complete medication regimen. Return to the care of Dr. Amid Shaheen.

Analysis

Review the medical record _Discharge Summary: PCP and HIV_ to answer the following questions.

1. How do you think the patient acquired the HIV infection?

   _____

2. What were the two diagnoses of the husband?

   _____

3. What four disorders in the medical history are significant for HIV?

   _____

4. What was the x-ray finding?

   _____

5. What two procedures are going to be performed to confirm the diagnosis of PCP pneumonia?

   _____

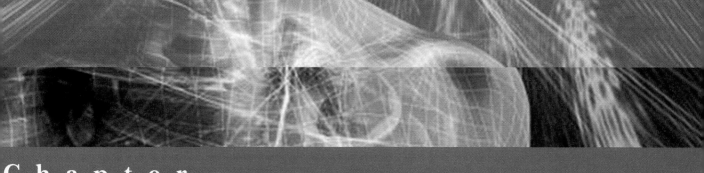

Chapter

10

Musculoskeletal System

CHAPTER OUTLINE

OBJECTIVES

Upon completion of this chapter, you will be able to:

- Locate and describe the structures of the musculoskeletal system.
- Recognize, pronounce, spell, and build words related to the musculoskeletal system.
- Describe pathological conditions, diagnostic and therapeutic procedures, and other terms related to the musculoskeletal system.

- Explain pharmacology related to the treatment of musculoskeletal disorders.
- Demonstrate your knowledge of this chapter by completing the learning and medical record activities.

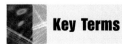

Key Terms

This section introduces important musculoskeletal system terms and their definitions. Word analyses are also provided.

Term	Definition
appendage ă-PĔN-dĭj	Any body part attached to a main structure *Examples of appendages include the arms and legs.*
articulation ăr-tĭk-ū-LĀ-shŭn	Place of union between two or more bones; also called *joint*
arthritis ăr-THRĪ-tĭs *arthr:* joint *-itis:* inflammation	Inflammation of a joint; usually accompanied by pain, swelling and, commonly, changes in structure *Types of arthritis include osteoarthritis, rheumatoid arthritis, gouty arthritis, and ankylosing spondylitis.*
cruciate ligaments KROO-shē-āt *cruci:* cross	Ligaments that cross each other forming an X within the notch between the femoral condyles *These ligaments help to prevent anterior-posterior displacement of the articular surfaces and to secure the articulating bones when standing.*
hematopoiesis hĕm-ă-tō-poy-Ē-sĭs *hemat/o:* blood *-poiesis:* formation, production	Production and development of blood cells, normally in the bone marrow
meatus mē-Ā-tŭs *meat:* opening, meatus *-us:* condition; structure	An opening or passage through any part of the body

Anatomy and Physiology

The musculoskeletal system includes muscles, bones, joints, and related structures, such as the tendons and connective tissue that function in the movement of body parts and organs.

Muscles

Muscle tissue is composed of contractile cells or fibers that provide movement of an organ or body part. Muscles contribute to posture, produce body heat, and act as a protective covering for internal organs. Muscles make up the bulk of the body and have the ability to contract, to relax, to be excited by a stimulus, and to return to their original size and shape. Regardless if muscles are attached to bones or to internal organs and blood vessels, the primary responsibility of muscles is movement. Apparent motion includes walking and talking. Less apparent motions provided by muscles are the passage and elimination of food through the digestive system, propulsion of blood through the arteries, and contraction of the bladder to eliminate urine. Review Figure 10–1 to familiarize yourself with the names and locations of selected muscles. These terms will appear when pathological conditions of muscles are discussed in both the textbook and medical reports.

There are three types of muscle tissue in the body:

- *Skeletal muscles,* also called *voluntary* or *striated muscles,* are muscles whose action is under voluntary control. Some examples of voluntary muscles are the muscles that move the eyeballs, tongue, and bones. Except for cardiac muscle, all striated muscles are voluntary.

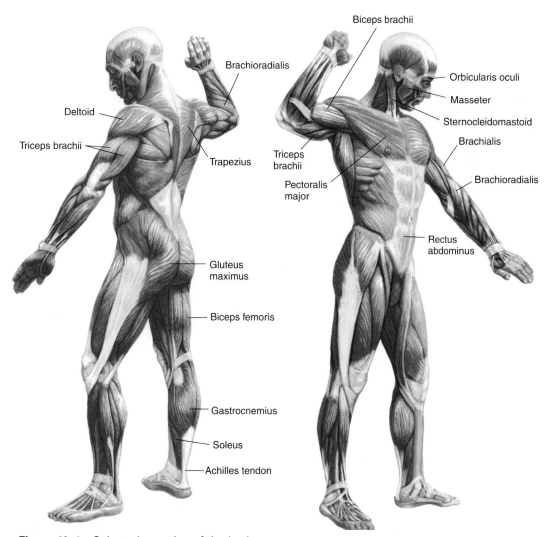

Figure 10–1   Selected muscles of the body.

- *Cardiac muscle,* found only in the heart, is unique for its branched interconnections, and it makes up most of the wall of the heart. It shares similarities with both skeletal and smooth muscles. Like skeletal muscle, it is striated, but it experiences rhythmic involuntary contractions like smooth muscle.
- *Smooth muscles (involuntary* or *visceral muscles)* are muscles whose action are involuntary. They are found principally in the visceral organs, the walls of arteries, the walls of respiratory passages, and in the urinary and reproductive ducts. The contraction of smooth muscle is controlled by the autonomic (involuntary) nervous system.

Figure 10–2 and Table 10–1 illustrate body movements produced by actions of muscles. Most are identified in pairs and provide opposing functions.

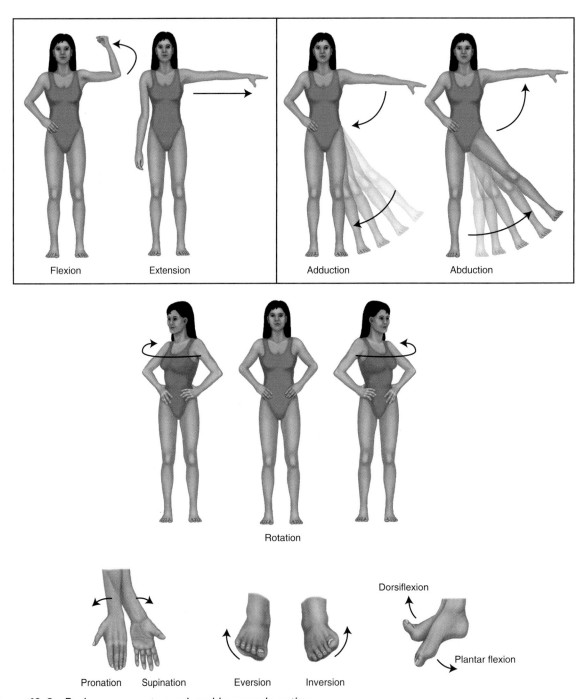

Figure 10–2   Body movements produced by muscle action.

Table 10–1   BODY MOVEMENTS PRODUCED BY MUSCLE ACTION

This chart lists body movements and the muscles used to produce them. With the exception of rotation, these movements are grouped in pairs of opposing functions.

Motion	Action
Adduction	Moves closer to the midline
Abduction	Moves away from the midline
Flexion	Decreases the angle of a joint
Extension	Increases the angle of a joint
Rotation	Moves a bone around its own axis
Pronation	Turns the palm down
Supination	Turns the palm up
Inversion	Moves the sole of the foot inward
Eversion	Moves the sole of the foot outward
Dorsiflexion	Elevates the foot
Plantar flexion	Lowers the foot (points the toes)

Attachments

Muscles attach to bones either by fleshy or fibrous attachments. In **fleshy attachments,** muscle fibers arise directly from bone. Although these fibers distribute force over wide areas, they are weaker than a fibrous attachment. In **fibrous attachments,** the connective tissue converges at the end of the muscle to become continuous and indistinguishable from the periosteum. When the fibrous attachment spans a large area of a particular bone, the attachment is called an *aponeurosis.* Such attachments are found in the lumbar region of the back. In some instances, this connective tissue penetrates the bone itself. When connective tissue fibers form a cord or strap, it is referred to as a *tendon.* This localizes a great deal of force in a small area of bone. Ligaments are composed of connective tissue and attach one bone to another.

 It is time to review muscle structures by completing Learning Activity 10–1.

Bones

Bones provide the framework of the body, protect internal organs, store calcium and other minerals, and produce blood cells within bone marrow. Together with other soft tissue, most vital organs are enclosed and protected by bones. For example, the bones of the skull protect the brain; the rib cage protects the heart and lungs. In addition to support and protection, the skeletal system carries out a number of other important functions. Movement is possible because bones provide points of attachment for muscles, tendons, and ligaments. As muscles contract, tendons and ligaments pull on bones and cause skeletal movement. Bone marrow, found within the larger bones, is responsible for **hematopoiesis,** continuously producing millions of blood cells to replace those that have been destroyed. Bones serve as a storehouse for minerals, particularly phosphorus and calcium. When the body experiences a need for a certain mineral, such as calcium during pregnancy, and a sufficient dietary supply is not available, calcium is withdrawn from the bones.

Bone Types

The four principal types of bones are short bones, flat bones, irregular bones, and long bones:

- *Short bones* are somewhat cube-shaped. They consist of a core of spongy bone, also known as *cancellous bone,* that is enclosed in a thin surface layer of compact bone. Examples of short bones include the bones of the ankles, wrists, and toes.
- *Irregular bones* include the bones that cannot be classified as short or long because of their complex shapes. Examples of irregular bones include vertebrae and the bones of the middle ear.
- *Flat bones* are exactly what their name suggests. They provide broad surfaces for muscular attachment or protection for internal organs. Examples of flat bones include bones of the skull, shoulder blades, and sternum.
- *Long bones* are found in the extremities of the body, such as the legs, arms, and fingers. (See Figure 10–3.) The parts of a long bone include:
  - The (1) **diaphysis** is the shaft or long, main portion of a bone.
  - The two ends of the bones, the (2) **distal epiphysis** and (3) **proximal epiphysis,** have a somewhat bulbous shape to provide space for muscle and ligament attachments near the joints. The epiphyses (singular, *epiphysis*) are made up largely of (4) **spongy bone** surrounded by a layer of compact bone. Red bone marrow is found within the porous chamber of spongy bone. This marrow is richly supplied with blood and

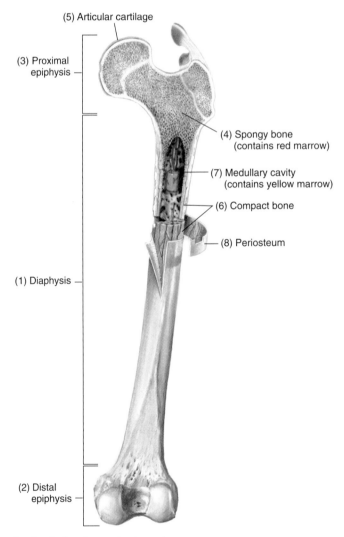

Figure 10–3 Longitudinal structure of a long bone.

consists of immature and mature blood cells in various stages of development. In an adult, the production of red blood cells (**erythropoiesis**) occurs in red bone marrow. Red bone marrow is also responsible for the formation of white blood cells (**leukopoiesis**) and platelets. Both ends of the epiphysis are covered by (5) **articular cartilage,** a type of elastic connective tissue that provides a smooth surface for movement of joints.

- In long bones, the bone shaft, or diaphysis, consists of (6) **compact bone** forming a cylinder that surrounds a central canal called the (7) **medullary cavity.** This medullary cavity, or *marrow cavity,* contains fatty yellow marrow in adults and consists primarily of fat cells and a few scattered blood cells.
- The (8) **periosteum,** a dense, white, fibrous membrane, covers the remaining surface of the bone. It contains numerous blood and lymph vessels and nerves. In growing bones, the inner layer contains the bone-forming cells known as *osteoblasts.* Because blood vessels and osteoblasts are located here, the periosteum provides a means for bone repair and general bone nutrition. Bones that lose periosteum through injury or disease usually scale or die. The periosteum also serves as a point of attachment for muscles, ligaments, and tendons.

It is time to review bone structures by completing Learning Activity 10–2.

Surface Features of Bones

Surfaces of bones are rarely smooth. Rather, they consist of projections, depressions, and openings that provide sites for muscle and ligament attachment. They also provide pathways and openings for blood vessels, nerves, and ducts. Various types of projections are evident in bones, some of which serve as points of **articulation.** Surfaces of bones may be rounded, sharp, or narrow or have a large ridge. Depressions and openings are cavities and holes in a bone. The most common types of projections, depressions, and openings are summarized in Table 10–2.

Table 10–2   SURFACE FEATURES OF BONES

This chart lists the most common types of projections, depressions, and openings along with the bones involved, descriptions, and examples for each. Becoming familiar with these terms will help you identify parts of individual bones described in medical reports related to orthopedics.

Surface Type	Bone Marking	Description	Example
Projections • Nonarticulating surfaces • Sites of muscle and ligament attachment	• Trochanter • Tubercle • Tuberosity	• Very large, irregularly shaped process found only on the femur • Small, rounded process • Large, rounded process	• Greater trochanter of the femur • Tubercle of the femur • Tuberosity of the humerus
Articulating surfaces • Projections that form joints	• Condyle • Head	• Rounded, articulating knob • Prominent, rounded, articulating end of a bone	• Condyle of the humerus • Head of the femur
Depressions and openings • Sites for blood vessel, nerve, and duct passage	• Foramen • Fissure • Meatus • Sinus	• Rounded opening through a bone to accommodate blood vessels and nerves • Narrow, slitlike opening • Canal-like passageway into a bone • Cavity or hollow space in a bone	• Foramen of the skull through which cranial nerves pass • Fissure of the sphenoid bone • External auditory meatus of the temporal bone • Cavity of frontal sinus containing a duct that carries secretions to the upper part of the nasal cavity

Divisions of the Skeletal System

The skeletal system of a human adult consists of 206 individual bones. However, only the major bones are discussed. For anatomical purposes, the human skeleton is divided into the axial skeleton and appendicular skeleton. (See Figure 10–4.)

Axial skeleton. The axial skeleton is divided into three major regions: skull, rib cage, and vertebral column. It contributes to the formation of body cavities and provides protection for internal organs, such as the brain, spinal cord, and organs enclosed in the thorax. The axial skeleton is distinguished with bone color in Figure 10–4.

Skull. The bony structure of the skull consists of **cranial bones** and **facial bones.** (See Figure

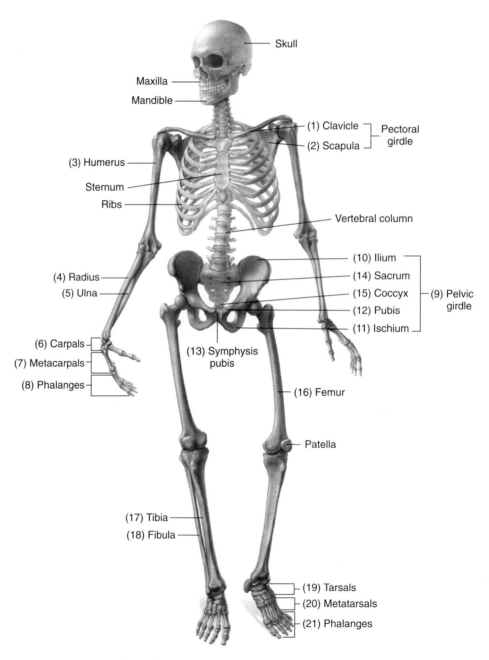

Figure 10–4   Anterior view of the skeleton.

10–5.) With the exception of one facial bone, all other bones of the skull are joined together by *sutures*. Sutures are the lines of junction between two bones, especially of the skull, and are usually immovable.

CRANIAL BONES. Eight bones, collectively known as the *cranium (skull),* enclose and protect the brain and the organs of hearing and equilibrium. Cranial bones are connected to muscles to provide head movements, chewing motions, and facial expressions.

An infant's skull contains membranous areas called *fontanels* or "soft spots" where the bone-making process is not yet complete. Their chief function is to allow a small compression of the skull during the delivery process. With age they ossify and become fixed.

The (1) **frontal bone** forms the anterior portion of the skull (forehead) and the roof of the bony cavities that contain the eyeballs. One (2) **parietal bone** is situated on each side of

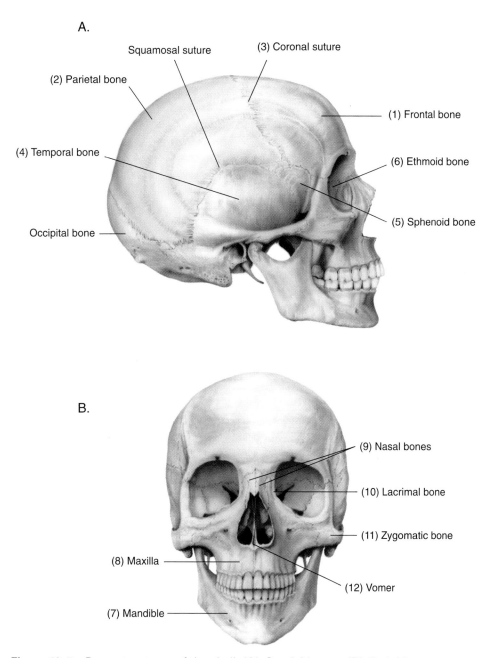

A.

Squamosal suture   (3) Coronal suture

(2) Parietal bone

(1) Frontal bone

(4) Temporal bone

(6) Ethmoid bone

(5) Sphenoid bone

Occipital bone

B.

(9) Nasal bones

(10) Lacrimal bone

(11) Zygomatic bone

(8) Maxilla

(12) Vomer

(7) Mandible

Figure 10–5 Bony structures of the skull. (A) Cranial bones. (B) Facial bones.

the skull just behind the frontal bone. Together, they form the upper sides and roof of the cranium. Each parietal bone meets the frontal bone along the (3) **coronal suture.** A single *occipital bone* forms the back and base of the skull. It contains an opening in its base through which the spinal cord passes. Two (4) **temporal bones,** one on each side of the skull, form part of the lower cranium. Each temporal bone has a complicated shape that contains various cavities and recesses associated with the internal ear, the essential part of the organ of hearing. The temporal bone projects downward to form the *mastoid process,* which provides a point of attachment for several neck muscles. The (5) **sphenoid bone,** located at the middle part of the base of the skull, forms a central wedge that joins with all other cranial bones, holding them together. A very light and spongy bone, the (6) **ethmoid bone,** forms most of the bony area between the nasal cavity and parts of the orbits of the eyes.

FACIAL BONES. All facial bones, with the exception of the (7) **mandible** (lower jaw bone), are joined together by sutures and are immovable. Movement of the mandible is needed for speaking and chewing **(mastication).** The (8) **maxillae,** paired upper jawbones, are fused in the midline by a suture. They form the upper jaw and hard palate (roof of the mouth). If the maxillary bones do not fuse properly before birth, a congenital defect called *cleft palate* results. The maxillae (singular, maxilla) and the mandible contain sockets for the roots of the teeth. Two thin and nearly rectangular bones, the (9) **nasal bones,** lie side by side and are fused medially, forming the shape and the bridge of the nose. Two paired (10) **lacrimal bones** are located at the corner of each eye. These thin, small bones unite to form the groove for the lacrimal sac and canals through which the tear ducts pass into the nasal cavity. The paired (11) **zygomatic bones** are located on the side of the face below the eyes and form the higher portion of the cheeks below and to the sides of the eyes. The zygomatic bone is commonly referred to as the *cheekbone.* The (12) **vomer** is a single, thin bone that forms the lower part of the nasal septum.

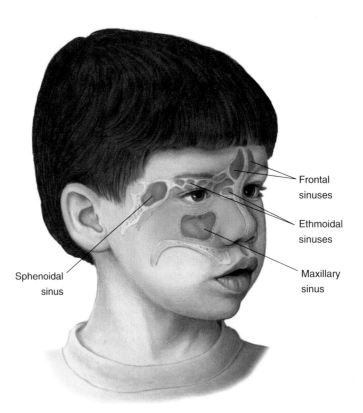

Frontal sinuses

Ethmoidal sinuses

Maxillary sinus

Sphenoidal sinus

Figure 10–6 Paranasal sinuses.

Other important structures, the **paranasal sinuses,** are cavities located within the cranial and facial bones. As their name implies, the frontal, ethmoidal, sphenoidal, and maxillary sinuses are named after the bones in which they are located. (See Figure 10–6.) The paranasal sinuses open into the nasal cavities and are lined with *ciliary epithelium* that is continuous with the mucosa of the nasal cavities. When sinuses are unable to drain properly, a feeling of being "stuffed up" ensues. This commonly occurs during upper respiratory infections or with allergies.

Thorax. The internal organs of the chest (thorax), including the heart and lungs, are enclosed and protected by a bony rib cage. The thorax consists of 12 pairs of ribs, all attached to the spine. (See Figure 10–7.) The first seven pairs, the (1) **true ribs,** are attached directly to the (2) **sternum** by a strip of (3) **costal cartilage.** The costal cartilage of the next five pairs of ribs is not fastened directly to the sternum, so these ribs are known as (4) **false ribs.** The last two pairs of false ribs are not joined, even indirectly, to the sternum but attach posteriorly to the thoracic vertebrae. These last two pairs of false ribs are known as (5) **floating ribs.**

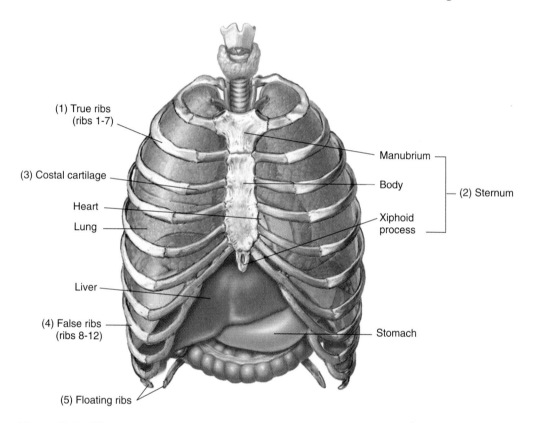

Figure 10–7 Thorax.

Vertebral column. The vertebral column of the adult is composed of 26 bones called *vertebrae* (singular, *vertebra*). The vertebral column supports the body and provides a protective bony canal for the spinal cord. A healthy, normal spine has four curves that help make it resilient and maintain balance. The cervical and lumbar regions curve forward, whereas the thoracic and sacral regions curve backward. Abnormal curves may be due to a congenital defect, poor posture, or bone disease. (See Figure 10–8.)

The vertebral column consists of five regions of bones, each deriving its name from its location within the spinal column. The seven (1) **cervical vertebrae** form the skeletal framework of the neck. The first cervical vertebra, the (2) **atlas,** supports the skull. The second cervical vertebra, the (3) **axis,** makes possible the rotation of the skull on the neck. Under the

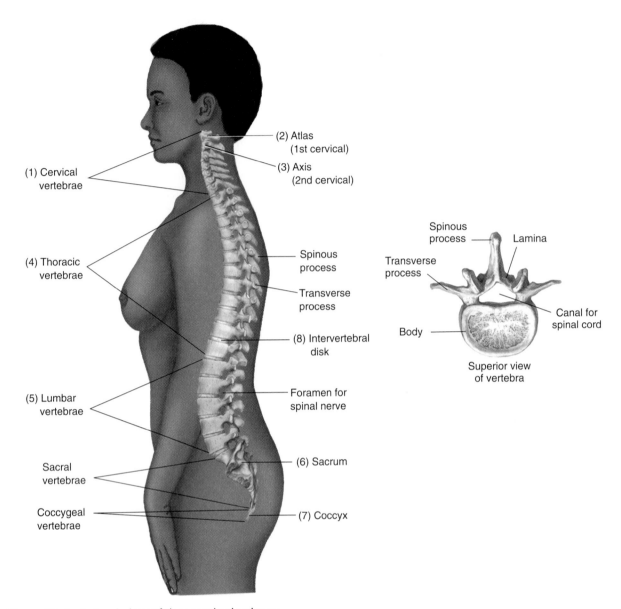

Figure 10–8   Lateral view of the vertebral column.

seventh cervical vertebra are twelve (4) **thoracic vertebrae,** which support the chest and serve as a point of articulation for the ribs. The next five vertebrae, the (5) **lumbar vertebrae,** are situated in the lower back area and carry most of the weight of the torso. Below this area are five sacral vertebrae, which are fused into a single bone in the adult and are referred to as the (6) **sacrum.** The tail of the vertebral column consists of four or five fragmented fused vertebrae referred to as the (7) **coccyx.**

Vertebrae are separated by flat, round structures, the (8) **intervertebral disks,** which are composed of a fibrocartilaginous substance with a gelatinous mass in the center (nucleus pulposus). When disk material protrudes into the neural canal, pressure on the adjacent nerve root causes pain. This condition is referred to as *herniation of an intervertebral disk,* **herniated nucleus pulposus (HNP),** *ruptured disk,* or *slipped disk.*

Appendicular skeleton. The appendicular skeleton consists of bones of the upper and lower limbs and their girdles that attach the limbs to the axial skeleton. The appendicular skeleton is distinguished with blue color in Figure 10–4. The difference between the axial and appendicular skeletons is that the axial skeleton protects internal organs, and provides central support for the body; the appendicular skeleton enables the body to move. The ability to walk, run, or catch a ball is possible because of the movable joints of the limbs that make up the appendicular skeleton.

Pectoral (shoulder) girdle. The pectoral girdle consists of two bones, the anterior (1) **clavicle** (collarbone) and the posterior (2) **scapula** (triangular shoulder blade). The primary function of the pectoral girdle is to attach the bones of the upper limbs to the axial skeleton and provide attachments for muscles that aid upper limb movements. The paired pectoral structures and their associated muscles form the shoulders of the body.

Upper limbs. The skeletal framework of each upper limb includes the arm, forearm, or hand. Anatomically speaking, the arm is only that part of the upper limb between the shoulder and elbow. Each limb or appendage consists of a (3) **humerus** (upper arm bone). The humerus articulates with the (4) **radius** and (5) **ulna** at the elbow. The radius and ulna form the skeleton of the forearm. The bones of the hand include eight (6) **carpals** (wrist); five radiating (7) **metacarpals** (palm); and ten radiating (8) **phalanges** (fingers).

Pelvic (hip) girdle. The (9) **pelvic girdle** is a basin-shaped structure that attaches the lower limbs to the axial skeleton. Along with its associated ligaments, it supports the trunk of the body, and provides protection for the visceral organs of the pelvis (lower organs of digestion and urinary and reproductive structures).

Male and female pelves (singular, *pelvis*) differ considerably in size and shape but share the same basic structures. Some of the differences are attributable to the function of the female pelvis during childbearing. The female pelvis is shallower than the male pelvis but wider in all directions. The female pelvis not only supports the enlarged uterus as the fetus matures but also provides a large opening to allow the infant to pass through during birth. Even so, female and male pelves are divided into the (10) **ilium,** (11) **ischium,** and (12) **pubis.** These three bones are fused together in the adult to form a single bone called the *innominate (hip) bone.* The bladder is located behind the (13) **symphysis pubis;** the rectum is in the curve of the (14) **sacrum** and (15) **coccyx.** In the female, the uterus, fallopian tubes, ovaries, and vagina are located between the bladder and the rectum.

Lower limbs. The lower limbs support the complete weight of the erect body and are subjected to exceptional stresses, especially in running or jumping. To accommodate for these types of forces, the lower limb bones are stronger and thicker than comparable bones of the upper limbs. The difference between the upper and lower limb bones is that the lighter bones of the upper limbs are adapted for mobility and flexibility; the massive bones of the lower limbs are specialized for stability and weight bearing. There are three parts of each lower limb: the thigh, the leg, and the foot.

The thigh consists of a single bone called the (16) **femur.** It is the largest, longest, and strongest bone in the body. The leg is formed by two parallel bones: the (17) **tibia** and the (18) **fibula.** The seven (19) **tarsals** (ankle bones) resemble metacarpals (wrist bones) in structure. Lastly, the bones of the foot include the (20) **metatarsals,** which consists of five small long bones numbered 1 to 5 beginning with the great toe on the medial side of the foot, and the much smaller (21) **phalanges** (toes).

Joints or Articulations

To allow for body movements, bones must have points where they meet **(articulate).** These articulating points form joints that have various degrees of mobility. Some are freely movable **(diarthroses),** others are only slightly movable **(amphiarthroses),** and the remaining are totally immovable **(synarthroses).** All three types are necessary for smooth, coordinated body movements.

Joints that allow movement are called synovial joints. The ends of the bones that comprise these joints are encased in a sleevelike extension of the periosteum called the *joint capsule.* This capsule binds the articulating bones to each other. In most synovial joints, the capsule is strengthened by ligaments that lash the bones together, providing additional strength to the joint capsule. A membrane called the *synovial membrane* surrounds the inside of the capsule. It secretes a lubricating fluid **(synovial fluid)** within the entire joint capsule. The ends of each of the bones are covered with a smooth layer of cartilage that serves as a cushion.

It is time to review skeletal structures by completing Learning Activity 10–3.

Medical Word Elements

This section introduces combining forms, suffixes, and prefixes related to the musculoskeletal system. Word analyses are also provided.

Element	Meaning	Word Analysis
COMBINING FORMS		
Skeletal System		
General		
ankyl/o	stiffness; bent, crooked	ankyl/osis (ăng-kǐ-LŌ-sǐs): immobility and stiffness of a joint *-osis:* abnormal condition; increase (used primarily with blood cells) *Ankylosis may be the result of trauma, surgery, or disease and most commonly occurs in rheumatoid arthritis.*
arthr/o	joint	arthr/itis (ăr-THRĪ-tǐs): inflammation of a joint *-itis:* inflammation
kyph/o	hill, mountain	kyph/osis (kǐ-FŌ-sǐs): humpback posture *-osis:* abnormal condition; increase (used primarily with blood cells)
lamin/o	lamina (part of vertebral arch)	lamin/ectomy (lăm-ǐ-NĔK-tō-mē): excision of the lamina *-ectomy:* excision, removal *Laminectomy is usually performed to relieve compression of the spinal cord or to remove a lesion or herniated disk.*
lord/o	curve, swayback	lord/osis (lor-DŌ-sǐs): swayback posture *-osis:* abnormal condition; increase (used primarily with blood cells)
myel/o	bone marrow; spinal cord	myel/o/pathy (mī-ě-LŎP-ă-thē): any pathological condition of the spinal cord *-pathy:* disease

Element	Meaning	Word Analysis
orth/o	straight	orth/o/ped/ist (or-thō-PĒ-dĭst): physician who specializes in the treatment of musculoskeletal disorders *ped:* foot; child *–ist:* specialist *Initially, an orthopedist corrected deformities and straightened children's bones. In today's medical practice, however, the orthopedist treats musculoskeletal disorders and associated structures in persons of all ages.*
oste/o	bone	oste/oma (ŏs-tē-Ō-mă): benign bony tumor *-oma:* tumor
ped/o **ped/i**	foot; child	ped/o/graph (PĔD-ō-grăf): imprint of the foot on paper ped/i/cure (PĔD-ĭ-kūr): care of feet
scoli/o	crooked, bent	scoli/osis (skō-lē-Ō-sĭs): abnormal curvature of the spine *-osis:* abnormal condition; increase (used primarily with blood cells)
thorac/o	chest	thorac/o/dynia (thō-răk-ō-DĬN-ē-ă): chest pain *-dynia:* pain
Specific Bones **acromi/o**	acromion (projection of scapula)	acromi/al (ăk-RŌ-mē-ăl): relating to the acromion *-al:* pertaining to, relating to
brachi/o	arm	brachi/algia (brā-kē-ĂL-jē-ă): pain in the arm *-algia:* pain
calcane/o	calcaneum (heel bone)	calcane/o/dynia (kăl-kăn-ō-DĬN-ē-ă): pain in the heel when standing or walking *-dynia:* pain
carp/o	carpus (wrist bone)	carp/o/ptosis (kăr-pŏp-TŌ-sĭs): wrist drop *-ptosis:* prolapse, downward displacement
cephal/o	head	cephal/ad (SĔF-ă-lăd): toward the head *-ad:* toward
cervic/o	neck; cervix uteri (neck of uterus)	cervic/o/dynia (sĕr-vĭ-kō-DĬN-ē-ă): pain or cramp of the neck; also called *cervical neuralgia* *-dynia:* pain
clavicul/o	clavicle (collarbone)	clavicul/ar (klă-VĬK-ū-lăr): pertaining to the clavicle *-ar:* pertaining to, relating to
cost/o	ribs	cost/ectomy (kŏs-TĔK-tō-mē): excision or resection of a rib *-ectomy:* excision, removal
crani/o	cranium (skull)	crani/o/tomy (krā-nē-ŎT-ō-mē): incision of the cranium *-tomy:* incision

(Continued)

Element	Meaning	Word Analysis	(Continued)
dactyl/o	fingers; toes	dactyl/o/megaly (dăk-tĭ-lō-MĔG-ă-lē): abnormally large size of fingers and toes *-megaly:* enlargement	
femor/o	femur (thigh bone)	femor/al (FĔM-or-ăl): pertaining to the femur *-al:* pertaining to, relating to	
fibul/o	fibula (smaller bone of lower leg)	fibul/o/calcane/al (fĭb-ū-lō-kăl-KĀ-nē-ăl): pertaining to the fibula and calcaneus *calcane:* calcaneum (heel bone) *-al:* pertaining to, relating to	
humer/o	humerus (upper arm bone)	humer/o/scapul/ar (hū-mĕr-ō-SKĂP-ū-lăr): concerning the humerus and scapula *scapul:* scapula (shoulder blade) *-ar:* pertaining to, relating to	
ili/o	ilium (lateral, flaring portion of hip bone)	ili/o/pelv/ic (ĭl-ē-ō-PĔL-vĭk): concerning the iliac area of the pelvis *pelv:* pelvis *-ic:* pertaining to, relating to	
ischi/o	ischium (lower portion of hip bone)	ischi/o/dynia (ĭs-kē-ō-DĬN-ē-ă): pain in the ischium *-dynia:* pain	
lumb/o	loins (lower back)	lumb/o/dynia (lŭm-bō-DĬN-ē-ă): pain in the lumbar region of the back; also called *lumbago* *-dynia:* pain	
metacarp/o	metacarpus (hand bone)	metacarp/ectomy (mĕt-ă-kăr-PĔK-tō-mē): surgical excision or resection of one or more metacarpal bones *-ectomy:* excision, removal	
metatars/o	metatarsus (foot bone)	metatars/algia (mĕt-ă-tăr-SĂL-jē-ă): pain that emanates from the heads of the metatarsus and worsens with weight bearing or palpation *-algia:* pain	
patell/o	patella (kneecap)	patell/ectomy (păt-ĕ-LĔK-tō-mē): removal of the patella *-ectomy:* excision, removal	
pelv/i	pelvis	pelv/i/metry (pĕl-VĬM-ĕt-rē): act or process of determining the dimension of the bony birth canal *-metry:* act of measuring	
pod/o	foot	pod/iatry (pō-DĪ-ă-trē): treatment and prevention of conditions of the feet *-iatry:* medicine, treatment	
phalang/o	phalanges (bones of fingers and toes)	phalang/ectomy (făl-ăn-JĔK-tō-mē): excision of one or more phalanges *-ectomy:* excision, removal	

Element	Meaning	Word Analysis
pub/o	pelvis bone (anterior part of pelvic bone)	pub/o/coccyg/eal (pū-bō-kŏk-SĬJ-ē-ăl): pertaining to the pubis and the coccyx *coccyg:* coccyx (tailbone) *-eal:* pertaining to, relating to
radi/o	radiation, x-ray; radius (lower arm bone on thumb side)	radi/al (RĀ-dē-ăl): pertaining to the radius *-al:* pertaining to, relating to
spondyl/o (used to make words about conditions of structure)	vertebrae (backbone)	spondyl/itis (spŏn-dĭl-Ī-tĭs): inflammation of the vertebrae *-itis:* inflammation
vertebr/o (used to make words that describe structure for anatomy)		inter/vertebr/al (ĭn-tĕr-VĔRT-ĕ-brĕl): relating to the area between two adjacent vertebrae *inter-:* between *-al:* pertaining to, relating to
stern/o	sternum (breastbone)	stern/ad (STĔR-năd): toward the sternum *-ad:* toward
tibi/o	tibia (larger bone of lower leg)	tibi/o/femor/al (tĭb-ē-ō-FĔM-or-ăl) pertaining to the tibia and femur *femor:* femur *-al:* pertaining to, relating to

Muscular System

Element	Meaning	Word Analysis
leiomy/o	smooth muscle (visceral)	leiomy/oma (lī-ō-mi-Ō-mă): tumor consisting principally of smooth muscle tissue *-oma:* tumor
muscul/o	muscle	muscul/ar (MŬS-kū-lăr): pertaining to muscles *-ar:* pertaining to, relating to
my/o		my/oma (mi-Ō-mă): tumor containing muscle tissue
rhabd/o	rod-shaped (striated)	rhabd/oid (RĂB-doyd): resembling a rod *-oid:* resembling
rhabdomy/o	rod-shaped (striated) muscle	rhabdomy/oma (răb-dō-mi-Ō-mă): tumor composed of striated muscular tissue *-oma:* tumor

Related Structures

Element	Meaning	Word Analysis
chondr/o	cartilage	chondr/itis (kŏn-DRĪ-tĭs): inflammation of cartilage *-itis:* inflammation

(Continued)

Element	Meaning	Word Analysis	(Continued)
fasci/o	band, fascia (fibrous membrane supporting and separating muscles)	fasci/o/plasty (FĂSH-ē-ō-plăs-tē): surgical repair of fascia -*plasty:* surgical repair	
fibr/o	fiber, fibrous tissue	fibr/oma (fī-BRŌ-mă): encapsulated tumor consisting of fibrous connective tissue -*oma:* tumor	
synov/o	synovial membrane, synovial fluid	synov/ectomy (sĭn-ō-VĔK-tō-mē): removal of a synovial membrane -*ectomy:* excision, removal	
ten/o	tendon	ten/o/desis (tĕn-ŎD-ĕ-sĭs): surgical binding or fixation of a tendon -*desis:* binding, fixation (of a bone or joint)	
tend/o		tend/o/plasty (TĔN-dō-plăs-tē): surgical repair of a tendon -*plasty:* surgical repair	
tendin/o		tendin/itis (tĕn-dĭn-Ī-tĭs): inflammation of a tendon -*itis:* inflammation	

SUFFIXES

Element	Meaning	Word Analysis	
-asthenia	weakness, debility	my/asthenia (mī-ăs-THĒ-nē-ă): muscle weakness and abnormal fatigue *my:* muscle	
-blast	embryonic cell	my/o/blast (MĪ-ō-blăst): embryonic cell that develops into a muscle cell *my/o:* muscle	
-clasia	to break; surgical fracture	oste/o/clasia (ŏs-tē-ō-KLĀ-zē-ă): surgical fracture of a bone to remedy a deformity; bony tissue absorption and destruction; also called *osteoclasis* *oste/o:* bone	
-clast		oste/o/clast (ŎS-tē-ō-klăst): device used to fracture a bone to correct a deformity; large multinuclear cell formed in the bone marrow of growing bones	
-desis	binding, fixation (of a bone or joint)	arthr/o/desis (ăr-thrō-DĒ-sĭs): binding together of a joint *arthr/o:* joint	
-malacia	softening	chondr/o/malacia (kŏn-drō-măl-Ā-shē-ă): softening of the articular cartilage, usually involving the patella *chondr/o:* cartilage	
-physis	growth	epi/physis (ĕ-PĬF-ĭ-sĭs): end of a long bone; upper, growing part of a bone *epi-:* above, upon	

Element	Meaning	Word Analysis
-porosis	porous	oste/o/porosis (ŏs-tē-ō-pŏ-RŌ-sĭs): disorder characterized by loss of bone density *oste/o:* bone *Osteoporosis may cause pain, especially in the lower back; pathological fractures; loss of stature; and various deformities.*
-scopy	visual examination	arthr/o/scopy (ăr-THRŎS-kō-pē): endoscopic examination of the interior of a joint *arthr/o:* joint *Arthroscopy is performed by inserting small surgical instruments to remove and repair damaged tissue, such as cartilage fragments or torn ligaments.*
PREFIXES		
a-	without, not	a/trophy (ĂT-rō-fē): wasting; decrease in size of an organ or tissue *-trophy:* development, nourishment
sub-	under, below	sub/patell/ar (sŭb-pă-TĔL-ăr): beneath the patella *patell:* patella (kneecap) *-ar:* pertaining to, relating to
supra-	above; excessive; superior	supra/cost/al (soo-pră-KŎS-tăl): above the ribs *cost:* ribs *-al:* pertaining to, relating to
syn-	union, together, joined	syn/dactyl/ism (sĭn-DĂK-tĭl-ĭzm): fusion of two or more fingers or toes *dactyl:* fingers, toes *-ism:* condition

 It is time to review medical word elements by completing Learning Activity 10–4.

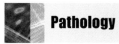 **Pathology**

Joints are especially vulnerable to constant wear and tear. Repeated motion, disease, trauma, and aging affect joints as well as muscles and tendons. Overall, disorders of the musculoskeletal system are more likely to be caused by injury than disease. Other disorders of structure and bone strength—such as osteoporosis, which occurs primarily in elderly women—affect the health of the musculoskeletal system.

For diagnosis, treatment, and management of musculoskeletal disorders, the medical services of a specialist may be warranted. *Orthopedics* is the branch of medicine concerned with the prevention, diagnosis, care, and treatment of musculoskeletal disorders. The physician who specializes in the diagnoses and treatment of musculoskeletal disorders is known as an *orthopedist*. These professionals employ medical, physical, and surgical methods to restore function that has been lost as a result of musculoskeletal injury or disease. Another physician who specializes in treating joint disease is the *rheumatologist*. Still another physician, the *osteopathic physician (DO)*, maintains that good health requires proper alignment of bones, muscles, ligaments, and nerves. Like the MD, osteopathic physicians combine manipulative procedures with state-of-the-art methods of medical treatment, including prescribing drugs and performing surgeries.

Bone Disorders

Disorders involving the bones include fractures, infections, osteoporosis, and spinal curvatures.

Fractures

When a bone is broken, it is called a *fracture*. The different types of fractures are classified by extent of damage. (See Figure 10–9.) A (1) **closed, or simple, fracture** is one in which the bone is broken but no external wound exists. An (2) **open, or compound, fracture** involves a broken bone and an external wound that leads to the site of fracture. Fragments of bone often protrude through the skin. A (3) **complicated fracture** is one in which a broken bone has injured some internal organ, such as when a broken rib pierces a lung. In a (4) **comminuted fracture,** the bone has broken or splintered into pieces. An (5) **impacted fracture** occurs when the bone is broken and one end is wedged into the interior of the other bone. An (6) **incomplete fracture** is when the line of fracture does not include the whole bone. A (7) **greenstick fracture** occurs when one side of a long bone is broken and the other side is bent. It occurs in children because their bones contain more collagen than adult bones and tend to splinter rather than break completely. A (8) **Colles fracture,** a break at the lower end of the radius, occurs just above the wrist. It causes displacement of the hand and usually occurs as a result of flexing a hand to cushion a fall. A **hairline fracture** is a minor fracture in which all portions of the bone are in perfect alignment. The fracture is seen on radiographic examination as a very thin hairline between the two segments but not extending entirely through the bone. **Pathological (spontaneous) fractures** are usually caused by a disease process such as a neoplasm or osteoporosis.

Unlike other repairs of the body, bones sometimes require months to heal. Several factors influence the rate at which fractures heal. Some fractures need to be immobilized to ensure that bones unite soundly in a suitable position. In most cases this is achieved with bandages, casts, traction, or a fixation device. Certain fractures, particularly those with bone fragments, require surgery to reposition and fix bones securely, so that surrounding tissues heal. In addition to promoting healing, immobilization prevents further injury and reduces pain.

Some bones have a natural tendency to heal more rapidly than others. For instance, the long bones of the arms usually mend twice as fast as those of the legs. Age also plays an important role in bone fracture healing rate; older patients require more time for healing. In addition, an adequate blood supply to the injured area and the nutritive state of the individual are crucial to the healing process.

Infections

Infection of the bone and bone marrow is called *osteomyelitis*. It may be acute or chronic. Bone infections are primarily caused by pus-forming **(pyogenic)** bacteria. The disease usually begins with local trauma to the bone causing a blood clot **(hematoma).** Bacteria from an acute infection in another area of the body find their way to the injured bone and establish the infection.

Most bone infections are more difficult to effectively treat than soft tissue infections. Eventually, some bone infections result in destruction **(necrosis)** of the bone and stiffening, or

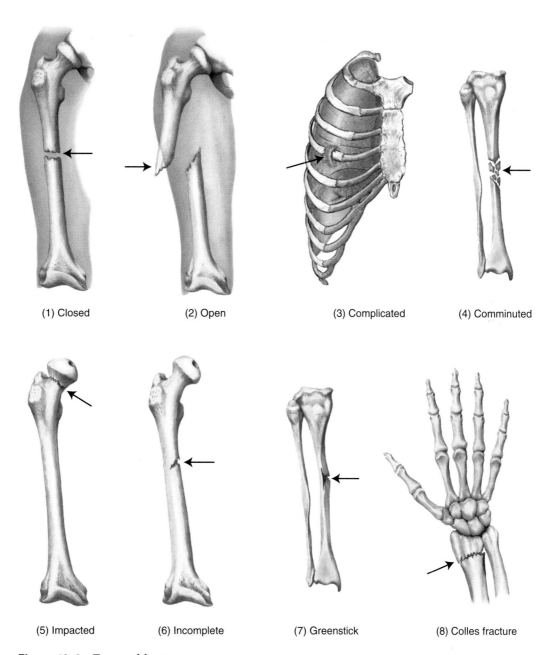

(1) Closed   (2) Open   (3) Complicated   (4) Comminuted

(5) Impacted   (6) Incomplete   (7) Greenstick   (8) Colles fracture

Figure 10–9 Types of fractures.

freezing, of the joints **(ankylosis).** Osteomyelitis may be acute or chronic. With early treatment, prognosis for acute osteomyelitis is good; prognosis for the chronic form of the disease is poor.

Paget disease, also known as *osteitis deformans,* is a chronic inflammation of bones, resulting in thickening and softening of bones. It can occur in any bone but most commonly affects the long bones of the legs, the lower spine, the pelvis, and the skull. This disease is found in the population older than age 40. Although a variety of causes have been proposed, a slow virus (not yet isolated) is currently thought to be the most likely cause.

Osteoporosis

Osteoporosis is a common metabolic bone disorder in the elderly, particularly in post-menopausal women and especially women older than age 60. It is characterized by decreased bone density that occurs when the rate of bone resorption (loss of substance) exceeds the rate of bone formation. Among the many causes of osteoporosis are disturbances of protein metabolism, protein deficiency, disuse of bones due to prolonged periods of immobilization, estrogen deficiencies associated with menopause, a diet lacking vitamins or calcium, and long-term administration of high doses of corticosteroids.

Patients with osteoporosis commonly complain of bone pain, typically in the back, which may be caused by repeated microscopic fractures. Thin areas of porous bone are also evident. Deformity associated with osteoporosis is usually the result of pathological fractures.

Spinal Curvatures

Any persistent, abnormal deviation of the vertebral column from its normal position may cause a spinal curvature. Three common deviations are *scoliosis, kyphosis,* and *lordosis.* (See Figure 10–10.)

An abnormal lateral curvature of the spine, either to the right or left, is called *scoliosis.* Some rotation of a portion of the vertebral column may also occur. Scoliosis, or *C-shaped curvature of the spine,* may be congenital, caused by chronic poor posture during childhood while the vertebrae are still growing, or the result of one leg being longer than the other. Treatment depends on the severity of the curvature and may vary from exercises, physical therapy, and back braces to surgical intervention. Untreated scoliosis may result in pulmonary insufficiency (curvature may decrease lung capacity), back pain, sciatica, disk disease, or even degenerative arthritis.

An abnormal curvature of a portion of the spine is called *kyphosis,* more commonly known as *humpback* or *hunchback.* Rheumatoid arthritis, rickets, poor posture, or chronic respiratory diseases may cause kyphosis. Treatment consists of spine-stretching exercises, sleeping with a board under the mattress, and wearing a brace to straighten the kyphotic curve; surgery is rarely required.

An abnormal, inward curvature of a portion of the spine is called *lordosis,* more

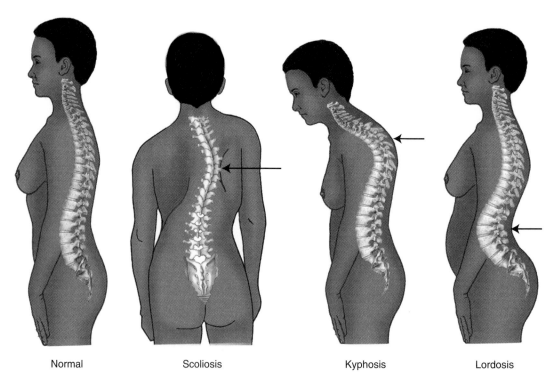

| Normal | Scoliosis | Kyphosis | Lordosis |

Figure 10–10 Spinal curvatures.

commonly known as *swayback*. It may be caused by increased weight of the abdominal contents, resulting from obesity or excessive weight gain during pregnancy. Kyphosis and lordosis also occur in combination with scoliosis. Scoliosis also occurs in combination with kyphosis and lordosis.

Joint Disorders

Arthritis, a general term for many joint diseases, is an inflammation of a joint usually accompanied by pain, swelling and, commonly, changes in structure. Because of their location and constant use, joints are prone to stress injuries and inflammation. The main types of arthritis include rheumatoid arthritis, osteoarthritis, and gouty arthritis, or gout.

Rheumatoid arthritis (RA), a systemic disease characterized by inflammatory changes in joints and their related structures, results in crippling deformities. (See Figure 10–11.) This form of arthritis is believed to be caused by an autoimmune reaction of joint tissue. It occurs most commonly in women between ages 23 and 35 but can affect people of any age group. Intensified aggravations **(exacerbations)** of this disease are commonly associated with periods of increased physical or emotional stress. In addition to joint changes, muscles, bones, and skin adjacent to the affected joint atrophy. There is no specific cure, but **nonsteroidal anti-inflammatory drugs (NSAIDs),** physical therapy, and orthopedic measures are used in treatment of less severe cases.

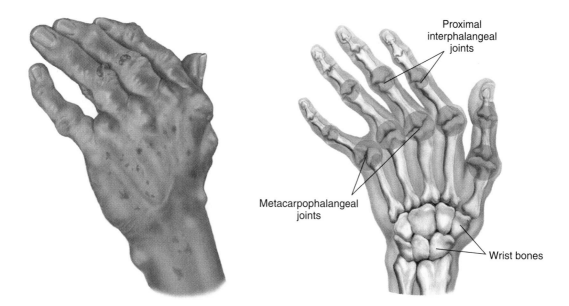

Figure 10–11 Rheumatoid arthritis.

Osteoarthritis, also called *degenerative joint disease (DJD),* is the most common type of connective tissue disease. Cartilage destruction and new bone formation at the edges of joints **(spurs)** are the most common pathologies seen with osteoarthritis. Even though osteoarthritis is less crippling than rheumatoid arthritis, it may result in fusion of two bone surfaces, thereby completely immobilizing the joint. In addition, small, hard nodules may form at the distal interphalangeal joints of the fingers **(Heberden nodes).**

Gouty arthritis, also called *gout,* is a metabolic disease caused by the accumulation of uric acid crystals in blood. These crystals may become deposited in joints and soft tissue near joints, causing painful swelling and inflammation. Although the joint chiefly affected is the big toe, any joint may be involved. Commonly, renal calculi **(nephrolithiasis)** form because of uric acid crystals collecting in the kidney.

Muscle Disorders

Disorders involving the muscles include muscular dystrophy and myasthenia gravis.

Muscular Dystrophy

Muscular dystrophy, a genetic disease, is characterized by gradual **atrophy** and weakening of muscle tissue. There are several types of muscular dystrophy. The most common type, *Duchenne dystrophy,* affects children, boys more commonly than girls. It is transmitted as a sex-linked disease passed from mother to son. As muscular dystrophy progresses, the loss of muscle function affects not only skeletal muscle but also cardiac muscle. At present, there is no cure for this disease, and most children with muscular dystrophy die before the age of 20 years.

Myasthenia Gravis

Myasthenia gravis (MG), a neuromuscular disorder, causes fluctuating weakness of certain skeletal muscle groups (of the eyes, face and, to a lesser degree, the limbs). It is characterized by destruction of the receptors in the synaptic region that respond to acetylcholine, a substance that transmits nerve impulses **(neurotransmitter).** As the disease progresses, the muscle becomes increasingly weak and may eventually cease to function altogether. Women tend to be affected slightly more than men. Initial symptoms include a weakness of the eye muscles and difficulty swallowing **(dysphagia).** Later, the individual has difficulty chewing and talking. Eventually, the muscles of the limbs may become involved.

Oncology

The two major types of malignancies that affect bone are those that arise directly from bone or bone tissue, called *primary bone cancer,* and those that arise in another region of the body and spread (metastasize) to bone, called *secondary bone cancer.* Primary bone cancers are very rare, but secondary bone cancers are quite prevalent. They are usually caused by malignant cells that have metastasized to the bone from the lungs, breast, or prostate.

Malignancies that originate from bone, fat, muscle, cartilage, bone marrow, and cells of the lymphatic system are called *sarcomas.* Three major types of sarcomas include *fibrosarcoma, osteosarcoma,* and *Ewing sarcoma.* Fibrosarcoma develops in cartilage and generally affects the pelvis, upper legs, and shoulders. The fibrosarcoma patient population is usually between ages 50 and 60. Osteosarcoma develops from bone tissue, and generally affects the knees, upper arms, and upper legs. The osteosarcoma patient population is usually between ages 20 and 25. Ewing sarcoma develops from primitive nerve cells in bone marrow. It usually affects the shaft of long bones but may occur in the pelvis or other bones of the arms or legs. This disease usually affects young boys between ages 10 and 20.

Signs and symptoms of sarcoma include swelling and tenderness, with a tendency toward fractures in the affected area. MRI, bone scan, and CT scan are diagnostic tests that assist in identifying bone malignances. All malignancies, including Ewing sarcoma, are staged and graded to determine the extent and degree of malignancy. This staging helps the physician determine an appropriate treatment modality. Generally, combination therapy is used, including chemotherapy for management of metastasis and radiation when the tumor is radiosensitive. In some cases, amputation is required.

Diagnostic, Symptomatic, and Related Terms

This section introduces diagnostic, symptomatic, and related terms and their meanings. Word analyses for selected terms are also provided.

Term	Definition
ankylosis ăng-kĭ-LŌ-sĭs *ankyl:* stiffness, bent, crooked *-osis:* abnormal condition, increase (used primarily with blood cells)	Stiffening and immobility of a joint as a result of disease, trauma, surgery, or abnormal bone fusion
carpal tunnel syndrome (CTS) KĂR-păl	Painful condition resulting from compression of the median nerve within the carpal tunnel (wrist canal through which the flexor tendons and the median nerve pass)
claudication klăw-dĭ-KĀ-shŭn	Lameness, limping
contracture kŏn-TRĂK-chūr	Fibrosis of connective tissue in skin, fascia, muscle, or joint capsule that prevents normal mobility of the related tissue or joint
crepitation krĕp-ĭ-TĀ-shŭn	Dry, grating sound or sensation caused by bone ends rubbing together, indicating a fracture or joint destruction
electromyography ē-lĕk-trō-mi-ŎG-ră-fē *electr/o:* electric *my/o:* muscle *-graphy:* process of recording	Use of electrical stimulation to record the strength of muscle contraction
exacerbation ĕks-ăs-ĕr-BĀ-shŭn	Increase in severity of a disease or of any of its symptoms
ganglion cyst GĂNG-lē-ŏn SĬST	Tumor of tendon sheath or joint capsule, commonly found in the wrist *The cyst is aspirated and injected with an anti-inflammatory agent.*
hypotonia hi-pō-TŌ-nē-ă *hypo-:* under, below, deficient *ton:* tension *-ia:* conditon	Loss of muscular tone or a diminished resistance to passive stretching
hemarthrosis hĕm-ăr-THRŌ-sĭs *hem:* blood *arthr:* joint *-osis:* abnormal condition; increase (used primarily with blood cells)	Effusion of blood into a joint cavity

(Continued)

Term	Definition	(Continued)

multiple myeloma
MŬL-tĭ-p'l
mī-ĕ-LŌ-mă
   myel: bone marrow; spinal cord
   -oma: tumor
	Primary malignant tumor that infiltrates the bone and red bone marrow
	Multiple myeloma is a progressive and typically fatal disease that causes multiple tumor masses, which commonly cause bone fractures.	

osteophyte ŎS-tē-ō-fit	Bony outgrowth that occasionally develops on the vertebra and may exert pressure on the spinal cord	
phantom limb FĂN-tŭm LĬM	Perceived sensation, following amputation of a limb, that the limb still exists *The sensation that pain exists in the removed part is known as phantom limb pain.*	
prosthesis prŏs-THĒ-sĭs	Replacement of a missing part by an artificial substitute, such as an artificial extremity	
rickets, rachitis RĬK-ĕts, ră-KĪ-tĭs	Form of osteomalacia in children caused by vitamin D deficiency	

sequestrum
sē-KWĔS-trŭm
   sequestr: separation
   -um: structure, thing
	Fragment of necrosed bone that has become separated from surrounding tissue	

spondylolisthesis spŏn-dĭ-lō-lĭs-THĒ-sĭs	Any forward slipping (subluxation) of a vertebra over the one below it	

spondylosis
spŏn-dĭ-LŌ-sĭs
   spondyl: vertebrae (backbone)
   -osis: abnormal condition; increase (used primarily with blood cells)
	Degeneration of the cervical, thoracic, and lumbar vertebrae and related tissues
	Spondylosis may cause pressure on nerve roots with subsequent pain or paresthesia in the extremities.	

sprain SPRĀN	Tearing of ligament tissue that may be slight, moderate, or complete *A complete tear of a major ligament is especially painful and disabling. Ligamentous tissue does not heal well because of poor blood supply. Treatment usually consists of surgical reconstruction of the severed ligament.*	
strain STRĀN	To exert physical force in a manner that may result in injury, usually muscular	
subluxation sŭb-lŭk-SĀ-shŭn	Partial or incomplete dislocation	

Term	Definition
talipes TĂL-ĭ-pēz	Any number of foot deformities, especially those occurring congenitally; also called *clubfoot* (See Figure 10–12.)

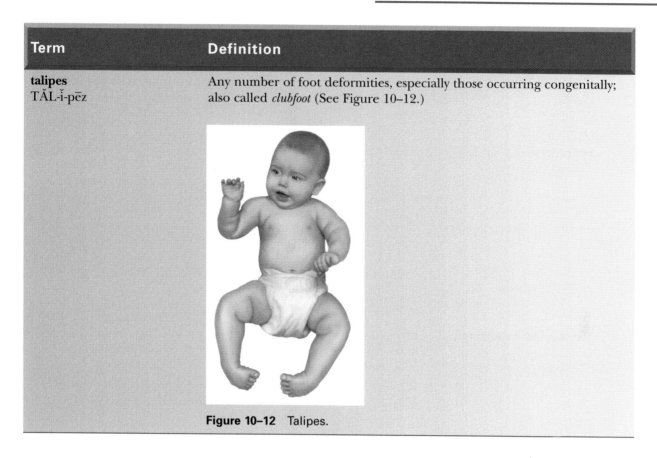

Figure 10–12   Talipes.

 It is time to review pathological, diagnostic, symptomatic, and related terms by completing Learning Activity 10–5.

 ## Diagnostic and Therapeutic Procedures

This section introduces procedures used to diagnose and treat musculoskeletal disorders. Descriptions are provided as well as pronunciations and word analyses for selected terms.

Procedure	Description
DIAGNOSTIC PROCEDURES	
Radiographic	
arthrography ăr-THRŎG-ră-fē *arthr/o:* joint *-graphy:* process of recording	Series of radiographs taken after injection of a radiopaque substance into a joint cavity, especially the knee or shoulder, to outline the contour of the joint

(Continued)

Procedure	Description	(Continued)
computed tomography (CT) scan kŏm-PŪ-tĕd tō-MŎG-ră-fē *tom/o:* to cut *-graphy:* process of recording	Imaging technique achieved by rotating an x-ray emitter around the area to be scanned and measuring the intensity of transmitted rays from different angles; formerly called *computerized axial tomography* (See Figure 4–4D.) *A bone scan is performed to evaluate skeletal involvement related to connective tissue disease; a joint scan is performed to determine joint damage throughout the entire body and is one of the most sensitive studies for early detection of joint disease.*	
dual energy x-ray absorptiometry (DEXA)	Technique to measure bone density for purposes of diagnosis and management of osteoporosis	
discography	Radiological examination of the intervertebral disk structures by injecting a contrast medium *Discography is used to diagnose suspected cases of herniated disk.*	
lumbosacral spinal radiography (LS spine) LŬM-bō-sā-krăl SPĪ-năl *lumb/o:* loins (lower back) *sacr:* sacrum *-al:* pertaining to, relating to *radi/o:* radiation, x-ray, radius (lower arm bone on thumb side) *-graphy:* process of recording	Radiography of the five lumbar vertebrae and the fused sacral vertebrae, including anteroposterior, lateral, and oblique views of the lower spine *The most common indication for lumbosacral spine radiography is lower back pain. It is used to identify or differentiate traumatic fractures, spondylosis, spondylolisthesis, and metastatic tumor.*	
myelography MĪ-ĕ-lŏg-ră-fē *myel/o:* bone marrow, spinal cord *-graphy:* process of recording	Radiography of the spinal cord after injection of a contrast medium to identify and study spinal distortions caused by tumors, cysts, herniated intervertebral disks, or other lesions	

THERAPEUTIC PROCEDURES

closed reduction	Manual correction of fractures without incision *Following reduction, the bone is immobilized with an external device to maintain proper alignment during the healing process.*	
casting	Application of a solid, stiff dressing formed with plaster of Paris or other material to a body part to immobilize it during the healing process	
splinting	Use of an orthopedic device to an injured body part for immobilization, stabilization, and protection during the healing process *A splint is constructed from wood, metal, or plaster of Paris and may be movable or immovable.*	
traction	Using weights and pulleys to align or immobilize a fracture and facilitate the healing process	

Procedure	Description
Surgical	
amputation ăm-pŭ-TĀ-shŭn	Partial or complete removal of a limb
arthrocentesis ăr-thrō-sĕn-TĒ-sĭs *arthr/o:* joint *-centesis:* surgical puncture	Puncture of a joint space to remove accumulated fluid
arthroclasia ăr-thrō-KLĀ-zē-ă *arthr/o:* joint *-clasia:* to break; surgical fracture	Surgical breaking of an ankylosed joint to provide movement
arthroscopy ăr-THRŎS-kō-pē *arthr/o:* joint *-scopy:* visual examination	Visual examination of a joint, especially the knee; used primarily to detect trauma or lesions and to obtain a biopsy of synovial tissue for microscopic examination
bursectomy bĕr-SĔK-tō-mē	Excision of bursa (padlike sac or cavity found in connective tissue, usually in the vicinity of joints)
bone grafting BŌN GRĂFT-ing	Implanting or transplanting bone tissue from another part of the body or from another person to serve as replacement for damaged or missing bone tissue
laminectomy lăm-ĭ-NĔK-tō-mē	Excision of the posterior arch of a vertebra *Laminectomy is most commonly performed to relieve the symptoms of a ruptured intervertebral (slipped) disk.*
open reduction	Treatment of bone fractures using surgery to place the bones in proper position
sequestrectomy sē-kwĕs-TRĔK-tō-mē	Excision of a sequestrum (segment of necrosed bone)
synovectomy sĭn-ō-VĔK-tō-mē	Excision of a synovial membrane

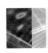

Pharmacology

Unlike other medications that treat specific disease, most pharmacological agents for musculoskeletal disorders are used to treat symptoms. (See Table 10–3.) Acute musculoskeletal conditions, such as strains, sprains, and "pulled muscles," are treated with analgesics and anti-inflammatory drugs. Nonsteroidal anti-inflammatory drugs (NSAIDs), salicylates, muscle relaxants, opioid analgesics, or narcotics are commonly used to treat pain either by anesthetizing (numbing) the area or by decreasing the inflammation. NSAIDs and salicylates are also used to treat arthritis, in addition to gold salts. Calcium supplements are used to treat hypocalcemia.

Table 10-3 DRUGS USED TO TREAT MUSCULOSKELETAL DISORDERS

This table lists common drug classifications used to treat musculoskeletal disorders, their therapeutic actions, and selected generic and trade names.

Classification	Therapeutic Action	Generic and Trade Names
calcium	Treats and prevents hypocalcemia *Over-the-counter calcium supplements are numerous and are contained in many antacids as a secondary therapeutic effect. They are used to prevent osteoporosis when normal diet is lacking adequate amounts of calcium.*	**calcium carbonate** KĂL-sē-ŭm KĂR-bŏn-āt 　*Alka-Mints Calcarb, Calci-Mix,* 　*Oystercal, Tums* **calcium citrate** KĂL-sē-ŭm SĬT-rāt 　*Cal-Citrate 250, Citracal, Citracal* 　*Liquitab*
gold salts	Treat rheumatoid arthritis by inhibiting activity within the immune system *Gold salts contain actual gold in capsules or in solution for injection. This agent prevents further disease progression but cannot reverse past damage.*	**auranofin** aw-RĂN-ă-fĭn 　*Ridaura* **aurothioglucose** aw-rō-thĭ-ō-GLOO-kōs 　*Solganal* **gold sodium thiomalate** GŌLD SŌ-dē-ŭm thĭ-ō-MĂ-lāt 　*Myochrysine*
nonsteroidal anti-inflammatory drugs (NSAIDs)	Relieve mild to moderate pain and reduce inflammation *NSAIDs have fewer GI adverse effects, such as ulcers, than aspirin. They are used to treat acute musculoskeletal conditions, such as sprains and strains, and inflammatory disorders, including rheumatoid arthritis, osteoarthritis, bursitis, gout, and tendinitis.*	**ibuprofen** ī-bū-PRō-fĕn 　*Advil, Excedrin IB, Medipren,* 　*Motrin, Nuprin* **naproxen** nă-PRŎK-sĕn 　*Aleve, Anaprox, Anaprox DS,* 　*EC-Naprosyn* **ketoprofen** kē-tō-PRō-fĕn 　*Actron, Orudis*

Table 10-3	DRUGS USED TO TREAT MUSCULOSKELETAL DISORDERS

Classification	Therapeutic Action	Generic and Trade Names

opioid analgesics	Relieve moderate to severe pain
	
	Opioid analgesics are narcotic drugs that may be derived from opium or synthetically produced. They provide preoperative and postoperative pain relief and sedation and are given by mouth, intramuscularly (I.M.), subcutaneously as a patch, or intravenously (I.V.). Because narcotics have a strong addictive quality, they are prescribed for short periods and used especially for severe back pain and postoperative orthopedic surgical procedures.
		fentanyl
		FĔN-tă-nĭl
		    Sublimaze, Duragesic, Actiq
		hydromorphone
		hĭ-drō-MOR-fōn
		    Dilaudid, Hydrostat IR, PMS Hydromorphone
		meperidine
		mĕ-PĔR-ĭ-dēn
		    Demerol
		morphine
		MOR-fēn
		    Astramorph, Duramorph, MS Contin, Roxanol
		propoxyphene hydrochloride
		prō-PŎK-sē-fēn hĭ-drō-KLŌ-rĭd
		    Darvon

salicylates	Relieve mild to moderate pain and reduce inflammation
	
	Salicylates have anti-inflammatory abilities and alleviate pain. Aspirin is in this drug classification and is known as acetylsalicylic acid (ASA), the oldest drug used to treat arthritis.
		aspirin
		ĂS-pĕr-ĭn
		    Acuprin, ASA, Aspergum, Bayer Aspirin
		magnesium salicylate
		măg-NĒ-zē-ŭm să-LĬS-ĭ-lāt
		    Doan's Regular Strength Tablets, Magan, Mobidin

skeletal muscle relaxants	Relieve muscle spasms and stiffness
	
	Skeletal muscle relaxants are also prescribed to treat conditions involving muscle spasticity, such as cerebral palsy, multiple sclerosis, stroke, and spinal cord injury.
		baclofen
		BĂK-lō-fĕn
		    Lioresal
		carisoprodol
		kăr-ĭ-sō-PRŌ-dŏl
		    Soma, Vanadom
		chlorzoxazone
		klor-ZŎK-să-zōn
		    Paraflex, Parafon Forte DSC, Relaxazone, Remular

Abbreviations

This section introduces musculoskeletal-related abbreviations and their meanings.

Abbreviation	Meaning
ACL	anterior cruciate ligament
AE	above the elbow
AK	above the knee
BE	below the elbow

(Continued)

Abbreviation	Meaning	(Continued)
BK	below the knee	
C1, C2, and so on	first cervical vertebra, second cervical vertebra, and so on	
Ca	calcium; cancer	
CDH	congenital dislocation of the hip	
CTS	carpal tunnel syndrome	
DJD	degenerative joint disease	
EMG	electromyography	
Fx	fracture	
HD	hemodialysis; hip disarticulation; hearing distance	
HNP	herniated nucleus pulposus (herniated disk)	
HP	hemipelvectomy	
IS	intracostal space	
I.M., IM	intramuscular; infectious mononucleosis	
I.V., IV	intravenous	
KD	knee disarticulation	
L1, L2, and so on	first lumbar vertebra, second lumbar vertebra, and so on	
MG	myasthenia gravis	
MS	musculoskeletal; multiple sclerosis; mental status; mitral stenosis	
NSAIDs	nonsteroidal anti-inflammatory drugs	
ORTH, ortho	orthopedics	
P	phosphorous; pulse	
PCL	posterior cruciate ligament	
RA	rheumatoid arthritis	
RF	rheumatoid factor	
ROM	range of motion	
SD	shoulder disarticulation	
THA	total hip arthroplasty	
THR	total hip replacement	
TKA	total knee arthroplasty	
TKR	total knee replacement	

 It is time to review procedures, pharmacology, and abbreviations by completing Learning Activity 10–6.

LEARNING ACTIVITIES

The following activities provide review of the musculoskeletal system terms introduced in this chapter. Complete each activity and review your answers to evaluate your understanding of the chapter.

Learning Activity 10–1

Identifying muscle structures

Label the following illustration using the terms listed below.

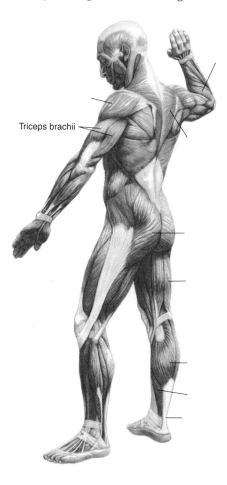
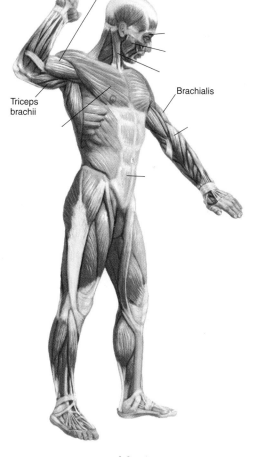

Achilles tendon	*gastrocnemius*	*rectus abdominus*
biceps brachii	*gluteus maximus*	*soleus*
biceps femoris	*masseter*	*sternocleidomastoid*
brachioradialis	*orbicularis oculi*	*trapezius*
deltoid	*pectoralis major*	

 Check your answers by referring to Figure 10–1 on page 265. Review material that you did not answer correctly.

Learning Activity 10–2

Identifying sections of a typical long bone (femur)

Label the following illustration using the terms listed below.

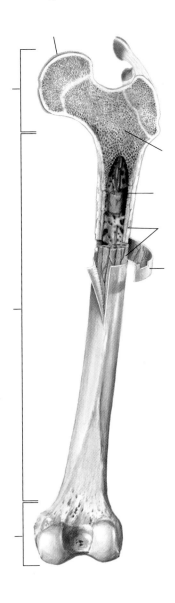

articular cartilage	*distal epiphysis*	*proximal epiphysis*
compact bone	*medullary cavity*	*spongy bone*
diaphysis	*periosteum*	

 Check your answers by referring to Figure 10–3 on page 268. Review material that you did not answer correctly.

Learning Activity 10–3

Identifying skeletal structures

Label the following illustration using the terms listed below.

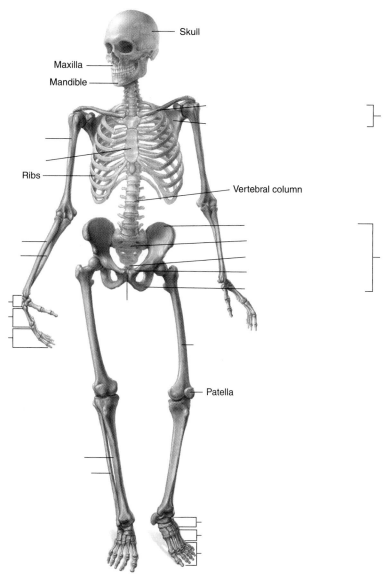

carpals	*ilium*	*phalanges*	*sternum*
clavicle	*ischium*	*pubis*	*symphysis pubis*
coccyx	*metacarpals*	*radius*	*tarsals*
femur	*metatarsals*	*sacrum*	*tibia*
fibula	*pectoral girdle*	*scapula*	*ulna*
humerus	*pelvic girdle*		

✓ Check your answers by referring to Figure 10–4 on page 270. Review material that you did not answer correctly.

Learning Activity 10–4

Building medical words

Use **oste/o** *(bone) to build words that mean:*

1. bone cells _____
2. pain in bones _____
3. disease of bones and joints _____
4. beginning or formation of bones _____

Use **cervic/o** *(neck) to build words that mean:*

5. pertaining to the neck _____
6. pertaining to the neck and arm _____
7. pertaining to the neck and face _____

Use **myel/o** *(bone marrow; spinal cord) to build words that mean:*

8. herniation of the spinal cord _____
9. sarcoma of bone marrow (cells) _____
10. softening of the spinal cord _____
11. resembling bone marrow _____

Use **stern/o** *(sternum) to build words that mean:*

12. pertaining to above the sternum _____
13. resembling the breastbone _____

Use **arthr/o** *(joint) or* **chondr/o** *(cartilage) to build words that mean:*

14. embryonic cell that forms cartilage _____
15. inflammation of a joint _____
16. inflammation of bones and joints _____

Use **pelv/i** *(pelvis) to build a word that means:*

17. instrument for measuring the pelvis _____

Use **my/o** *(muscle) to build words that mean:*

18. twitching of a muscle _____
19. any disease of muscle _____
20. rupture of a muscle _____

Build surgical words that mean:

21. excision of one or more of the phalanges (bones of a finger or toe) _____
22. incision of the thorax (chest wall) _____
23. excision of a vertebra _____
24. binding of a joint _____
25. repair of muscle (tissue) _____

 Check your answers in Appendix A. Review material that you did not answer correctly.

CORRECT ANSWERS _____ × 4 = _____ **% SCORE**

Learning Activity 10–5

Matching pathological, diagnostic, symptomatic, and related terms

Match the following terms with the definitions in the numbered list.

ankylosis	greenstick fracture	necrosis	scoliosis
chondrosarcoma	hematopoiesis	osteoporosis	sequestrum
claudication	hypotonia	phantom limb	spondylitis
comminuted fracture	kyphosis	prosthesis	spondylolisthesis
Ewing sarcoma	muscular dystrophy	pyogenic	subluxation
ganglion cyst	myasthenia gravis	rickets	talipes
gout			

1. _____ incomplete or partial dislocation
2. _____ softening of the bones caused by vitamin D deficiency
3. _____ slipped vertebrae
4. _____ limping
5. _____ degeneration of the muscles
6. _____ congenital deformity of the foot, which is twisted out of shape or position
7. _____ part of dead or necrosed bone that has become separated from surrounding tissue
8. _____ chronic neuromuscular disorder characterized by weakness manifested in ocular muscles
9. _____ an artificial part used for replacement of a missing limb
10. _____ tendon sheath or joint capsule tumor, frequently found in the wrist
11. _____ loss of muscular tonicity; diminished resistance of muscles to passive stretching
12. _____ type of sarcoma that attacks the shafts rather than the ends of long bones

13. _____ bone that is partially bent and partially broken; occurs in children

14. _____ exaggeration of the thoracic curve of the vertebral column; hunchback

15. _____ decrease in bone density; occurs in the elderly

16. _____ deviation of the spine to the right or left

17. _____ cartilaginous sarcoma

18. _____ bone that has splintered into pieces

19. _____ inflammation of the vertebrae

20. _____ metabolic disease caused by accumulation of uric acid, usually in the big toe

21. _____ development and production of blood cells, normally in the bone marrow

22. _____ formation of pus

23. _____ death of cells, tissues, or organs

24. _____ stiffening and immobility of a joint

25. _____ perceived sensation, following amputation, that the limb still exists

✓ Check your answers in Appendix A. Review material that you did not answer correctly.

CORRECT ANSWERS _____ × **4** = _____ **% SCORE**

Learning Activity 10–6

Matching procedures, pharmacology, and abbreviations

Match the following terms with the definitions in the numbered list.

ACL	*closed reduction*	*myelography*
amputation	*CPT*	*open reduction*
arthrodesis	*gold salts*	*relaxants*
arthrography	*HNP*	*salicylates*
arthroscopy	*laminectomy*	*sequestrectomy*

1. _____ radiograph of spinal cord after injection of a contrast medium
2. _____ treatment of bone fractures by use of surgery to place bones in proper position
3. _____ used to treat rheumatoid arthritis by inhibiting activity with the immune system
4. _____ painful disorder of the wrist and hand due to compression of the median nerve as it passes through the carpal tunnel
5. _____ excision of the posterior arch of a vertebra
6. _____ series of joint radiographs preceded by injection of a radiopaque substance or air into the joint cavity
7. _____ surgical immobilization of a joint
8. _____ partial or complete removal of a limb
9. _____ herniated nucleus pulposus
10. _____ relieve mild to moderate pain and reduce inflammation
11. _____ visual examination of a joint's interior, especially the knee
12. _____ excising a segment of necrosed bone
13. _____ anterior cruciate ligament
14. _____ relieve muscle spasms and stiffness
15. _____ manipulative treatment of bone fractures by placing the bones in proper position without incision

✓ Check your answers in Appendix A. Review any material that you did not answer correctly.

CORRECT ANSWERS _____ × 6.67 = _____ **% SCORE**

MEDICAL RECORD ACTIVITIES

The two medical records included in the activities that follow use common clinical scenarios to show how medical terminology is used to document patient care. Complete the terminology and analysis sections for each activity to help you recognize and understand terms related to the musculoskeletal system.

Medical Record Activity 10–1

Right knee arthroscopy and medial meniscectomy

Terminology

The terms listed in the chart come from the medical record *Right Knee Arthroscopy and Medial Meniscectomy* that follows. Use a medical dictionary such as *Taber's Cyclopedic Medical Dictionary*, the appendices of this book, or other resources to define each term. Then review the pronunciations for each term and practice by reading the medical record aloud.

Term	Definition
ACL	
arthroscopy ăr-THRŎS-kō-pē	
effusions ĕ-FŪ-zhŭnz	
intracondylar ĭn-tră-KŎN-dĭ-lăr	
Lachman test LĂK-măn	
meniscectomy mĕn-ĭ-SĔK-tō-mē	
MRI	
PCL	
synovitis sĭn-ō-VĪ-tĭs	

RIGHT KNEE ARTHROSCOPY AND MEDIAL MENISCECTOMY

POSTOPERATIVE DIAGNOSIS: Torn medial meniscus right knee

TYPE OF ANESTHESIA: General

INDICATIONS FOR PROCEDURE: This 42-year-old woman has jogged for the past 10 years an average of 25 miles each week. She has persistent posterior medial right knee pain with occasional effusions. The patient has MRI documented medial meniscal tear. She now presents for right knee arthroscopy and medial meniscectomy.

OPERATIVE FINDINGS: Examination of the knee under anesthesia showed a full range of motion; no effusion, no instability, and negative Lachman and negative McMurray sign tests. Arthroscopic evaluation showed a normal patellar femoral groove and normal intracondylar notch with normal ACL and PCL, some anterior synovitis, and a normal lateral meniscus and lateral compartment to the knee. The medial compartment of the knee showed an inferior surface, posterior and mid-medial meniscal tear that was flipped up on top of itself. This was resected, and then the remaining meniscus contoured back to a stable rim.

Analysis

Review the medical record *Right Knee Arthroscopy and Medial Meniscectomy* to answer the following questions.

1. Describe the meniscus and identify its location.

   _____

2. What is the probable cause of the tear in the patient's meniscus?

   _____

3. What does normal ACL and PCL refer to in the report?

   _____

4. Explain the McMurray sign test.

   _____

5. Because Lachman and McMurray tests were negative (normal), why was the surgery performed?

   _____

Medical Record Activity 10–2

Radiographic consultation: Tibial diaphysis nuclear scan

Terminology

The terms listed in the chart come from the medical record *Radiographic Consultation: Tibial Diaphysis Nuclear Scan*. Use a medical dictionary such as *Taber's Cyclopedic Medical Dictionary*, the appendices of this book, or other resources to define each term. Then review the pronunciations for each term and practice by reading the medical record aloud.

Term	Definition
buttressing BŬ-trĕs-ĭng	
cortical KOR-tĭ-kăl	
diaphysis dī-ĂF-ĭ-sĭs	
endosteal ĕn-DŎS-tē-ăl	
focal FŌ-kăl	
fusiform FŪ-zĭ-form	
NSAIDs	
nuclear scan NŪ-klē-ăr	
periosteal pĕr-ē-ŎS-tē-ăl	
resorption rē-SORP-shŭn	
tibial TĬB-ē-ăl	

RADIOGRAPHIC CONSULTATION: TIBIAL DIAPHYSIS NUCLEAR SCAN

Dear Dr. Hammuda:

We are pleased to provide the following in response to your request for consultation.

This is an 18-year-old male cross-country runner. He complains of pain for more than 1-month duration, with persistent symptoms over middle 1/3 of left tibia with resting. He finds no relief with NSAIDs.

FINDINGS: Nuclear scan reveals the following. There is focal, increased blood flow, blood pool, and delayed radiotracer accumulation within the left mid-posterior tibial diaphysis. The delayed spot planar images demonstrate focal fusiform uptake involving 50% to 75% of the tibial diaphysis width.

It is our opinion that with continued excessive, repetitive stress, the rate of resorption will exceed the rate of bone replacement. This will lead to weakened cortical bone with buttressing by periosteal and endosteal new bone deposition. If resorption continues to exceed replacement, a stress fracture will occur.

Analysis

Review the medical record *Radiographic Consultation: Tibial Diaphysis Nuclear Scan* to answer the following questions.

1. Where was the pain located?

   _____

2. What medication was the patient taking for pain and did it provide relief?

   _____

3. How was the blood flow to the affected area described by the radiologist?

   _____

4. How was the radiotracer accumulation described?

   _____

5. What will be the probable outcome with continued excessive repetitive stress?

   _____

6. What will happen if resorption continues to exceed replacement?

   _____

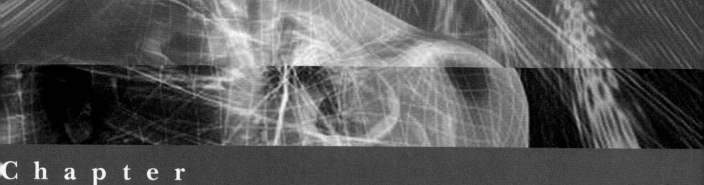

Chapter

11

Genitourinary System

CHAPTER OUTLINE

OBJECTIVES

Upon completion of this chapter, you will be able to:

- Locate and describe the urinary structures as well as the structures of the male reproductive system.

- Recognize, pronounce, spell, and build words related to the genitourinary system.

- Describe pathological conditions, diagnostic and therapeutic procedures, and other terms related to the genitourinary system.

- Explain pharmacology related to the treatment of urinary disorders as well as male reproductive disorders.

- Demonstrate your knowledge of this chapter by completing the learning and medical record activities.

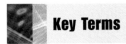

Key Terms

This section introduces important genitourinary system terms and their definitions. Word analyses are also provided.

Term	Definition
cortex KOR-tĕks	Outer layer of an organ or body structure
electrolytes ē-LĔK-trō-līts	Mineral salts (sodium, potassium, and calcium) that carry an electric charge in solution *A proper balance of electrolytes is essential to the normal functioning of the entire body but especially nerves, muscles, and heart.*
erythropoietin (EPO) ĕ-rĭth-rō-POY-ĕ-tĭn	Glycoprotein hormone produced by certain cells in the kidney *Erythropoietin responds to a decrease in oxygen concentration in blood by stimulating stem cells in the bone marrow to produce more erythrocytes (red blood cells).*
libido lĭ-BĒ-dō	Sexual desire or drive, either conscious or unconscious

meatus
 mē-Ā-tŭs
 	
   meat: opening, meatus
   -us: condition; structure
	An opening or passage through any part of the body

medulla mĕ-DŬL-lă	Inner or central portion of an organ
micturition mĭk-tū-RĬ-shŭn	The discharge of urine; urination
nitrogenous wastes nī-TRŎJ-ĕn-ŭs	Products of cellular metabolism that contain nitrogen *Nitrogenous wastes include urea, uric acid, creatine, creatinine, and ammonia.*
orifice OR-ĭ-fĭs	Opening, entrance, or outlet of any body cavity

percutaneous
 pĕr-kū-TĀ-nē-ŭs
 	
   per: through
   cutane: skin
   -ous: pertaining to, relating to
	Procedure performed through the skin, as in a biopsy

reflux RĒ-flŭks	Backward or return flow of a fluid, such as *vesicoureteral reflux*, where urine backs up into the renal pelvis
urea ū-RĒ-ă	Principal nitrogenous end product of protein metabolism excreted in urine and perspiration

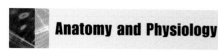

Anatomy and Physiology

The male and female urinary systems have similar structures. In the male, however, some of the urinary structures also have reproductive functions. Thus, the *genitourinary system* includes the urinary system of both the male and female and the reproductive system of the male.

Urinary System

The purpose of the urinary system is to regulate extracellular fluids (plasma, tissue fluid, and lymph) of the body by removing a variety of harmful substances from plasma while retaining useful products. Harmful substances, including **nitrogenous wastes** and excess **electrolytes** (sodium, potassium, and calcium), are excreted from the body as urine, while useful products are returned to the blood. Nitrogenous wastes are toxic to the body, and must be continuously eliminated or death will occur. Electrolyte concentration must remain fairly constant for proper functioning of nerves, heart, and muscles. The kidneys also secrete **erythropoietin,** a hormone that acts on bone marrow to stimulate production of red blood cells when blood oxygen levels are low.

Four major types of structures make up the urinary system:

- two kidneys
- two ureters
- bladder
- urethra (See Figure 11–1.)

The (1) **kidneys,** each about the size of a fist, are located in the abdominal cavity slightly above the waistline. Because they lie outside of the peritoneum, their location is said to be *retroperitoneal.* A concave medial border gives the kidney its beanlike shape. In a frontal section, two distinct areas are visible, an outer section, the (2) **renal cortex,** and a middle area, the (3) **renal medulla,** which contain portions of the microscopic filtering units of the kidney called *nephrons.* Near the medial border is the (4) **hilum (hilus),** an opening through which the (5) **renal artery** enters and the (6) **renal vein** exits the kidney. The renal artery carries blood that contains waste products to the nephrons for filtering. After waste products are removed, blood leaves the kidney by way of the renal vein.

Waste material, now in the form of urine, passes to a hollow chamber, the (7) **renal pelvis.** This cavity is an enlarged, funnel-shaped extension of the (8) **ureter** where the ureter merges with the kidney. Each ureter is a slender tube about 10 to 12 inches long that carries urine in peristaltic waves to the bladder. They pass behind the bladder and enter its base near the (9) **ureteral orifice.**

The (10) **urinary bladder,** an expandable hollow organ, acts as a temporary reservoir for urine. When empty, the bladder has small folds called *rugae* that allow expansion as the bladder fills. A triangular area at the base of the bladder called the *trigone* is delineated by the openings of the ureters and the urethra.

The base of the trigone forms the (11) **urethra,** the tube that discharges urine from the bladder. The length of the urethra is approximately $1\frac{1}{2}$ inches in women and about 7 to 8 inches in men. In the male, the urethra passes through the prostate gland and the penis. During **micturition,** urine is expelled through the urethral opening, the (12) **urinary meatus.**

Nephron

Microscopic examination of kidney tissue reveals the presence of approximately 1 million nephrons. (See Figure 11–2.) These microscopic structures are responsible for maintaining homeostasis by continually regulating the amount of water, salts, glucose, urea, and other minerals in blood. Substances removed by nephrons are nitrogenous wastes, including

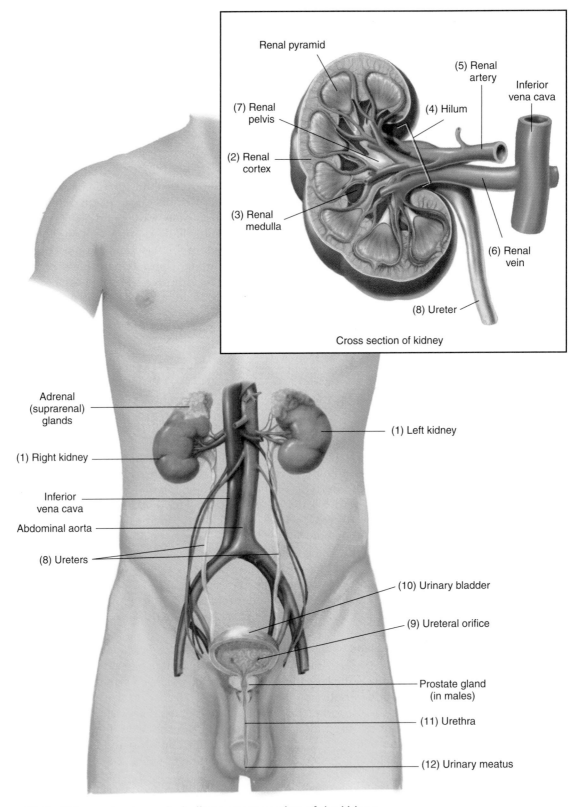

Figure 11–1   Urinary structures, including a cross-section of the kidney.

urea, uric acid, and creatinine, the end products of protein metabolism. Nephrons also remove excess electrolytes and many other products that exceed the amount tolerated by the body.

Each nephron includes a *renal corpuscle* and a *renal tubule.* The renal corpuscle is composed of a tuft of capillaries called the (1) **glomerulus** and a modified, funnel-shaped end of the renal tubule known as (2) **Bowman capsule.** This capsule encases the glomerulus. A larger (3) **afferent arteriole** carries blood to the glomerulus, and a smaller (4) **efferent arteriole** carries blood from the glomerulus. The difference in the size of these vessels provides the needed pressure to force small molecules out of the blood and into Bowman capsule. This process is nonselective, which means that all small molecules—including those needed by the body as well as waste molecules—enter the lumen of the tubule. As the efferent arteriole passes behind the renal corpuscle, it forms the (5) **peritubular capillaries.** These capillaries allow needed products filtered from the blood in Bowman capsule to re-enter the vascular system. Each renal tubule consists of four sections: the (6) **proximal convoluted tubule,** followed by the narrow (7) **loop of Henle,** then the larger (8) **distal tubule** and, finally, the (9) **collecting tubule.** The collecting tubule transports newly formed urine to the renal pelvis for excretion by the kidneys.

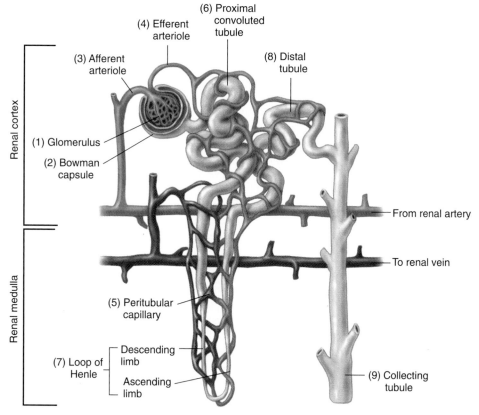

Figure 11–2 Nephron with its associated blood vessels.

The nephron performs three physiological activities as it produces urine:

- *Filtration* occurs in the renal corpuscle, where water, electrolytes, sugar, amino acids, and other small molecules are forced from the blood in the glomerulus into Bowman capsule as a result of increased pressure. The fluid that is formed is called *filtrate.*
- *Reabsorption* begins as filtrate passes through the four sections of the tubule. The tubule reclaims needed substances from the filtrate and returns them to the body for reuse. As filtrate travels the long and twisted pathway of the tubule, most of the water and some of the electrolytes and amino acids are returned to the peritubular capillaries, thus re-entering circulating blood.
- *Secretion* occurs when substances in the capillaries surrounding the distal and collecting tubule secrete ammonia, uric acid, and other substances directly into the tubule, a process that resembles reabsorption, but in the opposite direction. The remaining fluid that enters the collecting tubule is then called urine.

 It is time to review urinary system anatomy by completing Learning Activity 11–1.

Male Reproductive System

The purpose of the male reproductive system is to produce, maintain, and transport sperm, the male sex cell required for the fertilization of the egg. It also produces the male hormone, *testosterone,* which is essential to the development of sperm and male secondary sex characteristics.

The primary male reproductive organ consists of two (1) **testes** (singular, **testis**), located in an external sac called the (2) **scrotum.** (See Figure 11–3.) Within the testes are numerous small tubes that twist and coil to form (3) **seminiferous tubules,** which produce sperm. The testes also secrete testosterone, which develops and maintains secondary sex characteristics. Lying over the superior surface of each testis is a single, tightly coiled tube, the (4) **epididymis.** This structure stores sperm after it leaves the seminiferous tubules. The epididymis is the first duct through which sperm passes after its production in the testes. Tracing the duct upward, the epididymis forms the (5) **vas deferens (seminal duct** or **ductus deferens),** a narrow tube that passes through the inguinal canal into the abdominal cavity. The vas deferens extends over the top and down the posterior surface of the bladder, where it joins the (6) **seminal vesicle.** The union of the vas deferens with the duct from the seminal vesicle forms the (7) **ejaculatory duct.** The seminal vesicle contains nutrients that support sperm viability and secretes approximately 60% of the seminal fluid that is ultimately ejaculated during sexual intercourse (coitus). The ejaculatory duct passes at an angle through the (8) **prostate gland,** a triple-lobed organ fused to the base of the bladder. The prostate gland secretes a thin, alkaline substance that accounts for about 30% of seminal fluid. Its alkalinity helps protect sperm from the acidic environments of both the male urethra and the female vagina. The two pea-shaped (9) **bulbourethral (Cowper) glands** are located below the prostate and are connected by a small duct to the urethra. The bulbourethral glands provide alkaline fluid necessary for sperm viability. The (10) **penis** is the male organ of copulation. It is cylindrical and composed of erectile tissue that encloses the (11) **urethra.** The urethra expels both semen and urine from the body. During ejaculation, the sphincter at the base of the bladder closes, which not only stops the urine from being expelled with the semen, but also prevents semen from entering the bladder. The enlarged tip of the penis, the (12) **glans penis,** contains the (13) **urethral orifice (meatus).** A movable hood of skin, called the (14) **prepuce,** or *foreskin,* covers the glans penis.

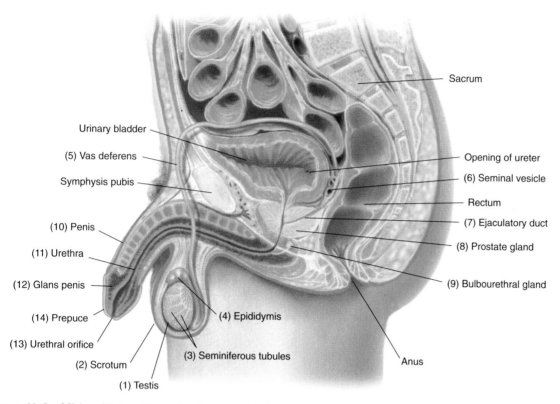

Figure 11–3 Midsagittal section of male reproductive structures shown through the pelvic cavity.

 It is time to review male reproductive anatomy by completing Learning Activity 11–2.

 Medical Word Elements

This section introduces combining forms, suffixes, and prefixes related to the genitourinary system. Word analyses are also provided.

Element	Meaning	Word Analysis
COMBINING FORMS		
Urinary System		
cyst/o	bladder	cyst/o/scope (SĬST-ō-skōp): instrument used to examine and treat lesions of the bladder and ureters *-scope:* instrument for examining
vesic/o		vesic/o/cele (VĚS-ĭ-kō-sēl): herniation of the bladder into the vagina; also called *cystocele* *-cele:* hernia, swelling

(Continued)

Element	Meaning	Word Analysis	(Continued)
glomerul/o	glomerulus	glomerul/o/pathy (glō-měr-ū-LŎP-ă-thē): any disease of the renal glomerulus *-pathy:* disease	
lith/o	stone, calculus	lith/o/tripsy (LĬTH-ō-trĭp-sē): crushing of a stone *-tripsy:* crushing	
meat/o	opening, meatus	meat/o/tomy (mē-ă-TŎT-ō-mē): incision of the urinary meatus to enlarge the opening *-tomy:* incision	
nephr/o	kidney	nephr/o/pexy (NĔF-rō-pĕks-ē): fixation of a floating or dropped kidney *-pexy:* fixation (of an organ)	
ren/o		ren/al (RĒ-năl): pertaining to the kidney *-al:* pertaining to, relating to	
peritone/o	peritoneum	peritone/o/clysis (pĕr-ĭ-tō-nē-ō-KLĪ-sĭs): introduction of a fluid into the peritoneal cavity *-clysis:* irrigation, washing	
pyel/o	renal pelvis	pyel/o/plasty (PĪ-ĕ-lō-plăs-tē): surgical repair of the renal pelvis *-plasty:* surgical repair	
ur/o	urine	ur/o/lith (Ū-rō-lĭth): concretion or stone in any part of the urinary tract *-lith:* stone, calculus	
ureter/o	ureter	ureter/ectasis (ū-rē-tĕr-ĔK-tă-sĭs): dilation of the ureter *-ectasis:* dilation, expansion	
urethr/o	urethra	urethr/o/stenosis (ū-rē-thrō-stĕn-Ō-sĭs): narrowing or stricture of the urethra *-stenosis:* narrowing, stricture	

Male Reproductive System

Element	Meaning	Word Analysis	
andr/o	male	andr/o/gen/ic (ăn-drō-JĔN-ĭk): pertaining to or causing masculinization *gen:* forming, producing, origin *-ic:* pertaining to, relating to	
balan/o	glans penis	balan/o/plasty (BĂL-ă-nō-plăs-tē): surgical repair of the glans penis *-plasty:* surgical repair	
epididym/o	epididymis	epididym/o/tomy (ĕp-ĭ-dĭd-ĭ-MŎT-ō-mē): incision of the epididymis *-tomy:* incision	

Element	Meaning	Word Analysis
orch/o	testis (plural, testes)	orch/itis (or-KĪ-tĭs): inflammation of one or both of the testes -*itis:* inflammation
orchi/o		orchi/algia (or-kē-ĂL-jē-ă): pain in the testes -*algia:* pain
orchid/o		orchid/o/ptosis (or-kĭd-ŏp-TŌ-sĭs): downward displacement of the testes -*ptosis:* prolapse, downward displacement
test/o		test/ectomy (tĕs-TĔK-tō-mē): excision of a testis -*ectomy:* excision, removal
prostat/o	prostate gland	prostat/o/megaly (prŏs-tă-tō-MĔG-ă-lē): enlargement of the prostate gland -*megaly:* enlargement
spermat/o	spermatozoa, sperm cells	spermat/o/cele (spĕr-MĂT-ō-sēl): cystic tumor of the epididymis containing spermatozoa -*cele:* hernia, swelling
sperm/o		sperm/ic (SPĔR-mĭk): pertaining to sperm cells -*ic:* pertaining to, relating to
vas/o	vessel; vas deferens; duct	vas/ectomy (văs-ĔK-tō-mē): removal of all or part of the vas deferens -*ectomy:* excision, removal
varic/o	dilated vein	varic/o/cele (VĂR-ĭ-kō-sēl): dilated or enlarged vein of the spermatic cord -*cele:* hernia, swelling
vesicul/o	seminal vesicle	vesicul/itis (vĕ-sĭk-ū-LĪ-tĭs): inflammation of the seminal vesicle -*itis:* inflammation
Other		
albumin/o	albumin, protein	albumin/oid (ăl-BŪ-mĭ-noyd): resembling albumin -*oid:* resembling
azot/o	nitrogenous compounds	azot/emia (ăz-ō-TĒ-mē-ă): presence of nitrogenous products, especially urea in the blood -*emia:* blood condition *Nitrogenous products are toxic, and if not removed from the body death will result.*
bacteri/o	bacteria	bacteri/uria (băk-tē-rē-Ū-rē-ă): presence of bacteria in urine -*uria:* urine

(Continued)

Element	Meaning	Word Analysis	(Continued)

crypt/o	hidden	crypt/orchid/ism (krĭpt-OR-kĭd-ĭzm): failure of the testes to descend into the scrotum
		
		   orchid: testis (plural, testes)
		   -ism: condition	

gonad/o	gonads, sex glands	gonad/o/pathy (gŏn-ă-DŎP-ă-thē): any disease of the sex glands *-pathy:* disease	

kal/i	potassium (an electrolyte)	hypo/kal/emia (hī-pō-kă-LĒ-mē-ă): abnormally low concentration of potassium in the blood
		
		   hypo-: under, below
		   -emia: blood condition
		
		Hypokalemia may result from excessive urination, which depletes potassium from the body.	

keton/o	ketone bodies (acids and acetone)	keton/uria (kē-tō-NŪ-rē-ă): presence of ketone bodies in the urine *-uria:* urine	
noct/o	night	noct/uria (nŏk-TŪ-rē-ă): excessive and frequent urination after going to bed *-uria:* urine *Nocturia is associated with prostate disease, urinary tract infection, and uncontrolled diabetes.*	

olig/o	scanty	olig/o/sperm/ia (ŏl-ĭ-gō-SPĔR-mē-ă): temporary or permanent deficiency of spermatozoa in semen
		
		   sperm: spermatozoa, sperm cells
		   -ia: condition	

py/o	pus	py/o/rrhea (pī-ō-RĒ-ă): flow or discharge of pus *-rrhea:* discharge, flow	
SUFFIXES			
-cide	killing	sperm/i/cide (SPĔR-mĭ-sīd): agent that kills or destroys sperm, especially when used as a contraceptive; also called *spermaticide* *sperm/i:* spermatozoa, sperm cells	
-genesis	forming, producing, origin	lith/o/genesis (lĭth-ō-JĔN-ĕ-sĭs): formation or production of stones or calculi *lith/o:* stone, calculus	
-iasis	abnormal condition (produced by something specified)	lith/iasis (lĭth-Ī-ă-sĭs): abnormal condition or presence of stones or calculi *lith/o:* stone, calculus	

Element	Meaning	Word Analysis
-ism	condition	an/orch/ism (ăn-OR-kĭzm): congenital absence of one or both testes *an-:* without, not *orch:* testis (plural, testes)
-spadias	slit, fissure	hypo/spadias (hī-pō-SPĀ-dē-ăs): congenital defect in which the urethra opens on the underside of the glans penis instead of the tip *hypo-:* under, below
-uria	urine	poly/uria (pŏl-ē-Ū-rē-ă): excessive formation and excretion of urine *poly-:* many, much
PREFIXES		
dia-	through, across	dia/lysis (dī-ĂL-ĭ-sĭs): procedure that uses a membrane to separate and selectively remove substances from a solution *-lysis:* separation; destruction; loosening
retro-	backward, behind	retro/peritone/al (rĕt-rō-pĕr-ĭ-tō-NĒ-ăl): pertaining to the area behind or outside of the peritoneum *peritone:* peritoneum *-al:* pertaining to, relating to

 It is time to review medical word elements by completing Learning Activity 11–3.

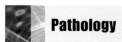 **Pathology**

Pathology of the urinary system includes a range of disorders from those that are asymptomatic to those that manifest an array of signs and symptoms. Causes for these disorders include congenital anomalies, infectious diseases, trauma, or conditions that secondarily involve the urinary structures. Many times, asymptomatic diseases are initially diagnosed when a routine urinalysis shows abnormalities. Forms of glomerulonephritis and chronic urinary tract infection are two such disorders. Symptoms specific to urinary disorders include changes in urination pattern or output and dysuria. Endoscopic tests, radiological evaluations, and laboratory tests that evaluate renal function are typically required to diagnose disorders of the urinary system.

Signs and symptoms of male reproductive disorders include pain, swelling, erectile dysfunction, and loss of **libido.** Characteristics of infectious diseases, especially those transmitted through sexual activity, commonly include pain, discharge, or lesions as well as a vague feeling of fullness or discomfort in the perineal or rectal area. A complete evaluation of the genitalia, reproductive history, and past and present genitourinary infections and disorders is necessary to identify disorders associated with male reproductive structures.

For diagnosis, treatment, and management of genitourinary disorders, the medical services of a specialist may be warranted. *Urology* is the branch of medicine concerned with male and female urinary disorders and diseases of the male reproductive system. The physician who specializes in the diagnoses and treatment of genitourinary disorders is known as a *urologist*.

Pyelonephritis

One of the most common forms of kidney disease is *pyelonephritis*, also called *kidney infection* or *complicated urinary tract infection*. In this disorder, bacteria invade the renal pelvis and kidney tissue, often as a consequence of a bladder infection that has ascended to the kidney via the ureters. When the infection is severe, lesions form in the renal pelvis, causing bleeding. The microscopic examination of urine reveals the following: large quantities of bacteria **(bacteriuria)**, white blood cells **(pyuria)**, and, when lesions are present, red blood cells **(hematuria)**. The onset of the disease is usually acute, with symptoms including chills, fever, nausea, and vomiting.

Glomerulonephritis

Any condition that causes the glomerular walls to become inflamed is referred to as *glomerulonephritis*. One of the most common causes of glomerular inflammation is a reaction to the toxins given off by pathogenic bacteria, especially streptococci, that have recently infected another part of the body, usually the throat. Glomerulonephritis is also associated with autoimmune diseases, such as systemic lupus erythematosus, polyarthritis, scleroderma, and diabetes.

When the glomerular membrane is inflamed, it becomes highly permeable. Red blood cells and protein pass through the glomerulus and enter the tubule as urine is being produced. In some cases, protein solidifies in the nephron tubules and forms solid masses that take the shape of the tubules in which they develop. These masses are called *casts*. They commonly pass out of the kidney by way of the urine and may be visible when urine is examined microscopically. The clinical picture for this disease includes blood and protein in the urine **(hematuria and proteinuria)**, and red cells casts, along with hypertension, edema, and impaired renal function. Most patients with acute glomerulonephritis associated with a streptococcal infection recover with no residual kidney damage.

Nephrolithiasis

Stones may form in any part of the urinary tract, but most arise in the kidney; this condition is called *nephrolithiasis*. (See Figure 11–4.) They commonly form when dissolved urine salts begin to solidify. As these stones increase in size, they obstruct urinary structures. As they lodge in the ureters, they cause intense pulsating pain called *colic*. Because urine is hindered from flowing into the bladder, it flows backward **(refluxes)** into the renal pelvis and the tubules, causing them to dilate. This distention is called *hydronephrosis*. Calculi are pulverized using concentrated ultrasound waves or x-rays, called *shockwaves*, directed at the stones from a machine outside the body **(extracorporeal shockwave lithotripsy [ESWL])**. (See Figure 11–5.) For excessively large stones or patients who have contraindications for the procedure, the alternative treatment is stone removal through a small incision in the skin **(percutaneous nephrolithotomy)**.

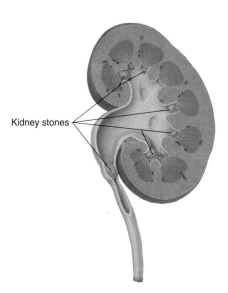

Figure 11–4   Kidney stones in the calices and ureter.

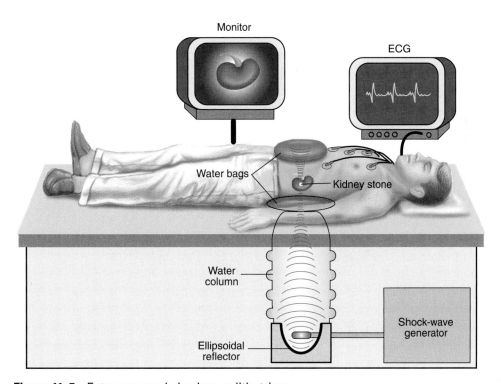

Figure 11–5   Extracorporeal shockwave lithotripsy.

Bladder Neck Obstruction

Any blockage of the bladder outlet is referred to as *bladder neck obstruction (BNO)*. Its causes include an enlarged prostate gland and obstructive masses, such as calculi, blood clots, and tumors. The resulting bladder distention may lead to hydronephrosis accompanied by bladder infection **(cystitis).** The patient experiences a need to void but can only void small quantities at a time **(retention with overflow).** Correction of BNO includes surgery that relieves or removes the obstruction.

Benign Prostatic Hyperplasia

Benign prostatic hyperplasia (BPH), sometimes called *nodular hyperplasia* or *benign prostatic hypertrophy,* is commonly associated with the aging process. (See Figure 11–6.) As the prostate gland enlarges, it decreases the urethral lumen, thus inhibiting complete voiding. Inability to empty the bladder completely may cause cystitis and, ultimately, nephritis. Surgical removal of the prostate may be necessary. Surgical removal may be done through the perineum **(perineal prostatectomy),** urethra **(transurethral resection of the prostate [TURP]),** or an abdominal opening above the pubis and directly over the bladder **(suprapubic prostatectomy).**

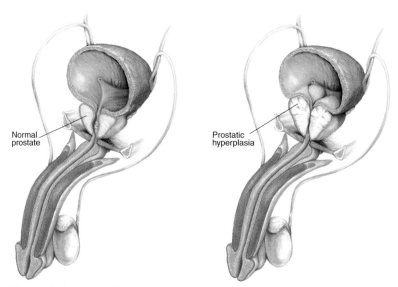

Normal prostate

Prostatic hyperplasia

Figure 11–6   Prostatic hyperplasia.

Cryptorchidism

Failure of the testes to descend into the scrotal sac prior to birth is called *cryptorchidism*. In many infants born with this condition, the testes descend spontaneously by the end of the first year. If this does not occur, correction of the disorder involves surgical suspension of the testes **(orchiopexy)** in the scrotum. This procedure is usually done before the child reaches age 2. Because an inguinal hernia commonly accompanies cryptorchidism, the hernia may be sutured **(herniorrhaphy)** at this time.

Acute Tubular Necrosis

In acute tubular necrosis (ATN), the tubular portion of the nephron is injured through a decrease in blood supply or the presence of toxic substances (usually after ingestion of toxic chemical agents). Two major causes of ATN are ischemia and nephrotoxic injury. Ischemia may be the result of circulatory collapse, severe hypotension, hemorrhage, dehydration, or other disorders that affect blood supply. Signs and symptoms of ATN include scanty urine production **(oliguria)** and increased blood levels of calcium **(hypercalcemia).** When tubular damage is not severe, the disorder is reversible.

Oncology

The second most common form of cancer in men is carcinoma of the prostate. In the United States, the disease is rarely found in men younger than age 50; however, the incidence dramatically increases with age. Susceptibility to the disease is influenced, to a large extent, by race. Incidence is least in Asians, moderate in whites, and high in blacks. Symptoms include difficulty starting urination **(hesitancy)** and stopping the urinary stream, dysuria, urinary frequency, and hematuria. By the time these symptoms develop and the patient seeks treatment, the disease is quite advanced and long-term survival is not likely. Early presymptomatic tests include a blood test for *prostate-specific antigen (PSA)* and periodic *digital rectal examination (DRE)*.

Like other forms of cancer, prostatic carcinomas are staged and graded to determine metastatic potential, response to treatment, survival, and appropriate forms of therapy. Because prostatic cancer is stimulated by testosterone, surgical removal of the testes **(bilateral orchiectomy)** and administration of estrogens temporarily arrest metastatic prostatic cancer.

Diagnostic, Symptomatic, and Related Terms

This section introduces diagnostic, symptomatic, and related terms and their meanings. Word analyses for selected terms are also provided.

Term	Definition
URINARY SYSTEM	
anuria ăn-Ū-rē-ă *an-:* without, not *-uria:* urine	Absence of urine production or urinary output *Anuria may be obstructive, in which there is blockage proximal to the bladder, or unobstructive, which is caused by severe damage to the nephrons of the kidneys.*
azotemia ăz-ō-TĒ-mē-ă *azot:* nitrogenous compounds *-emia:* blood condition	Retention of excessive amounts of nitrogenous compounds (urea, creatinine, and uric acid) in the blood; also called *uremia*
chronic renal failure KRŎ-nĭk RĒ-năl	Renal failure that occurs over a period of years, in which the kidneys lose their ability to maintain volume and composition of body fluids with normal dietary intake *Chronic renal failure is the result of decreased numbers of functioning nephrons in the kidneys.*
dysuria dĭs-Ū-rē-ă *dys-:* bad; painful; difficult *-uria:* urine	Painful or difficult urination *Dysuria is a symptom of numerous conditions.*
enuresis ĕn-ū-RĒ-sĭs *en-:* in, within *ur:* urine *-esis:* condition	Involuntary discharge of urine; also called *incontinence* *Enuresis that occurs during the night is called* nocturnal enuresis; *during the day,* diurnal enuresis.
fistula FĬS-tū-lă	Abnormal passage from a hollow organ to the surface or from one organ to another
frequency FRĒ-kwĕn-sē	Voiding at frequent intervals
hesitancy HĔZ-ĭ-tĕn-sē	Involuntary delay in initiating urination

Term	Definition
nephrotic syndrome ně-FRŎT-ĭk *nephr/o:* kidney *-tic:* pertaining to, relating to	Loss of large amounts of plasma protein, usually albumin, by way of urine, due to increased permeability of the glomerular membrane *Hypoproteinemia, edema, and hyperlipidemia are commonly associated with nephrotic syndrome.*
nocturia nŏk-TŪ-rē-ă *noct:* night *-uria:* urine	Excessive or frequent urination after going to bed *Nocturia is typically caused by excessive fluid intake, uncontrolled diabetes mellitus, urinary tract infections, prostate disease, impaired renal function, or the use of diuretics.*
oliguria ōl-ĭg-Ū-rē-ă *olig:* scanty *-uria:* urine	Diminished capacity to form and pass urine so that the end products of metabolism cannot be excreted efficiently *Oliguria is usually caused by fluid and electrolyte imbalances, renal lesions, or urinary tract obstruction.*
urgency ŪR-jĕn-sē	Feeling of the need to void immediately *Urinary urgency commonly occurs in urinary tract infections (UTIs).*
urolithiasis ū-rō-lĭ-THĪ-ă-sĭs *ur/o:* urine *lith:* stone, calculus *-iasis:* abnormal condition (produced by something specified)	Presence of stones in any urinary structure *Urolithiasis is commonly treated by pulverizing the stones with extracorporeal shockwave lithotripsy.*
Wilms tumor VĬLMZ TOO-mĕr	Rapidly developing malignant neoplasm of the kidney that usually occurs in children *Diagnosis of Wilms tumor is established by an excretory urogram with tomography. The tumor is well encapsulated in the early stage but may metastasize to other sites, such as lymph nodes and lungs.*
Male Reproductive System	
anorchidism ăn-OR-kĭ-dĭzm *an-:* without, not *orchid:* testis (plural, testes) *-ism:* condition	Congenital absence of one or both testes; also called *anorchia* or *anorchism* *Treatment for anorchidism requires replacement of the male hormone testosterone. Boys affected with anorchidism will need testosterone for puberty to occur.*
aspermia ă-SPĔR-mē-ă *a-:* without, not *sperm:* spermatozoa, sperm cells *-ia:* condition	Failure to form or ejaculate semen

(Continued)

Term	Definition	(Continued)
balanitis băl-ă-NĪ-tĭs *balan:* glans penis *-itis:* inflammation	Inflammation of the skin covering the glans penis *Uncircumcised men with poor personal hygiene are prone to this disorder.*	
epispadias ĕp-ĭ-SPĀ-dē-ăs *epi-:* above, upon *-spadias:* slit, fissure	Malformation in which the urethra opens on the dorsum of the penis	
erectile dysfunction ĕ-RĔK-tĭl	Repeated inability to get or keep an erection firm enough for sexual intercourse *Any disorder that causes injury to the nerves or impairs blood flow in the penis has the potential to cause erectile dysfunction.*	
hydrocele HĪ-drō-sēl *hydr/o:* water *-cele:* hernia, swelling	Accumulation of serous fluid in a saclike cavity, especially the testes and associated structures *Hydrocele is common in male newborns but usually resolves within the first year.*	
hypospadias hī-pō-SPĀ-dē-ăs *hypo-:* under, below, deficient *-spadias:* slit, fissure	Developmental anomaly in which the urethra opens on the underside of the penis or, in extreme cases, on the perineum	
phimosis fĭ-MŌ-sĭs *phim:* muzzle *-osis:* abnormal condition; increase (used primarily with blood cells)	Stenosis or narrowing of preputial orifice so that the foreskin cannot be retracted over the glans penis	
sterility stĕr-ĬL-ĭ-tē	Inability to produce offspring; in the male, inability to fertilize the ovum	
varicocele VĂR-ĭ-kō-sēl *varic/o:* dilated vein *-cele:* hernia, swelling	Swelling and distention of veins of the spermatic cord	

It is time to review pathological, diagnostic, symptomatic, and related terms by completing Learning Activity 11–4.

Diagnostic and Therapeutic Procedures

This section introduces procedures used to diagnose and treat genitourinary system disorders. Descriptions are provided as well as pronunciations and word analyses for selected terms.

Procedure	Description
DIAGNOSTIC PROCEDURES	
Clinical	
digital rectal examination (DRE)	Screening test that assesses the rectal wall surface for lesions or abnormally firm areas that might indicate cancer *In DRE, the physician inserts a gloved, lubricated finger into the rectum. In the male, the physician also evaluates the size and consistency of the prostate.*
electromyography ē-lĕk-trō-mī-ŎG-ră-fē *electr/o:* electricity *my/o:* muscle *-graphy:* process of recording	Measures the contraction of muscles that control urination using electrodes placed in the rectum and urethra *Electromyography determines whether incontinence is due to weak muscles or other causes.*
testicular self-examination (TSE)	Self-examination of the testes for abnormal lumps or swellings in the scrotal sac *TSE is increasingly recommended by physicians to detect abnormalities, especially cancer, when the disease is easily treatable. Testicular cancer is the number one cancer killer in men ages 20 to 30.*
Endoscopic	
endoscopy ĕn-DŎS-kō-pē *endo-:* in, within *-scopy:* examination	Visual examination of a cavity or canal using a specialized lighted instrument called an *endoscope* *The organ, cavity, or canal being examined dictates the name of the endoscopic procedure. (See Figure 4–5.) A camera and video recorder are commonly used during the procedure to provide a permanent record.*
cystoscopy sĭs-TŎS-kō-pē *cyst/o:* bladder *-scopy:* examination	Insertion of a cystoscope into the urethra to examine the urinary bladder, obtain biopsies of tumors or other growths, and remove polyps
nephroscopy nĕ-FRŎS-kō-pē *nephr/o:* kidney *-scopy:* examination	Examination of the inside of the kidney(s) using a specialized three-channel endoscope that enables visualization of the kidney and irrigation *The nephroscope is passed through a small incision made in the renal pelvis. Kidney pathology and congenital deformities may also be observed.*
urethroscopy ū-rē-THRŎS-kō-pē *urethr/o:* urethra *-scopy:* examination	Visual examination of the urethra, typically for lithotripsy or TURP

(Continued)

Procedure	Description	(Continued)
Laboratory		
blood urea nitrogen (BUN) ū-RĒ-ă NĪ-trō-jĕn	Test that determines the amount of urea nitrogen, a waste product of protein metabolism, present in a blood sample *Because urea is cleared from the bloodstream by the kidneys, the BUN test can be used as an indicator of kidney function.*	
culture and sensitivity (C&S) KŬL-tūr, sĕn-sĭ-TĬ-vĭ-tē	Test that determines the causative organism of a disease and how the organism responds to various antibiotics *C&S tests are performed on urine, blood, and body secretions.*	
prostate specific antigen (PSA) PRŎS-tāt spĕ-SĬF-ĭk ĂN-tĭ-jĕn	Blood test used to detect prostatic disorders, especially prostatic cancer *PSA is a substance produced by the prostate and is normally found in a blood sample in small quantities. The level is elevated in prostatitis, benign prostatic hyperplasia, and tumors of the prostate.*	
semen analysis SĒ-mĕn ă-NĂL-ĭ-sĭs	Test that analyzes a semen sample for volume, sperm count, motility, and morphology to evaluate fertility or verify sterilization after a vasectomy	
urinalysis (UA) ū-rĭ-NĂL-ĭ-sĭs	Battery of tests performed on a urine specimen, including physical observation, chemical tests, and microscopic evaluation *Urinalysis not only provides information on the urinary structures but may also be the first indicator of such system disorders as diabetes and liver and gallbladder disease.*	
Radiographic		
cystography sĭs-TŎG-ră-fē *cyst/o:* bladder *-graphy:* process of recording	Radiographic examination of the urinary bladder using a contrast medium *Cystography is used to diagnose tumors or defects in the bladder wall, vesicoureteral reflux, stones, or other pathological conditions of the bladder.*	
cystometrography sĭs-tō-mĕ-TRŎG-ră-fē *cyst/o:* bladder *metr/o:* uterus (womb); measure *-graphy:* process of recording	Procedure that assesses volume and pressure in the bladder at varying stages of filling using saline and a contrast medium introduced into the bladder through a catheter *Cystometrography is the primary test used to investigate stress incontinence and urge incontinence.*	

Procedure	Description

cystourethrography
sĭs-tō-ū-rē-THRŎG-ră-fē
 	
  cyst/o: bladder
  urethr/o: urethra
  -graphy: process of recording
	Radiographic evaluation of the urinary bladder and urethra after administration of a contrast medium

voiding (VCUG)	Cystourethrography with additional radiological examination of the bladder and urethra performed before, during, and after voiding *Voiding cystourethrography is performed to determine the cause of repeated bladder infections or stress incontinence and to identify congenital or acquired structural abnormalities of the bladder and urethra.*
kidney, ureter, bladder (KUB) radiography	Radiographic examination to determine the location, size, and shape of the kidneys in relationship to other organs in the abdominopelvic cavity *KUB radiography identifies stones and calcified areas and does not require a contrast medium.*

pyelography
 	
  pyel/o: renal pelvis
  -graphy: process of recording
	Radiographic examination of the ureters and renal pelvis

intravenous (IVP)
  ĭn-tră-Vē-nŭs
 	
    intra-: in, within
    ven: vein
    -ous: pertaining to, relating to
	Radiographic examination of the ureters and renal pelvis after I.V. injection of a contrast medium; also called *excretory urography (EU)* or *intravenous urography (IVU)*
	
	IVP detects kidney stones, an enlarged prostate, internal injuries after an accident or trauma, and tumors in the kidneys, ureters, and bladder.

computed tomography (CT) scan kŏm-PŪ-tĕd tō-MŎG-ră-fē	Imaging technique that rotates an x-ray emitter around the area to be scanned and measures the intensity of transmitted rays from different angles *In the genitourinary system, CT scans are used to diagnose tumors, cysts, inflammation, abscesses, perforation, bleeding, and obstructions of the kidneys, ureters, and bladder.*
nuclear scan, renal	Test used to evaluate blood flow, structure, and functions of the kidneys after I.V. injection of a mildly radioactive substance *A monitor is used to track the radioactive substance as it passes through the kidney.*
ultrasound ŬL-tră-sŏwnd	Test that uses high-frequency sound waves (ultrasound) and displays the reflected "echoes" on a monitor; also called *sonography, echography,* or *echo*
scrotal SKRŌ-tăl	Use of ultrasound to assess patency of the vas deferens and other structures

(Continued)

Procedure	Description	(Continued)

THERAPEUTIC PROCEDURES

Clinical

dialysis
dī-ĂL-ĭ-sĭs

   dia-: through, across
   -lysis: separation;
   destruction; loosening

Passage of a solute through a membrane

hemodialysis
hē-mō-dī-ĂL-ĭ-sĭs

   hem/o: blood
   dia-: through, across
   -lysis: separation;
   destruction; loosening

Removal of toxic substances from the blood by shunting blood from the body through a semipermeable membranous tube (See Figure 11–7.)

At the completion of the process of hemodialysis, the cleansed blood is returned to the body.

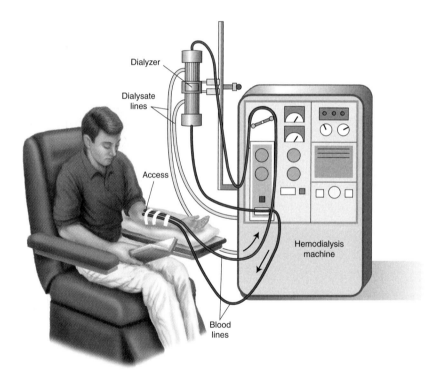

Figure 11–7   Hemodialysis.

Procedure	Description
peritoneal pĕr-ĭ-tō-NĒ-ăl *peritone:* peritoneum *-al:* pertaining to, relating to	Removal of toxic substances from the body by perfusing the peritoneal cavity with a warm, sterile chemical solution (See Figure 11–8.) *In peritoneal dialysis, the lining of the peritoneal cavity is used as the dialyzing membrane. Dialyzing fluid remains in the peritoneal cavity for 1 to 2 hours and then is removed. The procedure is repeated as often as necessary.*
lithotripsy LĬTH-ō-trĭp-sē *lith/o:* stone, calculus *-tripsy:* crushing **extracorporeal shockwave (ESWL)** ĕks-tră-kor-POR-ē-ăl SHŎK-wāv	Procedure for eliminating a stone within the urinary system or gallbladder by mechanically crushing the stone through a surgical incision or using a noninvasive method such as ultrasonic shockwaves to shatter it Use of shockwaves as a noninvasive method to break up stones in the gallbladder or biliary ducts *In ESWL, ultrasound is used to locate the stone or stones and to monitor the destruction of the stones. The patient is usually placed on a course of oral dissolution drugs to ensure complete removal of all stones and stone fragments. (See Figure 11–5.)*

(Continued)

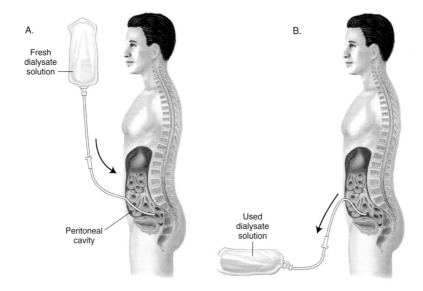

A.
Fresh dialysate solution
Peritoneal cavity

B.
Used dialysate solution

Figure 11–8   Peritoneal dialysis. (A) Introducing dialysis fluid into the peritoneal cavity. (B) Draining dialysate with waste products from peritoneal cavity.

Procedure	Description	(Continued)

Surgical

Procedure	Description
circumcision sĕr-kŭm-SĬ-zhŭn	Removal of all or part of the foreskin, or prepuce, of the penis
nephrolithotomy, percutaneous (PCNL) nĕf-rō-lĭth-ŎT-ō-mē	Removal of a stone from the kidney through a very small incision in the skin *Percutaneous nephrolithotomy is performed when ESWL is not possible, such as when the stone measures larger than 2 cm. It is less complicated than an open operation, allows a quicker recovery time, and has virtually replaced the open method.*
nephropexy NĔF-rō-pĕks-ē *nephr/o:* kidney *-pexy:* fixation (of an organ)	Fixation of a floating or mobile kidney
orchidectomy or-kĭ-DĔK-tō-mē *orchid:* testis (plural, testes) *-ectomy:* excision, removal	Removal of one or both testes; also called *orchiectomy* *Orchidectomy may be indicated for serious disease or injury to the testis or to control cancer of the prostate by removing a source of androgenic hormones.*
resection of the prostate rē-SĔK-shŭn	Partial excision of the prostate gland
transurethral trăns-ū-RĒ-thrăl *trans-:* through, across *urethr:* urethra *-al:* pertaining to, relating to	Procedure to remove prostatic tissue by cauterization or cryosurgery *Transurethral resection of the prostate (TURP) is performed using an endoscope passed through the urethra.*
urethrotomy ū-rē-THRŎT-ō-mē *urethr/o:* urethra *-tomy:* incision	Incision of a urethral stricture *Urethrotomy corrects constrictions of the urethra that make voiding difficult.*

Procedure	Description

vasectomy
văs-ĔK-tō-mē
 	
   vas: vessel; vas deferens; duct
   -ectomy: excision, removal
	Excision of all or a segment of the vas deferens (See Figure 11–9.)
	
	Bilateral vasectomy is the most successful method of male contraception. Although the procedure is considered permanent, with advances in microsurgery, vasectomy is sometimes reversible.

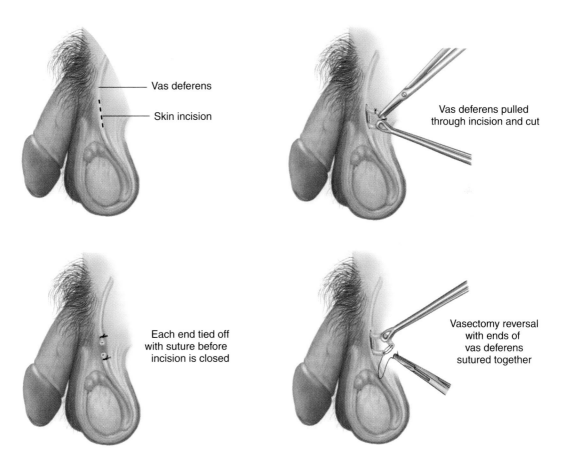

Vas deferens

Skin incision

Vas deferens pulled through incision and cut

Each end tied off with suture before incision is closed

Vasectomy reversal with ends of vas deferens sutured together

Figure 11–9   Vasectomy and reversal.

Pharmacology

This section discusses urinary and male reproductive pharmacologic agents. Urinary tract drugs include antibiotics, diuretics, antidiuretics, urinary antispasmodics, and potassium supplements, commonly taken concurrently with many diuretics to counteract potassium depletion. (See Table 11–1.) Pharmacologic agents are used to treat conditions of the male reproductive system including hypogonadism, erectile disfunction, and reproductive concerns and disorders.

Table 11–1   DRUGS USED TO TREAT GENITOURINARY DISORDERS

This table lists common drug classifications used to treat urinary and male reproductive disorders, their therapeutic actions, and selected generic and trade names.

Classification	Therapeutic Action	Generic and Trade Names
Urinary System		

antibiotics	Inhibit or kill bacterial microorganisms
	
	The most common disorder of the urinary system is urinary tract infection (UTI).
		ciprofloxacin
		sip-rō-FLŎCKS-ă-sĭn
		  Cipro
		levofloxacin
		lē-vō-FLŎKS-ă-sĭn
		  Levaquin
		norfloxacin
		nor-FLŎKS-ă-sĭn
		  Noroxin

antidiuretics	Reduce or control excretion of urine	**vasopressin** văs-ō-PRĔS-ĭn *Pitressin, Pressyn*

antispasmodics	Decrease spasms in the urethra and bladder by relaxing the smooth muscles lining their walls, thus allowing normal emptying of the bladder
	
	Bladder spasms can result from such conditions as UTI and catheterization.
		neostigmine
		nē-ō-STĬG-mĭn
		  Prostigmin
		
		oxybutynin
		ŏk-sē-BŪ-ti-nĭn
		  Ditropan

diuretics	Promote the excretion of urine
	
	Diuretics are grouped by their action and are used to treat edema hypertension, heart failure, and various renal and hepatic diseases.
		bumetanide
		bū-MĔT-ă-nĭd
		  Bumex
		furosemide
		fū-RŌ-sē-mid
		  Lasix
		spironolactone
		spī-rō-nō-LĂK-tōn
		  Aldactone

potassium supplements	Treat or prevent hypokalemia *Potassium supplements are commonly used with diuretics to counteract their potassium-wasting effect. Dietary sources of potassium are usually insufficient to replace potassium lost because of the diuretic.*	**potassium chloride** pō-TĂS-ē-ŭm KLŌ-rĭd *K-Dur, K-Tab*

Table 11–1   DRUGS USED TO TREAT GENITOURINARY DISORDERS

Classification	Therapeutic Action	Generic and Trade Names
Male Reproductive System		

androgens	Increase testosterone levels
	
	Androgens are used to correct hormone deficiency in hypogonadism and treat delayed puberty in males. In females, they are used to suppress tumor growth in some forms of breast cancer.
		testosterone base
		těs-TŎS-těr-ōn
		  Andro, Histerone, Testamone
		testosterone cypionate
		těs-TŎS-těr-ōn SĬP-ē-ō-nāt
		  Andronate, depAndro, Depotest

anti-impotence agents	Treat erectile dysfunction by promoting increased blood flow to the corpus cavernosum to maintain an erection sufficient to allow sexual intercourse	**sildenafil citrate** sǐl-DĔN-ă-fǐl SĬT-răt *Viagra*
spermicides	Chemically destroy sperm before they are able to enter the uterus *Spermicides are available in foam, jelly, gel, and suppositories and are used within the female vagina for contraception. If used within an hour of sexual intercourse, spermicide effectiveness is estimated at about 70% to 80%.*	**nonoxynol 9, octoxynol 9** nŏn-ŎK-sǐ-nŏl, ŏk-TŎKS-ǐ-nŏl *Semicid, Koromex, Ortho-Gynol*

Abbreviations

This section introduces genitourinary-related abbreviations and their meanings.

Abbreviation	Meaning
AGN	acute glomerulonephritis
ARF	acute renal failure
ATN	acute tubular necrosis
BNO	bladder neck obstruction
BPH	benign prostatic hyperplasia; benign prostatic hypertrophy
BUN	blood urea nitrogen
C&S	culture and sensitivity
cath	catheterization; catheter
cysto	cystoscopy

(Continued)

Abbreviation	Meaning	*(Continued)*
DRE	digital rectal examination	
ED	erectile dysfunction; emergency department	
ESRD	end-stage renal disease	
ESWL	extracorporeal shockwave lithotripsy	
EU	excretory urography; also called *intravenous pyelography (IVP)* or *intravenous urography (IVU)*	
GU	genitourinary	
HD	hemodialysis; hip disarticulation; hearing distance	
IVP	intravenous pyelography; also called *excretory urography (EU)* or *intravenous urography (IVU)*	
IVU	intravenous urography (IVU); also called *excretory urography (EU)* or *intravenous pyelography (IVP)*	
K	potassium (an electrolyte)	
KUB	kidney, ureter, bladder	
Na	sodium (an electrolyte)	
PCNL	percutaneous nephrolithotomy	
pH	symbol for degree of acidity or alkalinity	
PSA	prostate-specific antigen	
RP	retrograde pyelography	
sp. gr.	specific gravity	
TSE	testicular self-examination	
TURP	transurethral resection of the prostate (for prostatectomy)	
UA	urinalysis	
VCUG	voiding cystourethrography	

It is time to review procedures, pharmacology, and abbreviations by completing Learning Activity 11–5

LEARNING ACTIVITIES

The activities that follow provide review of the genitourinary system terms introduced in this chapter. Complete each activity and review your answers to evaluate your understanding of the chapter.

Learning Activity 11-1

Identifying urinary structures

Label the following illustration using the terms listed below.

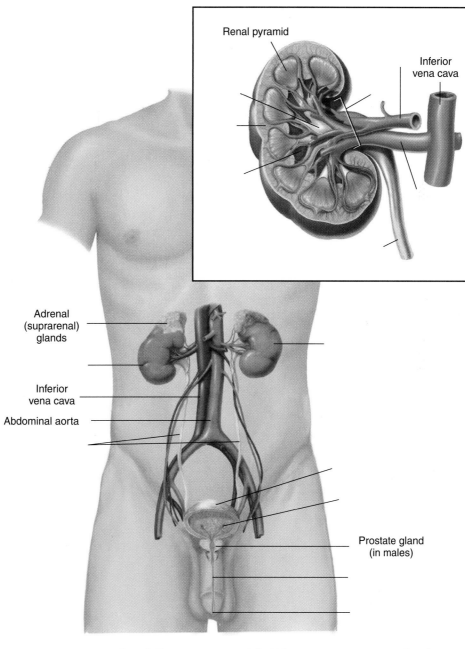

hilum	*renal medulla*	*right kidney*	*ureteral orifice*
left kidney	*renal pelvis*	*ureters*	*urinary bladder*
renal artery	*renal vein*	*urethra*	*urinary meatus*
renal cortex			

 Check your answers by referring to Figure 11–1 on page 310. Review material that you did not answer correctly.

Learning Activity 11–2

Identifying male reproductive structures

Label the following illustration using the terms listed below.

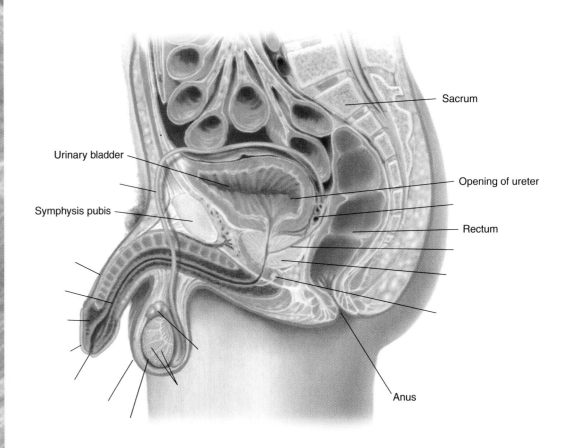

Sacrum

Urinary bladder

Opening of ureter

Symphysis pubis

Rectum

Anus

bulbourethral gland	*prepuce*	*testis*
ejaculatory duct	*prostate gland*	*urethra*
epididymis	*scrotum*	*urethral orifice*
glans penis	*seminal vesicle*	*vas deferens*
penis	*seminiferous tubules*	

✓ Check your answers by referring to Figure 11–3 on page 313. Review material that you did not answer correctly.

Learning Activity 11–3

Building medical words

*Use **nephr/o** (kidney) to build words that mean:*

1. stone in the kidney _____
2. abnormal condition of pus in the kidney _____
3. abnormal condition of water in the kidney _____

*Use **pyel/o** (renal pelvis) to build words that mean:*

4. dilation of the renal pelvis _____
5. disease of the renal pelvis _____

*Use **ureter/o** (ureter) to build words that mean:*

6. dilation of the ureter _____
7. calculus in the ureter _____

*Use **cyst/o** (bladder) to build words that mean:*

8. inflammation of the bladder _____
9. instrument to view the bladder _____

*Use **vesic/o** (bladder) to build words that mean:*

10. herniation of the bladder _____
11. pertaining to the bladder and prostate _____

*Use **urethr/o** (urethra) to build words that mean:*

12. narrowing or stricture of the urethra _____
13. instrument used to incise the urethra _____

*Use **ur/o** (urine) to build words that mean:*

14. radiography of urinary (structures) _____
15. disease of the urinary (tract) _____

*Use the suffix **-uria** (urine) to build words that mean:*

16. difficult or painful urination _____
17. scanty urination _____

*Use **orchid/o** or **orchi/o** (testes) to build words that mean:*

18. disease of the testes _____
19. pain in the testes _____

*Use **balan/o** (glans penis) to build a word that means:*

20. discharge from the glans penis _____

Build surgical words that mean:

21. excision of the testes _____

22. surgical repair of the glans penis _____

23. excision of (all or a segment of) the vas deferens _____

24. incision of the renal pelvis _____

25. fixation of the bladder _____

✓ Check your answers in Appendix A. Review material that you did not answer correctly.

CORRECT ANSWERS _____ × 4 = _____ **% SCORE**

Learning Activity 11–4

Matching pathological, diagnostic, symptomatic, and related terms

Match the following terms with the definitions in the numbered list.

anorchism	epispadias	oliguria
anuria	fistula	orchiopexy
aspermia	herniorrhaphy	phimosis
azotemia	hesitancy	pyuria
balanitis	hydrocele	sterility
benign prostatic hyperplasia	nephrotic syndrome	urgency
enuresis	nocturia	

1. _____ need to void immediately

2. _____ abnormal passage from a hollow organ to the surface or between organs

3. _____ complete absence of one or both testes

4. _____ absence of urine production

5. _____ metabolic wastes in the blood that contain nitrogen

6. _____ fixation of testes in cryptorchidism

7. _____ nonmalignant enlargement of the prostate

8. _____ difficulty starting urination

9. _____ scanty urine production

10. _____ loss of large amounts of plasma protein resulting in systemic edema

11. _____ stenosis of the preputial orifice

12. _____ inability to produce offspring

13. _____ malformation in which the urethra opens on the dorsum of penis

14. _____ lack of or failure to ejaculate semen

15. _____ pus in the urine

16. _____ suture of hernia
17. _____ excessive urination at night
18. _____ involuntary passage of urine
19. _____ accumulation of fluid in a saclike cavity
20. _____ inflammation of skin covering the penis

✓ Check your answers in Appendix A. Review any material that you did not answer correctly.

CORRECT ANSWERS _____ ×5 = _____ **% SCORE**

Learning Activity 11–5

Matching procedures, pharmacology, and abbreviations

Match the following terms with the definitions in the numbered list.

androgens	diuretics	potassium supplements
antibiotics	ESWL	resection
C&S	KUB	semen analysis
circumcision	orchiectomy	urethrotomy
cystoscopy	peritoneal dialysis	vasectomy

1. _____ radiograph that shows the size, shape, and location of the kidneys in relationship to other organs in the abdominopelvic cavity
2. _____ test used to verify sterility after vasectomy
3. _____ visual examination of the urinary bladder
4. _____ inhibit or kill bacterial microorganisms
5. _____ laboratory test that evaluates effect of an antibiotic on an organism
6. _____ drug used to promote the excretion of urine
7. _____ incision of a urethral stricture
8. _____ noninvasive test used to pulverize urinary or bile stones
9. _____ removal of toxic substances by perfusing the peritoneal cavity
10. _____ partial excision of a structure
11. _____ most effective form of male contraception
12. _____ surgical removal of the testes
13. _____ surgical removal of all or part of the foreskin
14. _____ used to increase testosterone levels
15. _____ used to treat or prevent the hypokalemia commonly associated with use of diuretics

✓ Check your answers in Appendix A. Review material that you did not answer correctly.

CORRECT ANSWERS _____ × 6.67 = _____ **% SCORE**

MEDICAL RECORD ACTIVITIES

The two medical records included in the activities that follow use common clinical scenarios to show how medical terminology is used to document patient care. Complete the terminology and analysis sections for each activity to help you recognize and understand terms related to the genitourinary system.

Medical Record Activity 11–1

Operative report: Ureterocele

Terminology

The terms listed in the chart come from the medical record *Operative Report: Ureterocele* that follows. Use a medical dictionary such as *Taber's Cyclopedic Medical Dictionary*, the appendices of this book, or other resources to define each term. Then review the pronunciations for each term and practice by reading the medical record aloud.

Term	Definition
calculus KĂL-kū-lŭs	
cystolithotripsy sĭs-tō-LĬTH-ō-trĭp-sē	
cystoscope SĬST-ō-skōp	
fulguration fŭl-gŭ-RĀ-shŭn	
hematuria hē-mă-TŪ-rē-ă	
resectoscope rē-SĔK-tō-skōp	
transurethral trăns-ū-RĒ-thrăl	
ureterocele ū-RĒ-tĕr-ō-sēl	
urethral sound ū-RĒ-thrăl	

OPERATIVE REPORT: URETEROCELE

PREOPERATIVE DIAGNOSIS: Hematuria with left ureterocele and ureterocele calculus

POSTOPERATIVE DIAGNOSIS: Hematuria with left ureterocele and ureterocele calculus

OPERATION: Cystoscopy, transurethral incision of ureterocele, extraction of stone, and cystolithotripsy

ANESTHESIA: General

PROCEDURE: The patient was prepped and draped and placed in the lithotomy position. The urethra was calibrated with ease, using a #26 French Van Buren urethral sound. A #24 resectoscope was inserted with ease. The prostate and bladder appeared normal, except for the presence of a left ureterocele, which was incised longitudinally; a large calculus was extracted from the ureterocele. There was minimal bleeding and no need for fulguration. The stone was crushed with the Storz stone-crushing instrument, and the fragments were evacuated. The bladder was emptied and the procedure terminated.

Analysis

Review the medical record *Operative Report: Ureterocele* to answer the following questions.

1. Why did the doctor perform a cystoscopy?

   _____

2. What was the name and size of the urethral sound used in the procedure?

   _____

3. What is the function of the urethral sound?

   _____

4. In what direction was the ureterocele incised?

   _____

5. Was fulguration required? Why or why not?

   _____

Medical Record Activity 11–2

Operative report: Extracorporeal shockwave lithotripsy

Terminology

The terms listed in the chart come from the medical record *Operative Report: Extracorporeal Shockwave Lithotripsy* that follows. Use a medical dictionary such as *Taber's Cyclopedic Medical Dictionary*, the appendices of this book, or other resources to define each term. Then review the pronunciations for each term and practice by reading the medical record aloud.

Term	Definition
calculus KĂL-kū-lŭs	
calyx KĀ-lĭx	
cystoscope SĬST-ō-skōp	
cystoscopy sĭs-TŎS-kō-pē	
dorsal lithotomy DOR-săl lĭth-ŎT-ō-mē	
ESWL	
extracorporeal ĕks-tră-kor-POR-ē-ăl	
fluoroscopy floo-or-ŎS-kō-pē	
lithotripsy LĬTH-ō-trĭp-sē	
Lt	
shockwave	
staghorn calculus STĂG-horn KĂL-kū-lŭs	
stent STĔNT	

OPERATIVE REPORT: EXTRACORPOREAL SHOCKWAVE LITHOTRIPSY

PREOPERATIVE DIAGNOSIS: Lt renal calculus

POSOPERATIVE DIAGNOSIS: Lt renal calculus

PROCEDURE: Extracorporeal shockwave lithotripsy, cystoscopy with double-J stent removal

INDICATION FOR PROCEDURE: This 69-year-old male had undergone ESWL on 5/15/xx, with double-J stent placement to allow stone fragments to pass from the calyx to the bladder. At that time, approximately 50% of a partial staghorn calculus was fragmented. He now presents for the fragmenting of the remainder of the calculus and removal of the double-J stent.

PROCEDURE: The patient was brought to the lithotripsy unit and placed in the supine position on the lithotripsy table. After induction of anesthesia, fluoroscopy was used to position the patient in the focal point of the shockwaves. Being well positioned, he was given a total of 4,000 shocks with a maximum power setting of 3.0. After confirming complete fragmentation via fluoroscopy, the patient was transferred to the cystoscopy suite.

The patient was placed in the dorsal lithotomy position and draped and prepped in the usual manner. A cystoscope was inserted into the bladder through the urethra. Once the stent was visualized, it was grasped with the grasping forceps and removed as the scope was withdrawn. The patient tolerated the procedure well and was transferred to Recovery.

Analysis

Review the medical record *Operative Report: Extracorporeal Shockwave Lithotripsy* to answer the following questions.

1. What previous procedures were performed on the patient?

   _____

2. Why is this current procedure being performed?

   _____

3. What imaging technique was used for positioning the patient to ensure that the shock-waves would strike the calculus?

   _____

4. In what position was the patient placed in the cystoscopy suite?

   _____

5. How was the double-J stent removed?

   _____

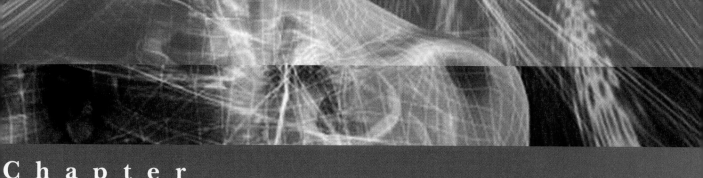

Chapter

12

Female Reproductive System

CHAPTER OUTLINE

OBJECTIVES

Upon completion of this chapter, you will be able to:

- Locate and describe the structures of the female reproductive system.
- Recognize, pronounce, spell, and build words related to the female reproductive system.

- Describe pathological conditions, diagnostic and therapeutic procedures, and other terms related to the female reproductive system.
- Explain pharmacology related to the treatment of female reproductive disorders.
- Demonstrate your knowledge of this chapter by completing the learning and medical record activities.

Key Terms

This section introduces important female reproductive system terms and their definitions. Word analyses are also provided.

Term	Definition
fulguration fŭl-gū-RĀ-shŭn	Destruction of tissue using a high-frequency electrical current *Fulguration of the oviducts via laparoscopy permits gynecologic sterilization.*
genitalia jĕn-ĭ-TĀL-ē-ă	The sex, or reproductive, organs visible on the outside of the body *Female genitalia include the vulva, mons pubis, labia majora, labia minora, clitoris, and Bartholin glands. The male genitalia include the penis, scrotum, and testicles.*
gestation jĕs-TĀ-shŭn	The length of time from conception to birth *The human gestational period typically extends approximately 280 days from the last menstrual period. A gestation (pregnancy) of less than 37 weeks is regarded as premature.*
glans GLĂNZ	Small, rounded mass or glandlike body; erectile tissue at the ends of the clitoris and the penis
lactation lăk-TĀ-shŭn	Production and release of milk by mammary glands
orifice OR-ĭ-fĭs	Mouth; entrance or outlet of any anatomic structure
puerperium pū-ĕr-PĒ-rē-ŭm	Time after childbirth that lasts approximately 6 weeks, during which the anatomic and physiological changes brought about by pregnancy resolve and a woman adjusts to the new or expanded responsibilities of motherhood and nonpregnant life
viable VĪ-ă-b'l	Capable of sustaining life; denotes a fetus sufficiently developed to live outside of the uterus *A viable infant is one who at birth weighs at least 500 g or is 24 weeks or more of gestational age. Because an infant is determined viable does not mean the baby is born alive.*

Anatomy and Physiology

The female reproductive system is composed of internal and external organs of reproduction. The internal organs include the (1) **ovaries,** (2) **fallopian tubes,** (3) **uterus,** (4) **vagina,** and external genitalia. The external genitalia are collectively known as the vulva. Included in these structures are the (5) **labia minora,** (6) **labia majora,** (7) **clitoris,** and (8) **Bartholin glands.** (See Figure 12–1.)

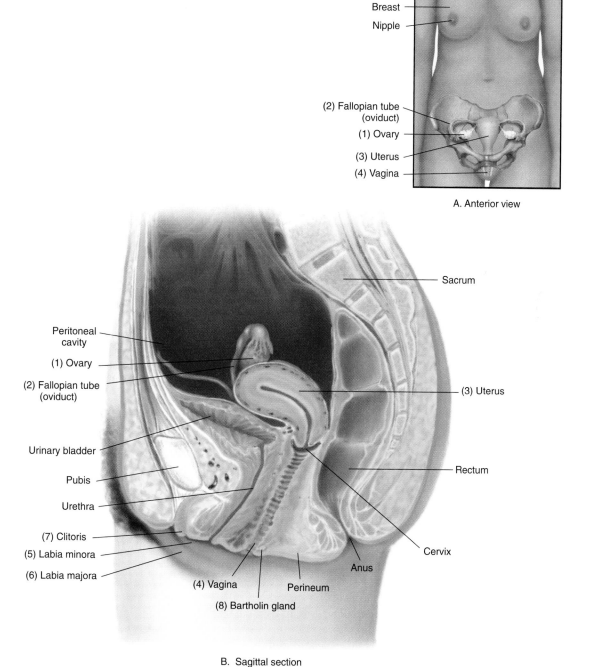

A. Anterior view

B. Sagittal section

Figure 12–1 Female reproductive system. (A) Anterior view. (B) Sagittal section showing organs within the pelvic cavity.

The organs of the female reproductive system are designed to produce **ova** (female reproductive cells), transport the cells to the site of fertilization, provide a favorable environment for a developing fetus through pregnancy and childbirth, and produce female sex hormones. Hormones play an important role in the reproductive process, with each providing its influence at critical times during preconception, fertilization, and **gestation.** (See Figure 12–2.)

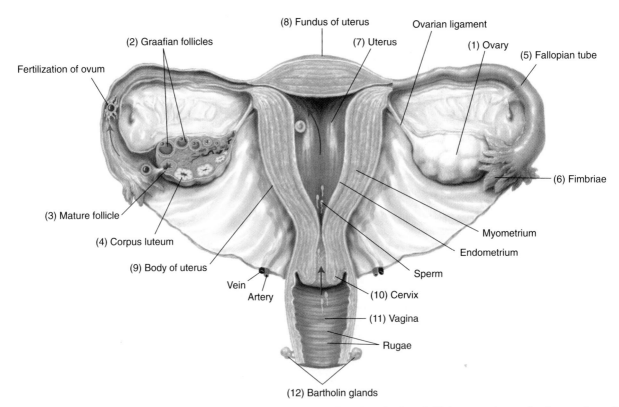

Figure 12–2   Anterior view of female reproductive system. The developing follicles are shown in the sectioned left cavity.

Female Reproductive Organs

Female reproductive organs include the ovaries, fallopian tubes, uterus, and vagina.

Ovaries

The (1) **ovaries** are almond-shaped glands located in the pelvic cavity, one on each side of the uterus. Each ovary contains thousands of tiny, saclike structures called (2) **graafian follicles.** Each of these structures contains an ovum. When an ovum matures, the (3) **mature follicle** moves to the surface of the ovary, ruptures, and releases the ovum, a process called *ovulation.* After ovulation, the empty follicle is transformed into a very different looking structure called the (4) **corpus luteum,** a small yellow mass that secretes estrogen and progesterone. The corpus luteum ultimately degenerates at the end of a nonfertile cycle. Estrogen and progesterone influence the menstrual cycle and menopause. In addition, both hormones prepare the uterus for implantation of the fertilized egg, help to maintain pregnancy, and promote growth of the placenta. Estrogen and progesterone also play an important role in development of secondary sex characteristics. (See Chapter 13, Endocrine System.)

Fallopian Tubes

Two (5) **fallopian tubes (oviducts, uterine tubes)** extend laterally from superior angles of the uterus. The (6) **fimbriae** are fingerlike projections that create wavelike currents (peristalsis) in fluid surrounding the ovary to move the ovum into the uterine tube. If the egg unites with a spermatozoon, the male reproductive cell, fertilization or conception takes place. If conception does not occur, the ovum disintegrates within 48 hours and is discharged through the vagina.

Uterus and Vagina

The (7) **uterus** contains and nourishes the embryo from the time the fertilized egg is implanted until the fetus is born. It is a muscular, hollow, inverted-pear–shaped structure located in the pelvic area between the bladder and rectum. The uterus is normally in a position of anteflexion (bent forward) and consists of three parts: the (8) **fundus,** the upper, rounded part; the (9) **body,** which is the central part; and the (10) **cervix,** also called the *neck of the uterus* or *cervix uteri,* the inferior constricted portion that opens into the vagina.

The (11) **vagina** is a muscular tube that extends from the cervix to the exterior of the body. Its lining consists of folds of mucous membrane that give the organ an elastic quality. During sexual excitement, the vaginal orifice is lubricated by secretions from (12) **Bartholin glands.** In addition to serving as the organ of sexual intercourse and receptor of semen, the vagina discharges menstrual flow. It also acts as a passageway for the delivery of the fetus. The **clitoris** (see Figure 12–1), located anterior to the vaginal orifice, is composed of erectile tissue that is richly innervated with sensory endings. The clitoris is similar in structure to the penis in the male, but is smaller and has no urethra. The area between the vaginal orifice and the anus is known as the **perineum.** (See Figure 12–1.) During childbirth, the obstetrician may decide to surgically incise the area to enlarge the vaginal opening for delivery. If the incision is made, the procedure is called an *episiotomy.*

Mammary Glands

Although mammary glands (breasts) are present in both sexes, they function only in females. (See Figure 12–3.) The breasts are not directly involved in reproduction but become important after delivery. Their biological role is to secrete milk for the nourishment of the newborn, a process called *lactation.* Breasts begin to develop during puberty as a result of periodic stimulation of the ovarian hormones estrogen and progesterone and are fully developed by age 16. Estrogen is responsible for the development of (1) **adipose tissue,** which enlarges the size of the breasts until they reach full maturity. Breast size is primarily determined by the amount of fat around the glandular tissue but is not indicative of functional ability. Each breast is composed of 15 to 20 lobules of milk-producing glands that are drained by a (2) **lactiferous duct,** which opens on the tip of the raised (3) **nipple.** Circling the nipple is a border of slightly darker skin called the (4) **areola.** During pregnancy, the breasts enlarge and remain so until lactation ceases. At menopause, breast tissue begins to atrophy.

Menstrual Cycle

The initial menstrual period, *menarche,* occurs at puberty (about age 12) and continues approximately 40 years, except during pregnancy. The duration of the menstrual cycle is approximately 28 days, during which time several phases occur. (See Table 12–1.)

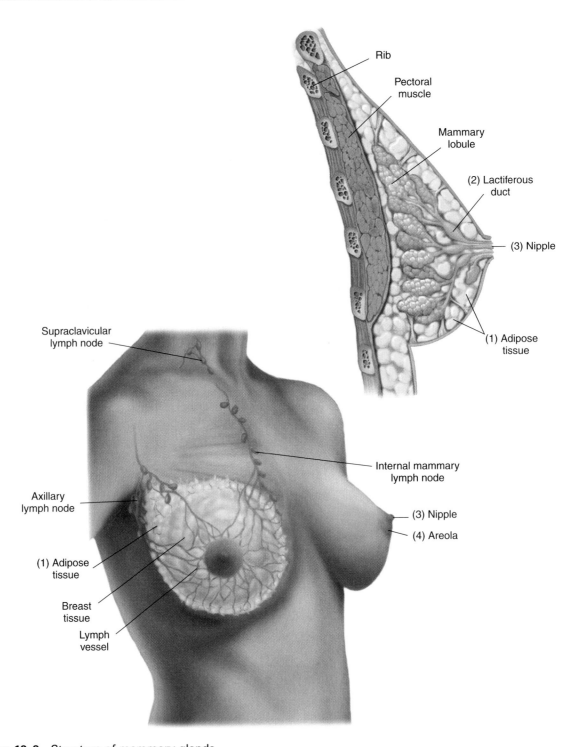

Figure 12–3   Structure of mammary glands.

Table 12-1   CHANGES IN THE MENSTRUAL CYCLE

The menstrual cycle consists of a series of phases, during which the uterine endometrium changes as it responds to changing levels of ovarian hormones. These changes are outlined in the table below. In addition, see Figure 12–4 for an illustration of these changes.

Phase	Description
Menstrual Days 1 to 5	The uterine endometrium sloughs off because of hormonal stimulation, a process that is accompanied by bleeding. The detached tissue and blood are discharged through the vagina as the menstrual flow.
Ovulatory Days 6 to 14	When menstruation ceases, the endometrium begins to thicken as new tissue is rebuilt. As the estrogen level rises, several ova begin to mature in the graafian follicles with only one ovum reaching full maturity. About the 14th day of the cycle the graafian follicle ruptures, releasing the egg, a process called *ovulation*. The egg then leaves the ovary and travels down the fallopian tube toward the uterus.
Postovulatory Days 15 to 28	The empty graafian follicle fills with a yellow material and is now called the corpus luteum. Secretions of estrogen and progesterone by the corpus luteum stimulate the building of the endometrium in preparation for the implantation of an embryo. If fertilization does not occur, the corpus luteum begins to degenerate as estrogen and progesterone levels decline.* With the decrease of hormone levels, the uterine lining begins to shed, the menstrual cycle starts over again, and the first day of menstruation starts.

*Some women experience a loose grouping of symptoms called *premenstrual syndrome (PMS)*. These symptoms usually occur about 5 days after the decline in hormones and include nervous tension, irritability, headaches, breast tenderness, and a feeling of depression.

Pregnancy

During pregnancy, the uterus changes its shape, size, and consistency. It increases greatly in size and muscle mass; houses the growing placenta, which nourishes the embryo-fetus; and expels the baby after gestation. To prepare and serve as the birth canal at the end of pregnancy, the vaginal canal elongates as the uterus rises in the pelvis. The mucosa thickens, secretions increase, and the vascularity and elasticity of the cervix and vagina become more pronounced.

The average pregnancy (**gestation**) lasts approximately 9 months and is followed by childbirth (**parturition**). Up to the 3rd month of pregnancy, the product of conception is referred to as the embryo. From the 3rd month to the time of birth, the unborn offspring is referred to as the fetus.

Pregnancy also causes enlargement of the breasts, sometimes to the point of pain. Many other changes occur throughout the body to accommodate the development and birth of the fetus. Toward the end of gestation, the myometrium begins to contract weakly at irregular intervals. At this time, the full-term fetus is usually positioned head down within the uterus.

Labor and Childbirth

Labor is the physiological process by which the fetus is expelled from the uterus. Labor occurs in three stages. The first is the **stage of dilation,** which begins with uterine contractions and terminates when there is complete dilation of the cervix (10 cm). The second is the **stage of expulsion,** which is the time from complete cervical dilation to birth of the baby. The last stage is the **placental stage,** or *afterbirth.* This stage begins shortly after childbirth, when the uterine contractions discharge the placenta from the uterus. (See Figure 12–5.)

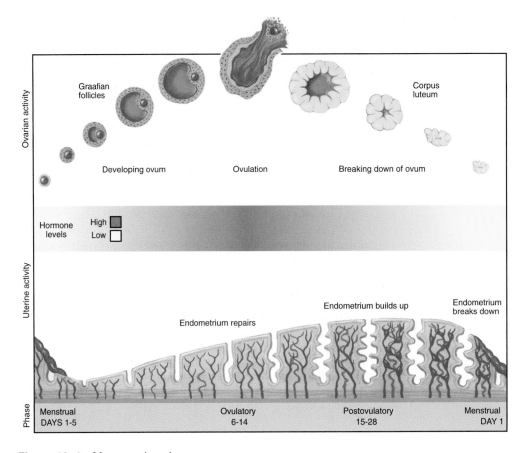

Figure 12–4   Menstrual cycle.

Menopause

Menopause is cessation of ovarian activity and diminished hormone production that occurs at about age 50. Menopause is usually diagnosed if absence of menses **(amenorrhea)** has persisted for 1 year. The period in which symptoms of approaching menopause occur is also known as *change of life* or *climacteric*.

Many women experience hot flashes and vaginal drying and thinning **(vaginal atrophy)** as estrogen levels fall. Although **hormone replacement therapy (HRT)** has become more controversial, it is still used to treat vaginal atrophy and porous bones **(osteoporosis),** and is believed to play a role in heart attack prevention. Restraint in prescribing estrogens for long periods in all menopausal women arises from concern that there is an increased risk that long-term usage will induce neoplastic changes in estrogen-sensitive aging tissue.

   It is time to review anatomy by completing Learning Activities 12–1 and 12–2.

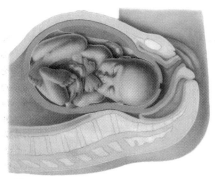

(1) Labor begins, membranes intact

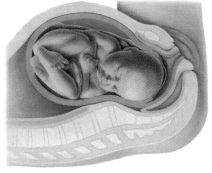

(2) Effacement of cervix,
which is now partially dilated

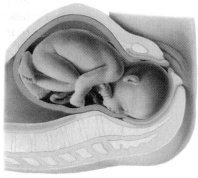

(3) When head reaches floor
of pelvis, it rotates

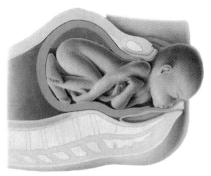

(4) Extension of the cervix allows head
to pass through

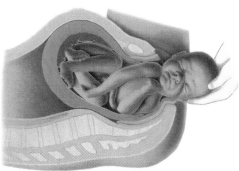

(5) Delivery of head, head rotates to
realign itself with body

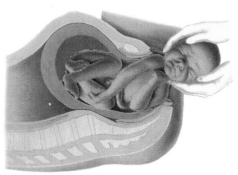

(6) Delivery of shoulders

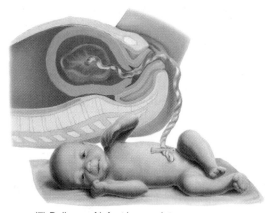

(7) Delivery of infant is complete,
uterus begins to contract

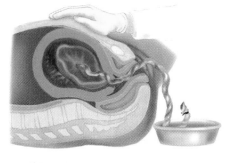

(8) Umbilical cord is cut, external massage
to uterus continues to stimulate
contractions, and placenta is delivered

Figure 12–5 Sequence of labor and childbirth.

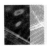

Medical Word Elements

This section introduces combining forms, suffixes, and prefixes related to the female reproductive system. Word analyses are also provided.

Element	Meaning	Word Analysis
COMBINING FORMS		
amni/o	amnion (amniotic sac)	amni/o/centesis (ăm-nē-ō-sĕn-TĒ-sĭs): transabdominal puncture of the amniotic sac *-centesis:* surgical puncture *Amniocentesis is performed under ultrasound guidance using a needle and syringe to remove amniotic fluid.*
cervic/o	neck; cervix uteri (neck of uterus)	cervic/itis (sĕr-vĭ-SĪ-tĭs): inflammation of the cervix *-itis:* inflammation
colp/o **vagin/o**	vagina	colp/o/scopy (kŏl-PŎS-kō-pē): visual examination of the vagina *-scopy:* visual examination vagin/o/cele (VĂJ-ĭn-ō-sēl): vaginal hernia; also called *colpocele* *-cele:* hernia, swelling
galact/o **lact/o**	milk	galact/o/cele (gă-LĂK-tō-sēl): cystic tumor of the female breast caused by occlusion of a milk duct; also called *lacto-cele* *-cele:* hernia, swelling lact/o/gen (LĂK-tō-jĕn): any substance that stimulates milk production *-gen:* forming, producing, origin
gynec/o	woman, female	gynec/o/logist (gī-nĕ-KŎL-ō-jĭst): physician specializing in treating disorders of the female reproductive system *-logist:* specialist in study of
hyster/o	uterus (womb)	hyster/ectomy (hĭs-tĕr-ĔK-tō-mē): surgical removal of the uterus *-ectomy:* excision, removal
mamm/o **mast/o**	breast	mamm/o/gram (MĂM-ō-grăm): radiograph of the breast *-gram:* record, writing mast/o/pexy (MĂS-tō-pĕks-ē): surgical fixation of the breast(s) *-pexy:* fixation (of an organ) *Mastopexy is a reconstructive, cosmetic surgical procedure performed to affix sagging breasts in a more elevated position, commonly improving their shape.*

Element	Meaning	Word Analysis
men/o	menses, menstruation	men/o/rrhagia (měn-ō-RĀ-jē-ă): excessive amount of menstrual flow over a longer duration than a normal period *-rrhagia:* bursting forth (of)
metri/o **uter/o**	uterus (womb)	endo/metri/al (ĕn-dō-MĒ-trē-ăl): pertaining to the lining of the uterus *endo-:* in, within *-al:* pertaining to, relating to uter/o/vagin/al (ū-tĕr-ō-VĂJ-i-năl): relating to the uterus and vagina *vagin/o:* vagina *-al:* pertaining to, relating to
metr/o	uterus (womb); measure	metr/o/ptosis (mē-trō-TŌ-sĭs): prolapse or downward displacement of the uterus *-ptosis:* prolapse, downward displacement
nat/o	birth	pre/nat/al (prē-NĀ-tăl): occurring before birth *pre-:* before, in front *-al:* pertaining to, relating to
oophor/o **ovari/o**	ovary	oophor/oma (ō-ŏf-ō-RŌ-mă): ovarian tumor *-oma:* tumor ovari/o/rrhexis (ō-vā-rē-ō-RĔK-sĭs): rupture of an ovary *-rrhexis:* rupture
perine/o	perineum	perine/o/rrhaphy (pěr-i-nē-OR-ă-fē): suture of the perineum *-rrhaphy:* suture *Perineorrhaphy is used to repair a laceration that occurs or is made surgically during the delivery of the fetus.*
salping/o	tube (usually fallopian or eustachian [auditory] tubes)	salping/o/plasty (săl-PĬNG-gō-plăs-tē): surgical repair of a fallopian tube *-plasty:* surgical repair

(Continued)

Element	Meaning	Word Analysis	(Continued)

SUFFIXES

Element	Meaning	Word Analysis
-arche	beginning	men/arche (mĕn-ĂR-kē): first menstrual period *men:* menses, menstruation
-cyesis	pregnancy	pseudo/cyesis (soo-dō-si-Ē-sĭs): condition in which a woman believes she is pregnant when she is not; also called *false pregnancy* *pseudo-:* false
-gravida	pregnant woman	multi/gravida (mŭl-tĭ-GRĂV-ĭ-dă): woman who has been pregnant more than once *multi-:* many, much
-para	to bear (offspring)	nulli/para (nŭl-ĬP-ă-ră): woman who has never produced a viable offspring *nulli-:* none
-salpinx	tube (usually fallopian or eustachian [auditory] tubes)	hem/o/salpinx (hē-mō-SĂL-pĭnks): collection of blood in a fallopian tube, commonly associated with a tubal pregnancy; also called *hematosalpinx* *hem/o:* blood
-tocia	childbirth, labor	dys/tocia (dĭs-TŌ-sē-ă): difficult childbirth *dys-:* bad; painful; difficult
-version	turning	retro/version (rĕt-rō-VĔR-shŭn): tipping back of an organ *retro-:* backward, behind *Retroversion of the uterus occurs in one of every four otherwise healthy women.*

Element	Meaning	Word Analysis
PREFIXES		
ante-	before, in front of	ante/version (ăn-tē-VĔR-zhŭn): tipping forward of an organ *-version:* turning
dys-	bad; painful; difficult	dys/men/o/rrhea (dĭs-mĕn-ō-RĒ-ă): pain associated with menstruation *men/o:* menses, menstruation *-rrhea:* discharge, flow
endo-	in, within	endo/metr/itis (ĕn-dō-mē-TRĪ-tĭs): inflammatory condition of the endometrium *metr:* uterus (womb); measure *-itis:* inflammation
multi-	many, much	multi/para (mŭl-TĬP-ă-ră): woman who has delivered more than one viable infant *-para:* to bear (offspring)
post-	after	post/nat/al (pōst-NĀ-tăl): occurring after birth *nat:* birth *-al:* pertaining to, relating to
primi-	first	primi/gravida (prī-mĭ-GRĂV-ĭ-dă): woman during her first pregnancy *-gravida:* pregnant woman

 It is time to review medical word elements by completing Learning Activity 12–3.

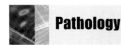

Pathology

Many female reproductive disorders are caused by infection, injury, or hormonal dysfunction. Although some disorders may be mild and correct themselves over time, others, such as those caused by infection, may require medical attention. Pain, itching, lesions, and discharge are signs and symptoms commonly associated with sexually transmitted diseases and must not be ignored. Other common problems of the female reproductive system are related to hormonal dysfunction that may cause menstrual disorders.

As a preventive measure, a pelvic examination should be performed regularly throughout life. This diagnostic procedure helps identify many pelvic abnormalities and diseases. Cytological and bacteriologic specimens are usually obtained at the time of examination.

Gynecology is the branch of medicine concerned with diseases of the female reproductive organs and the breast. **Obstetrics** is the branch of medicine that manages the health of a woman and her fetus during pregnancy, childbirth, and the puerperium. Because of the obvious overlap between gynecology and obstetrics, many practices include both specialties. The physician who simultaneously practices these specialties is called an **obstetrician/gynecologist.**

Menstrual Disorders

Menstrual disorders are usually caused by hormonal dysfunction or pathological conditions of the uterus and may produce a variety of symptoms. These disorders include:

- Menstrual pain and tension (**dysmenorrhea**) may be the result of uterine contractions, pathological growths, or such chronic disorders as anemia, fatigue, diabetes, and tuberculosis. The female hormone estrogen is used to treat dysmenorrhea and also to regulate menstrual abnormalities.
- Irregular uterine bleeding between menstrual periods (**metrorrhagia**) or after menopause is usually symptomatic of disease, including benign or malignant uterine tumors. Consequently, early diagnosis and treatment are warranted. Metrorrhagia is probably the most significant form of menstrual disorder.
- Profuse or prolonged bleeding during regular menstruation (**menorrhagia** or **hypermenorrhea**) may, during early life, be caused by endocrine disturbances. However, in later life, it is usually due to inflammatory diseases, fibroids, tumors, or emotional disturbances.
- Premenstrual syndrome (PMS) is a disorder with signs and symptoms that range from complaints of headache and fatigue to mood changes, anxiety, depression, uncontrolled crying spells, and water retention. Signs and symptoms involving almost every organ have been attributed to PMS. This syndrome occurs several days before the onset of menstruation and ends when menses begins or a short time after and appears to be related to hormones. The reason most individuals with PMS seek medical assistance is related to mood change. Simple changes in behavior, such as an increase in exercise and a reduction in caffeine, salt, and alcohol use, may be beneficial.

Endometriosis

Endometriosis is the presence of functional endometrial tissue in areas outside the uterus. (See Figure 12–6.) The endometrial tissue develops into what are called implants, lesions, or growths and can cause pain, infertility, and other problems. The ectopic tissue is usually confined to the pelvic area but may appear anywhere in the abdominopelvic cavity. Like normal endometrial tissue, the ectopic endometrium responds to hormonal fluctuations of the menstrual cycle.

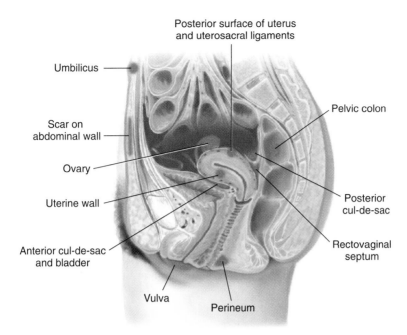

Posterior surface of uterus
and uterosacral ligaments

Umbilicus

Pelvic colon

Scar on
abdominal wall

Ovary

Uterine wall

Posterior
cul-de-sac

Anterior cul-de-sac
and bladder

Rectovaginal
septum

Vulva

Perineum

Figure 12–6 Endometriosis.

Pelvic and Vaginal Infections

Pelvic inflammatory disease (PID) is a general term for inflammation of the uterus, fallopian tubes, ovaries, and adjacent pelvic structures and is usually caused by bacterial infection. The infection may be confined to a single organ or it may involve all the internal reproductive organs. The disease-producing organisms (pathogens) generally enter through the vagina during coitus, induced abortion, childbirth, or the postpartum period. As an ascending infection, the pathogens spread from the vagina and cervix to the upper structures of the female reproductive tract. Two of the most common causes of PID are gonorrhea and chlamydia, both of which are sexually transmitted diseases (STDs). Unless treated promptly, PID may result in scarring of the narrow fallopian tubes and of the ovaries, causing sterility. The widespread infection of the reproductive structures can also lead to fatal septicemia. Because regions of the uterine tubes have an internal diameter as small as the width of a human hair, the scarring and closure of the tubes is one of the major causes of female infertility.

Vaginitis

The vagina is generally resistant to infection because of the acidity of vaginal secretions. Occasionally, however, localized infections and inflammations occur from viruses, bacteria, or yeast. If confined to the vagina, these infections are called vaginitis. Although symptoms may be numerous and varied, including painful intercourse, the most common symptoms are genital itching and a foul-smelling vaginal discharge. It is not uncommon for vaginitis to be accompanied by urethral inflammation (urethritis) because of the proximity of the urethra to the vagina. Two of the most common types of vaginitis are candidiasis and trichomoniasis.

Candidiasis, also called *moniliasis,* is caused by *Candida albicans,* a yeast that is present as part of the normal flora of the vagina. Steroid therapy, diabetes, or pregnancy may cause a change in the vaginal environment that disrupts the normal flora and promotes the overgrowth of this organism, resulting in a yeast **(fungal)** infection. The use of antibiotics may also disrupt the normal balance of microorganisms in the vagina by destroying friendly bacteria, thus allowing the overpopulation of yeast. Antifungal agents (**mycostatics**) that suppress the growth of fungi are used to treat this disease. Trichomoniasis, caused by the protozoan *Trichomonas vaginalis,* is now known to be one of the most common causes of sexually transmitted lower genital tract infections. Trichomoniasis is discussed more fully in the sexually transmitted disease section that follows.

Sexually Transmitted Disease

Sexually transmitted disease (STD), also called venereal disease, is any of several contagious diseases acquired as a result of sexual activity with an infected partner. As many as 20 different STDs have been identified, of which the newest and most serious is acquired immunodeficiency syndrome (AIDS). (For a full description of AIDS, see Chapter 9, Blood, Lymph, and Immune Systems.) In the United States, the widespread occurrence of STDs is regarded as an epidemic. As a group, STDs are the single most important cause of reproductive disorders. Until recently, gonorrhea and syphilis were the most common STDs but, over the past few decades, chlamydia has become the most widespread STD. Viral diseases such as genital herpes and genital warts are also increasing in prevalence. The current STDs of medical concern are gonorrhea, syphilis, chlamydia, genital herpes, genital warts, and trichomoniasis. Each is described, along with signs and symptoms for males and females.

Gonorrhea

Gonorrhea is caused by the bacterium *Neisseria gonorrhoeae* and involves the mucosal surface of the genitourinary tract and, possibly, the rectum and pharynx. This disease may be acquired through sexual intercourse and through orogenital and anogenital contact. Some women do not experience pain or manifest overt clinical symptoms (**asymptomatic**) until the disease has spread to the ovaries (**oophoritis**) and uterine tubes (**salpingitis**), causing PID. The most common symptom of gonorrhea in women is a greenish-yellow cervical discharge. The organism may infect the eyes of the newborn during vaginal delivery, which may result in blindness. As a precaution, silver nitrate is instilled in the eyes of newborns immediately after delivery as a preventive measure to ensure that this infection does not occur. The most common sign of gonorrhea in males is a discharge of pus from the penis. Other signs and symptoms include inflammation of the urethra (**urethritis**), which may cause painful urination (**dysuria**). If left untreated, the disease may infect the bladder (**cystitis**) and inflame the joints (**arthritis**). In addition, sterility may result from formation of scars that close the reproductive tubes of both sexes. Both sex partners must be treated because the infection can recur.

Syphilis

Although less common than gonorrhea, syphilis is the more serious of the two diseases. It is caused by infection with the bacterium *Treponema pallidum.* Syphilis is a chronic, infectious, multisystemic disease acquired through sexual contact or at birth (congenitally). A primary sore (chancre) develops at the point where the bacteria entered the body. The chancre is an ulcerated sore with hard edges that contains contagious organisms for 10 days to 3 months. In pregnancy, the fetus is infected from the mother through the placenta. However, the vast majority of cases are contracted through sexual activity. The danger of transmission is greatest in the early stage of syphilis. If left untreated, the end result is systemic infection that commonly leads to blindness, insanity, and eventual death.

Chlamydia

Chlamydia, caused by infection with the bacterium *Chlamydia trachomatis,* is the most prevalent and one of the most damaging STDs in the United States. In women, chlamydial infections are associated with mucopurulent discharge and inflammation of the cervix uteri (cervicitis) that may lead to PID. Chlamydia can be transmitted to the newborn baby during the birth process and cause a form of conjunctivitis or pneumonia. In men, chlamydial infections are associated with a whitish discharge from the penis that may lead to urethritis or epididymitis. Chlamydia in men, women, and babies can be successfully treated with antibiotics. However, many cases are asymptomatic, especially in women, and the disease commonly remains untreated until irreversible damage to the reproductive structures has occurred.

Genital Herpes

Genital herpes causes red, blisterlike, painful lesions that closely resemble the common fever blister or cold sore that appears on the lips and around the mouth. Although both diseases are caused by the herpes simplex virus (HSV), genital herpes is associated with type 2 (HSV-2), and the oral herpes is associated with type 1 (HSV-1). Regardless, both forms can cause oral and genital infection through oral-genital sexual activity. The fluid in the blisters is highly infectious and contains the active virus. However, this disease is associated with a phenomenon called viral shedding. During viral shedding, the virus is present on the skin of the infected patient, and can be transmitted to sexual partners, even when no lesions are present. Individuals with herpes infection may have only one episode or may have repeated attacks that usually lessen in severity over the years. The disease may be transmitted to a baby during the birth process and, although rare, may lead to death of the infant. In females, the lesions appear around the vaginal area, buttocks, and thighs. In men, lesions appear on the glans, foreskin, or penile shaft.

Genital Warts

Genital warts (condylomas) are caused by the human papilloma virus (HPV). Of the 100 identified types of HPV, only about 30 are spread through sexual contact. The warts may be very small and almost unnoticeable or may be large and appear in clusters. In females, the lesions may be found on the vulva, in the vagina, or on the cervix. In males, the lesions commonly appear on the penis or around the rectum. Many warts disappear without treatment, but there is no way to determine which ones will resolve. When treatment is required, surgical excision or freezing the wart is the usual method. HPV infection has been found to increase the risk of certain cancers, including penile, vaginal, cervical, and anal cancer. The virus is linked to 80% of all cases of invasive cervical cancer. Thus, women who have been diagnosed with HPV infection are urged to have Pap smears every 6 months after diagnosis. There is also a much greater incidence of miscarriages in individuals with HPV disease.

Trichomoniasis

Trichomoniasis, caused by the protozoan *Trichomonas vaginalis,* affects both males and females but symptoms are more common in females. In women, it causes vaginitis, urethritis, and cystitis. Signs and symptoms include a frothy, yellow-green vaginal discharge with a strong odor. The infection may also cause discomfort during intercourse and urination. Irritation and itching in the female genital area and, in rare cases, lower abdominal pain can also occur. When symptoms are present in males, they include irritation inside the penis, mild discharge, or slight burning after urination or ejaculation. Treatment is generally very effective but reinfection is common if sexual partners are not treated simultaneously.

Uterine Fibroids

About 30% to 40% of all women develop benign tumors called *fibroids* (also called *leiomyomas* or, more commonly, *myomas*). These benign tumors develop slowly between ages 25 and 40 and commonly enlarge in response to fluctuating endocrine stimulation after this period. Although some individuals are asymptomatic with these types of tumors, when present they include menorrhagia, backache, constipation, and urinary symptoms. In addition, such tumors commonly cause metrorrhagia and even sterility.

Treatment of uterine fibroid tumors depends on their size and location. If the patient plans to have children, treatment is as conservative as possible. As a rule, large tumors that produce pressure symptoms should be removed. Usually, the uterus is removed (**hysterectomy**), but the ovaries are preserved. (See Figure 12–10.) If the tumor is small, a myomectomy may be performed. However, when the tumor is producing excessive bleeding, both the uterus and the tumor are excised.

Oncology

The two most common forms of cancer involving the female reproductive system are breast cancer and cervical cancer.

Breast Cancer

Breast cancer, also called *carcinoma of the breast,* is the most common malignancy of women in the United States. This disease appears to be associated with ovarian hormonal function. In addition, a diet high in fats appears to increase the incidence of breast cancer. Other contributing factors include a family history of the disease and possibly the use of hormone replacement therapy (HRT). Women who have not borne children (**nulliparous**) or those who have had an early onset of menstruation (**menarche**) or late onset of menopause are also more likely to develop breast cancer. Because this type of malignancy is highly responsive to treatment when detected early, women are urged to practice breast self-examination monthly and to receive periodic mammography after age 40. Many breast malignancies are detected by the patient.

Cervical Cancer

Cancer of the cervix most commonly affects women between ages 40 and 49. Statistics indicate that infection associated with sexual activity has some relationship to the incidence of cervical cancer. First coitus at a young age, large number of sex partners, infection with certain sexually transmitted viruses, and frequent intercourse with men whose previous partners had cervical cancer are all associated with increased risk of developing cervical cancer.

A cytological examination known as a *Papanicolaou (Pap) test* can detect cervical cancer before the disease becomes clinically evident. Abnormal cervical cytology routinely calls for colposcopy, which can detect the presence and extent of preclinical lesions requiring biopsy and histological examination. Treatment of cervical cancer consists of surgery, radiation, and chemotherapy. If left untreated, the cancer will eventually metastasize and lead to death.

Diagnostic, Symptomatic, and Related Terms

This section introduces diagnostic, symptomatic, and related terms and their meanings. Word analyses for selected terms are also provided.

Term	Definition
FEMALE REPRODUCTIVE SYSTEM	
adnexa ăd-NĔK-să	Accessory parts of a structure *Adnexa uteri are the ovaries and fallopian tubes.*
atresia ă-TRĒ-zē-ă	Congenital absence or closure of a normal body opening, such as the vagina
choriocarcinoma kō-rē-ō-kăr-sĭ-NŌ-mă *chori/o:* chorion *carcin:* cancer *-oma:* tumor	Malignant neoplasm of the uterus or at the site of an ectopic pregnancy *Although its actual cause is unknown, choriocarcinoma is a rare tumor that may occur after pregnancy or abortion.*
corpus luteum KOR-pŭs LŪ-tē-ŭm	Ovarian scar tissue that results from rupturing of a follicle during ovulation and becomes a small yellow body that produces progesterone after ovulation
contraceptive diaphragm kŏn-tră-SĔP-tĭv DĪ-ă-frăm	Contraceptive device consisting of a hemisphere of thin rubber bonded to a flexible ring; inserted into the vagina together with spermicidal jelly or cream up to 2 hours before coitus so that spermatozoa cannot enter the uterus, thus preventing conception
dyspareunia dĭs-pă-RŪ-nē-ă	Occurrence of pain during sexual intercourse
endocervicitis ĕn-dō-sĕr-vĭ-SĪ-tĭs *endo-:* in, within *cervic:* neck; cervix uteri (neck of the uterus) *-itis:* inflammation	Inflammation of the mucous lining of the cervix uteri *Endocervicitis is usually chronic, commonly due to infection, and accompanied by cervical erosion.*
fibroids FĪ-broyds *fibr:* fiber, fibrous tissue *-oids:* resembling	Benign uterine tumors composed of muscle and fibrous tissue; also called *leiomyomas (myomas)* and *fibromyoma uteri* *Myomectomy or hysterectomy may be indicated if the fibroids grow too large, causing such symptoms as metrorrhagia, pelvic pain, and menorrhagia.*
infertility ĭn-fĕr-TĬL-ĭ-tē	Inability or diminished ability to produce offspring
hormonal contraception hor-MŌ-năl kŏn-tră-SĔP-shŭn	Use of hormones to suppress ovulation and prevent conception
oral contraceptive pills (OCPs) OR-ăl kŏn-tră-SĔP-tĭv	Birth control pills containing estrogen and progesterone in varying proportions *When taken according to schedule, oral contraceptives are about 98% effective.*

(Continued)

Term	Definition	(Continued)
menarche mĕn-ĂR-kē *men:* menses, menstruation *-arche:* beginning	Beginning of menstrual function	
oligomenorrhea ŏl-ĭ-gō-mĕn-ō-RĒ-ă *olig/o:* scanty *men/o:* menses, menstruation *-rrhea:* discharge, flow	Scanty or infrequent menstrual flow	
perineum pĕr-ĭ-NĒ-ŭm	Region between the vulva and anus that constitutes the pelvic floor	
puberty PŪ-bĕr-tē	Period during which secondary sex characteristics begin to develop and the capability of sexual reproduction is attained	
pyosalpinx pī-ō-SĂL-pĭnks *py/o:* pus *-salpinx:* tube (usually fallopian or eustachian [auditory] tubes)	Pus in the fallopian tube	
retroversion rĕt-rō-VĔR-shŭn *retro-:* backward, behind *-version:* turning	Turning or state of being turned back, especially an entire organ, such as the uterus, being tipped from its normal position	
sterility stĕr-ĬL-ĭ-tē	Inability of the female to become pregnant or the male to impregnate the female	
vaginismus văj-ĭn-ĬZ-mŭs	Painful spasm of the vagina from contraction of the muscles surrounding the vagina	

OBSTETRICS

Term	Definition	
abruptio placentae ă-BRŬP-shē-ō plă-SĔN-tē	Premature separation of a normally situated placenta	
abortion ă-BOR-shŭn	Termination of pregnancy before the embryo or fetus is capable of surviving outside the uterus	
amnion ĂM-nē-ŏn	Membrane, continuous with and covering the fetal side of the placenta, that forms the outer surface of the umbilical cord *The fetus is suspended in amniotic fluid.*	
breech presentation	Common abnormality of delivery in which the fetal buttocks or feet present rather than the head	
Down syndrome, trisomy 21 DOWN SĬN-drōm, TRĪ-sō-mē	Congenital condition characterized by physical malformations and some degree of mental retardation *Trisomy (of chromosome) 21 usually occurs in 1 of 700 live births. The terms* Down syndrome *and* trisomy 21 *are preferred to the term* mongolism.	

Term	Definition
dystocia dĭs-TŌ-sē-ă *dys-:* bad; painful; difficult *-tocia:* childbirth, labor	Difficult labor, which may be produced by the large size of the fetus or the small size of the pelvic outlet
eclampsia ĕ-KLĂMP-sē-ă	Most serious form of toxemia during pregnancy *Signs of eclampsia include high blood pressure, edema, convulsions, renal dysfunction, proteinuria and, in severe cases, coma.*
ectopic pregnancy ĕk-TŌP-ĭk PRĔG-năn-sē	Pregnancy in which the fertilized ovum does not reach the uterine cavity but becomes implanted on any tissue other than the lining of the uterine cavity, such as a fallopian tube, an ovary, the abdomen, or even the cervix uteri (See Figure 12–7.) *Kinds of ectopic pregnancy include* abdominal pregnancy, ovarian pregnancy, *and* tubal pregnancy.
gravida GRĂV-ĭ-dă	Pregnant woman *The term* gravida *may be followed by numbers, indicating number of pregnancies, such as* gravida 1, 2, 3, 4 *or* I, II, III, IV, *and so forth.*
multigravida mŭl-tĭ-GRĂV-ĭ-dă *multi-:* many, much *-gravida:* pregnant woman	Woman who has been pregnant more than once
multipara mŭl-TĬP-ă-ră *multi-:* many, much *-para:* to bear (offspring)	Woman who has delivered more than one viable infant
para PĂR-ă	Woman who has given birth to one or more viable infants Para *followed by a Roman numeral or preceded by a Latin prefix (primi-, quadri-, and so forth) designates the number of times a pregnancy has culminated in a single or multiple birth. For example,* para I *and* primipara *refer to a woman who has given birth for the first time.* Para II *refers to a woman who has given birth a second time. Whether the births were multiple (twins, triplets) is irrelevant.*
parturition păr-tū-RĬSH-ŭn	Process of giving birth
pelvimetry pĕl-VĬM-ĕ-trē *pelv/i:* pelvis *-metry:* act of measuring	Measurement of the pelvic dimensions or proportions, which helps determine whether it will be possible to deliver a fetus through the normal route *Pelvimetry is performed by various methods, including manually or radiogically.*
placenta previa plă-SĔN-tă PRĒ-vē-ă	Condition in which the placenta is attached near the cervix and ruptures prematurely, with spotting as the early symptom *Prevention of hemorrhage may necessitate a cesarean delivery.*

(Continued)

Term	Definition	(Continued)
primigravida prī-mĭ-GRĂV-ĭ-dă *primi-:* first *-gravida:* pregnant woman	Woman pregnant for the first time	
primipara prī-MĬP-ă-ră *primi-:* first *-para:* to bear (offspring)	Woman who has given birth to one viable infant, her first child, indicated by the notation *para I* on the patient's chart	
puerperium pū-ĕr-PĒ-rē-ŭm	Period of 42 days after childbirth and expulsion of the placenta and membranes, during which the reproductive organs usually return to normal	

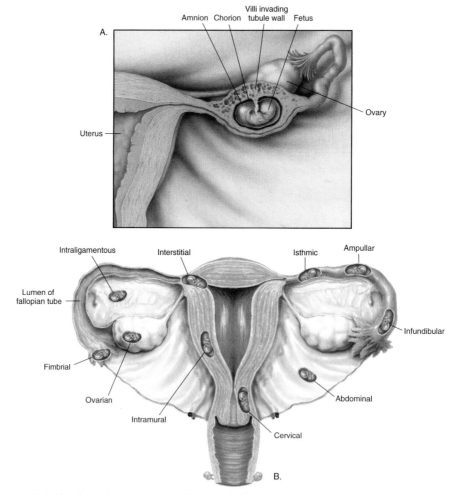

Figure 12–7 (A) Ectopic pregnancy (B) Sites of ectopic pregnancy.

 It is time to review pathological, diagnostic, symptomatic, and related terms by completing Learning Activity 12–4.

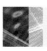

Diagnostic and Therapeutic Procedures

This section introduces procedures used to diagnose and treat female reproductive disorders. Descriptions are provided as well as pronunciations and word analyses for selected terms.

Procedure	Description
DIAGNOSTIC PROCEDURES	
Clinical	
amniocentesis ăm-nē-ō-sĕn-TĒ-sĭs *amni/o:* amnion (amniotic sac) *-centesis:* surgical puncture	Transabdominal puncture of the amniotic sac under ultrasound guidance using a needle and syringe to remove amniotic fluid (See Figure 12–8.) *The sample obtained in amniocentesis is chemically and cytologically studied to detect genetic and biochemical disorders and fetal maturity. The procedure also allows for transfusion of platelets or blood to the fetus and instillation of drugs for treating the fetus.*

(Continued)

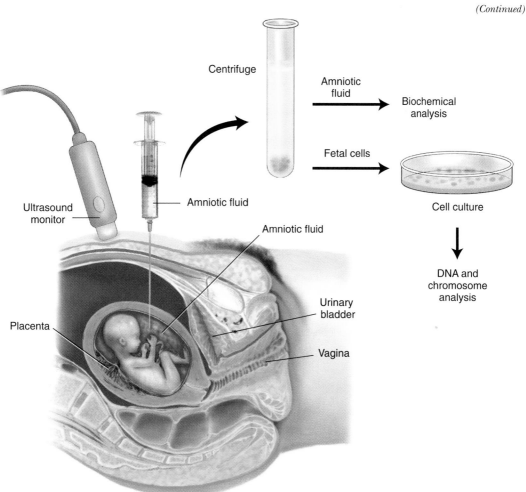

Figure 12–8 Amniocentesis.

Procedure	Description	(Continued)

| **insufflation**
ĭn-sŭ-FLĀ-shŭn | Delivery of pressurized air or gas into a cavity, chamber, or organ to allow visual examination, remove an obstruction, or apply medication
Insufflation is performed to increase the distance between structures so the physician can see more clearly and better diagnose possible disorders. |
| **tubal**
  TŪ-băl | Test for patency of the uterine tubes made by transuterine insufflation with carbon dioxide; also called *Rubin test* |

Endoscopic

| **colposcopy**
kŏl-PŎS-kō-pē

colp/o: vagina
-scopy: visual examination | Visual examination of the vagina and cervix with an optical magnifying instrument (colposcope)
Colposcopy is used chiefly to identify areas of cervical dysplasia in women with abnormal Papanicolaou smears and as an aid in biopsy or excision procedures, including cautery, cryotherapy, and loop electrosurgical excision. |
| **laparoscopy**
lăp-ăr-ŎS-kō-pē

lapar/o: abdomen
-scopy: visual examination | Visual examination of the abdominal cavity with a laparoscope through one or more small incisions in the abdominal wall, usually at the umbilicus (See Figure 12–9.)
Laparoscopy has become a standard technique for many routine surgical procedures, including gynecologic sterilization by fulguration of the oviducts or tubal ligation. |

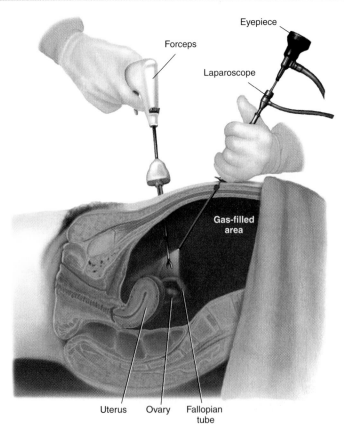

Figure 12–9 Laparoscopy.

Procedure	Description
Laboratory	
chorionic villus sampling (CVS) kor-ē-ŎN-ĭk VĬL-ŭs SĂM-plĭng	Sampling of placental tissues for prenatal diagnosis of potential genetic defects *The sample is obtained through a catheter inserted into the uterus. The advantage of CVS over amniocentesis is that it can be undertaken in the 1st trimester of pregnancy.*

endometrial biopsy
ĕn-dō-MĒ-trē-ăl BĪ-ŏp-sē
 	
  endo-: in, within
  metri: uterus(womb); measure
  -al: pertaining to, relating to
	Removal of a sample of uterine endometrium for microscopic study
	Endometrial biopsy is commonly used in fertility assessment to confirm ovulation and as a diagnostic tool to determine the cause of dysfunctional and postmenopausal bleeding.

Papanicolaou (Pap) test pă-pă-nĭ-kō-LĂ-oo	Cytological study used to detect abnormal cells sloughed from the cervix and vagina, usually obtained during routine pelvic examination *A Pap test is commonly used to diagnose and prevent cervical cancer. It may also be used to evaluate cells from any organ, such as the pleura and peritoneum, to detect changes that indicate malignancy.*
Radiographic	

mammography
măm-ŎG-ră-fē
 	
  mamm/o: breast
  -graphy: process of recording
	Radiographic examination of the soft tissues of the breast
	Mammography is used to identify various benign and malignant neoplastic processes and may identify a malignant lesion. The record produced by mammography is called a mammogram.

hysterosalpingography
hĭs-tĕr-ō-săl-pĭn-GŎG-ră-fē
 	
  hyster/o: uterus (womb)
  salping/o: tube (usually fallopian or eustachian [auditory] tubes)
  -graphy: process of recording
  -gram: record, writing
	Radiography of the uterus and uterine tubes (oviducts) following injection of a contrast medium
	Hysterosalpingography is used to determine pathology in the uterine cavity, evaluate tubal patency, and determine the cause of infertility. The record produced by hysterosalpingography is called hysterosalpingogram.

ultrasonography
ŭl-tră-sŏn-ŎG-ră-fē
 	
  ultra-: excess, beyond
  son/o: sound
  -graphy: process of recording
	Process by which high-frequency sound waves (ultrasound) produce and display an image from reflected "echoes" on a monitor; also called *ultrasound, sonography,* and *echo.* (See Figure 4–4B.)
	The record produced by ultrasonography is called ultrasonogram.

pelvic PĔL-vĭk	Ultrasound of the pelvic region used to evaluate abnormalities in the female reproductive system as well as the fetus in the obstetric patient

transvaginal
trănz-VĂJ-ĭ-năl
 	
  trans-: through, across
  vagin: vagina
  -al: pertaining to, relating to
	Ultrasound of the pelvic area performed with a probe inserted into the vagina, which provides sharper images of pathological and normal structures within the pelvis

(Continued)

Procedure	Description	(Continued)

THERAPEUTIC PROCEDURES

Surgical

cerclage sĕr-KLĂZH	Procedure in which a nonabsorbable ligature is applied around the cervix uteri to treat incompetent uterus, thus decreasing the chance of a spontaneous abortion
cesarean birth sē-SĀR-ē-ăn	Incision of the abdomen and uterus to remove the fetus; also called *C-section* *Cesarean birth is most commonly used in the event of cephalopelvic disproportion, presence of sexually transmitted disease organisms in the birth canal, fetal distress, and breech presentation.*

colpocleisis
kŏl-pō-KLĪ-sĭs
 	
   colp/o: vagina
   -cleisis: closure
	Surgical closure of the vaginal canal

conization kŏn-ĭ-ZĀ-shŭn	Excision of a cone-shaped piece of tissue, such as mucosa of the cervix, for histological examination
cordocentesis kor-dō-sĕn-TĒ-sĭs	Sampling of fetal blood drawn from the umbilical vein and performed under ultrasound guidance *Cord blood is evaluated in the laboratory to identify hemolytic diseases or genetic abnormalities.*
cryosurgery, cryocautery krī-ō-SĔR-jĕr-ē, krī-ō-KAW-tĕr-ē	Process of freezing tissue to destroy cells *Cryosurgery is used for chronic cervical infections and erosions because offending organisms may be entrenched in cervical cells and glands. The process destroys these infected areas and, in the healing process, normal cells are replenished. This procedure may also be used when a patient shows atypical or possible malignancy, as seen on a Pap smear.*
dilatation and curettage (D&C) dĭl-ă-TĀ-shŭn, kū-rĕ-TĂZH	Widening of the cervical canal with a dilator and scraping of the uterine endometrium with a curette *D&C is used to obtain a sample for cytological examination of tissue, control abnormal uterine bleeding, and treat incomplete abortion.*

episiorrhaphy
ĕ-pĭs-ē-OR-ă-fē
 	
   episi/o: vulva
   -rrhaphy: suture
	Repair of a lacerated vulva or an episiotomy

episiotomy
ĕ-pĭs-ē-ŎT-ō-mē
 	
   episi/o: vulva
   -tomy: incision
	Incision of the perineum from the vaginal orifice; usually done to prevent tearing of the tissue and to facilitate childbirth

Procedure	Description
hysterectomy hĭs-tĕr-ĔK-tō-mē *hyster:* uterus (womb) *-ectomy:* excision, removal	Excision of the uterus (See Figure 12–10.) *Indications for hysterectomy include abnormalities of the uterus and cervix (cancer, severe dysfunctional bleeding, large or bleeding fibroid tumors, prolapse of the uterus, or severe endometriosis). The approach to excision may be abdominal or vaginal.*
subtotal	Hysterectomy where the cervix, ovaries, and fallopian tubes remain
total (complete)	Hysterectomy where the cervix is removed but the ovaries and fallopian tubes remain
total (complete) plus bilateral salpingo-oophorectomy bī-LĂT-ĕr-ăl săl-pĭng-gō-ō-ŏf-ō-RĔK-tō-mē	Total hysterectomy, including uterus, cervix, fallopian tubes, and ovaries

(Continued)

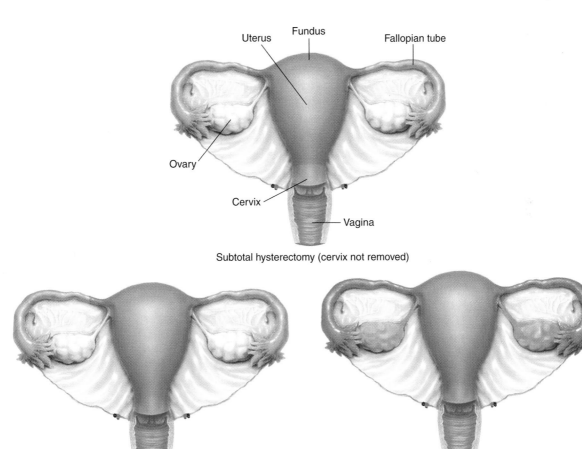

Subtotal hysterectomy (cervix not removed)

Total hysterectomy
(cervix removed)

Total hysterectomy
plus bilateral salpingo-
oophorectomy

Figure 12–10   Hysterectomy.

Procedure	Description	(Continued)
intrauterine device (IUD) ĭn-trā-Ū-tĕr-ĭn dĕ-VĪS	Plastic or metal object placed inside the uterus to prevent implantation of a fertilized egg in the uterine lining	
lumpectomy lŭm-PĔK-tō-mē	Excision of a small primary breast tumor that leaves the remainder of the breast intact	

mammoplasty, mastoplasty
MĂM-ă-plăs-tē,
MĂS-tō-plăs-tē
 	
  mamm/o: breast
  -plasty: surgical repair
	Surgical reconstruction of the breast(s), sometimes augmented by substances such as fat tissue or silicone to alter size and shape	

mastectomy
măs-TĔK-tō-mē
 	
  mast: breast
  -ectomy: excision, removal
	Excision of the breast	

radical RĂD-ĭ-kăl	Removal of the breast and any involved skin, pectoral muscles, axillary lymph nodes, and subcutaneous fat	

myomectomy
mī-ō-MĔK-tō-mē
 	
  my/o: muscle
  -ectomy: excision, removal
	Excision of a myomatous tumor, generally uterine	

salpingo-oophorectomy
săl-pĭng-gō-ō-ŏf-ō-RĔK-tō-mē
 	
  salping/o: tube (usually fallopian or eustachian [auditory] tubes)
  oophor: ovary
  -ectomy: excision, removal
	Excision of an ovary and fallopian tube
	
	A salpingo-oophorectomy is usually identified as right, left, or bilateral.	

tubal ligation TŪ-băl lĭ-GĀ-shŭn	Procedure that ties (ligates) the uterine tubes to prevent pregnancy *Tubal ligation is a form of sterilization surgery that is usually performed during laparoscopy.*	

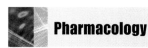

Pharmacology

Hormones perform a vital role in both reproduction and sexual development of the female. Hormone replacement therapy (HRT) is the use of synthetic or natural estrogens or a combination of estrogen and progestin to replace the decline or lack of natural hormones, a condition that accompanies hysterectomy and menopause. (See Table 12–2.) Such symptoms as vaginal dryness, hot flashes, and fatigue are commonly relieved or lessened using HRT. The medical profession is currently rethinking the use of hormone replacement in menopause because of an apparent increased risk of some disorders with extended use of the combination therapy. Use of estrogen alone for HRT is still in clinical trials but has not exhibited the strong contraindications of the combination form of HRT. Estrogen may be administered orally, transdermally, by injection, or as a topical cream (to treat vaginal symptoms only). Other hormones, including oxytocins and prostaglandins, are used for obstetric applications. In addition, pharmacological agents are available for birth control and family planning. These include oral contraceptives, implants, morning-after pills (abortifacients), and spermicides. (See Chapter 11, Genitourinary System.)

Table 12–2   DRUGS USED TO TREAT OBSTETRIC AND GYNECOLOGIC DISORDERS

This table lists common drug classifications used to treat obstetric and gynecologic disorders, their therapeutic actions, and selected generic and trade names.

Classification	Therapeutic Action	Generic and Trade Names

antifungals	Treat vaginal yeast infection
	
	Most antifungals used to treat yeast infections are applied topically in the form of ointments, suppositories, or vaginal tablets.
		miconazole
		mĭ-KŎN-ă-zōl
		  Monistat
		nystatin
		NĬS-tă-tĭn
		  Mycostatin, Nilstat

estrogens	Treat adverse symptoms of menopause, including hot flashes, vaginal dryness, and fatigue, through hormone replacement therapy (HRT) *HRT also reduces the risk of osteoporosis and helps keep cholesterol levels low.*	**conjugated estrogens** KŎN-jū-gā-tĕd ĔS-trō-jĕnz *Cenestin, Premarin*

oral contraceptives	Prevent pregnancy
	
	Oral contraceptives, or birth control pills, exert a hormonal influence to suppress ovulation and prevent pregnancy. Most contain a combination of estrogen and progestin and are highly effective (95% to 99%) in preventing pregnancy if taken as directed.
		desogestrel/ethinyl estradiol
		dĕz-ō-JĔS-trăl/ĔTH-ĭ-nĭl ĕs-tră-DĪ-ŏl
		  Desogen, Ortho-Cept
		ethinyl estradiol/ norgestrel
		ĔTH-ĭ-nĭl ĕs-tră-DĪ-ŏl/nor-JĔS-trĕl
		  Lo/Ovral, Ovral

oxytocics	Induce labor at term by increasing the strength and frequency of uterine contractions *Oxytocics are also used during the postpartum period to control bleeding after the expulsion of the placenta.*	**oxytocin** ŏk-sē-TŌ-sĭn *Pitocin, Syntocinon*

(Continued)

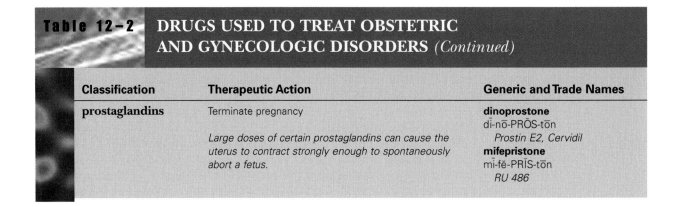

Classification	Therapeutic Action	Generic and Trade Names

prostaglandins	Terminate pregnancy
	
	Large doses of certain prostaglandins can cause the uterus to contract strongly enough to spontaneously abort a fetus.
		dinoprostone
		dī-nō-PRŎS-tōn
		  Prostin E2, Cervidil
		mifepristone
		mĭ-fĕ-PRĬS-tōn
		  RU 486

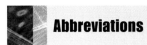

Abbreviations

This section introduces female reproductive-related abbreviations and their meanings.

Abbreviation	Meaning
GYNECOLOGIC	
AB; ab	abortion; antibodies
AI	artificial insemination
BSE	breast self-examination
D&C	dilatation (dilation) and curettage
DUB	dysfunctional uterine bleeding
FSH	follicle-stimulating hormone
G	gravida (pregnant)
GC	gonorrhea
GYN	gynecology
HRT	hormone replacement therapy
HSG	hysterosalpingography
HSV	herpes simplex virus
IUD	intrauterine device
LH	luteinizing hormone
LMP	last menstrual period

Abbreviation	Meaning
LSO	left salpingo-oophorectomy
OCPs	oral contraceptive pills
Pap	Papanicolaou smear
PID	pelvic inflammatory disease
PMP	previous menstrual period
PMS	premenstrual syndrome
RSO	right salpingo-oophorectomy
STD	sexually transmitted disease
TAH	total abdominal hysterectomy
TVH	total vaginal hysterectomy
VD	venereal disease
FETAL-OBSTETRIC	
CPD	cephalopelvic disproportion
CS, C-section	cesarean section
CVS	chorionic villus sampling
CWP	childbirth without pain
FECG; FEKG	fetal electrocardiogram
FHR	fetal heart rate
FHT	fetal heart tone
FTND	full-term normal delivery
IUGR	intrauterine growth rate; intrauterine growth retardation
IVF-ET	in vitro fertilization and embryo transfer
LBW	low birth weight
NB	newborn
OB	obstetrics
para 1, 2, 3	unipara, bipara, tripara (number of viable births)
UC	uterine contractions

It is time to review procedures, pharmacology, and abbreviations by completing Learning Activity 12–5.

LEARNING ACTIVITIES

The activities that follow provide review of the female reproductive system terms introduced in this chapter. Complete each activity and review your answers to evaluate your understanding of the chapter.

Learning Activity 12–1

Identifying female reproductive structures (lateral view)

Label the following illustration using the terms listed below.

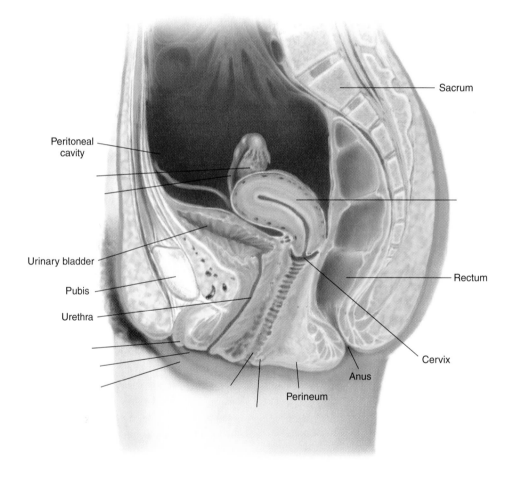

Bartholin gland	*labia majora*	*uterus*
clitoris	*labia minora*	*vagina*
fallopian tube	*ovary*	

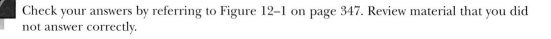

Check your answers by referring to Figure 12–1 on page 347. Review material that you did not answer correctly.

Identifying female reproductive structures (anterior view)

Label the following illustration using the terms listed below.

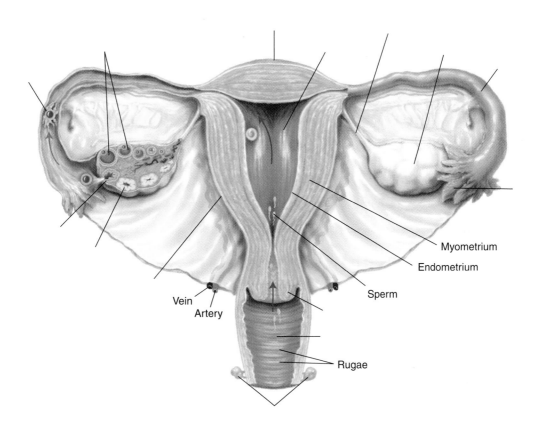

Myometrium

Endometrium

Sperm

Vein

Artery

Rugae

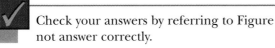

Bartholin glands	*fertilization of ovum*	*ovarian ligament*
body of the uterus	*fimbriae*	*ovary*
cervix	*fundus of uterus*	*uterus*
corpus luteum	*graafian follicles*	*vagina*
fallopian tube	*mature follicle*	

Check your answers by referring to Figure 12–2 on page 348. Review material that you did not answer correctly.

Learning Activity 12–3

Building medical words

Use **gynec/o** *(woman, female) to build words that mean:*

1. disease (specific to) women _____

2. physician who specializes in diseases of the female _____

Use **cervic/o** *(neck; cervix uteri) to build words that mean:*

3. inflammation of the cervix uteri and vagina _____

4. pertaining to the cervix uteri and bladder _____

Use **colp/o** *(vagina) to build words that mean:*

5. instrument used to examine the vagina _____

6. visual examination of the vagina _____

Use **vagin/o** *(vagina) to build words that mean:*

7. inflammation of the vagina _____

8. herniation of the vagina _____

Use **hyster/o** *(uterus) to build words that mean:*

9. myoma of the uterus _____

10. disease of the uterus _____

11. radiography of the uterus and oviducts _____

Use **metr/o** *(uterus) to build words that mean:*

12. hemorrhage from the uterus _____

13. inflammation around the uterus _____

Use **uter/o** *(uterus) to build words that mean:*

14. herniation of the uterus _____

15. relating to the uterus and cervix _____

16. pertaining to the uterus and bladder _____

Use **oophor/o** *(ovary) to build words that mean:*

17. inflammation of an ovary _____

18. inflammation of an ovary and oviduct _____

Use **salping/o** *(fallopian tube) to build words that mean:*

19. herniation of a fallopian tube _____

20. radiography of the uterine tubes _____

Build surgical words that mean:

21. fixation of (a displaced) ovary _____
22. excision of the uterus and ovaries _____
23. suturing the perineum _____
24. excision of the uterus, oviducts, and ovaries _____
25. puncture of the amnion (amniotic sac) _____

✓ Check your answers in Appendix A. Review material that you did not answer correctly.

CORRECT ANSWERS _____ × 4 = _____ **% SCORE**

Learning Activity 12–4

Matching pathological, diagnostic, symptomatic, and related terms

Match the following terms with the definitions in the numbered list.

asymptomatic	*dystocia*	*parturition*
atresia	*eclampsia*	*primigravida*
candidiasis	*gestation*	*primipara*
chancre	*leiomyoma*	*pruritus vulvae*
condylomas	*menarche*	*pyosalpinx*
congenital	*metrorrhagia*	*retroversion*
Down syndrome	*oligomenorrhea*	*viable*

1. _____ accumulation of pus in a uterine tube
2. _____ woman who has had one pregnancy that has resulted in a viable offspring
3. _____ pregnancy; 40 weeks in human beings
4. _____ primary syphilitic sore
5. _____ an entire organ, such as the uterus, that is tipped backward from its normal position
6. _____ present at birth
7. _____ difficult labor or childbirth
8. _____ congenital absence of a normal body opening, such as the vagina
9. _____ trisomy 21
10. _____ intense itching of the external female genitalia
11. _____ without symptoms
12. _____ irregular uterine bleeding between menstrual periods
13. _____ beginning of menstrual function

14. _____ benign uterine tumor composed of muscle and fibrous tissue

15. _____ infrequent menstrual flow

16. _____ process of giving birth

17. _____ most serious form of toxemia of pregnancy

18. _____ capable of living outside the uterus

19. _____ genital warts

20. _____ woman during her first pregnancy

✓ Check your answers in Appendix A. Review material that you did not answer correctly.

CORRECT ANSWERS _____ × 5 = _____ **% SCORE**

Learning Activity 12–5

Matching procedures, pharmacology, and abbreviations

Match the following terms with the definitions in the numbered list.

amniocentesis	*episiotomy*	*oxytocins*
antifungals	*estrogens*	*Pap test*
chorionic villus sampling	*hysterosalpingography*	*prostaglandins*
colpocleisis	*IUD*	*total abdominal hysterectomy (TAH)*
cordocentesis	*laparoscopy*	*tubal ligation*
cryocautery	*lumpectomy*	*ultrasonography*
D&C	*OCPs*	

1. _____ cytological study used to detect cancer in cells that an organ has shed

2. _____ radiography of the uterus and oviducts after a contrast medium is injected into those organs

3. _____ transabdominal puncture of the amniotic sac to remove amniotic fluid for biochemical and cytological study

4. _____ class of drugs used to treat vaginal yeast infections

5. _____ surgical closure of the vaginal canal

6. _____ procedure that widens the cervical canal with a dilator and scrapes the uterine endometrium with a curette

7. _____ excision of the entire uterus, including the cervix, through an abdominal incision

8. _____ tying the uterine tubes to prevent pregnancy

9. _____ birth control pills taken orally

10. _____ examination of the abdominal cavity using an endoscope

11. _____ incision of the perineum to facilitate childbirth

12. _____ noninvasive ultrasound technique used to produce images of internal structures in the body

13. _____ test to detect chromosomal abnormalities that can be done earlier than amniocentesis

14. _____ hormone replacement to reduce adverse symptoms of menopause

15. _____ agents used to induce labor and to rid uterus of unexpelled placenta or fetus that has died

16. _____ freezing tissue to destroy cells

17. _____ birth control method in which object is placed inside the uterus to prevent pregnancy

18. _____ sampling of fetal blood drawn from the umbilical vein

19. _____ excision of a small primary breast tumor

20. _____ agents used to terminate pregnancy

✓ Check your answers in Appendix A. Review any material that you did not answer correctly.

CORRECT ANSWERS _____ × **5** = _____ **% SCORE**

MEDICAL RECORD ACTIVITIES

The two medical records included in the activities that follow use common clinical scenarios to show how medical terminology is used to document patient care. Complete the terminology and analysis sections for each activity to help you recognize and understand terms related to the female reproductive system.

Medical Record Activity 12–1

Primary herpes 1 infection

Terminology

The terms listed in the chart come from the medical record *Primary Herpes 1 Infection* that follows. Use a medical dictionary such as *Taber's Cyclopedic Medical Dictionary*, the appendices of this book, or other resources to define each term. Then review the pronunciations for each term and practice by reading the medical record aloud.

Term	Definition
adenopathy ăd-ĕ-NŎP-ă-thē	
chlamydia klă-MĬD-ē-ă	
GC screen	
herpes lesions HĔR-pēz	
introitus ĭn-TRŌ-ĭ-tŭs	
labia LĀ-bē-ă	
LMP	
lt	
monilial mō-NĬL-ē-ăl	
OCPs	

Term	Definition
pruritus proo-RĪ-tŭs	
R/O	
rt	
vulvar VŬL-văr	
Wet prep WĔT PRĔP	

PRIMARY HERPES 1 INFECTION

PRESENT ILLNESS: A 24-year-old patient started having some sore areas around the labia, both rt and lt side. She stated that the last few days she started having a brownish discharge. She has pruritus and pain of her vulvar area with adenopathy and pm fever, and blisters. Apparently her partner had a cold sore and they had oral-genital sex.

The patient has been using condoms since last seen in April. She has not missed any OCPs. LMP 5/15/xx. Patient has what looks like herpes lesions and ulcers all over vulva and introitus area. Rt labia appears as an ulcerlike lesion; it appears to be almost like an infected follicle. Speculum inserted, a brown discharge noted. GC screen, chlamydia screen, and general culture obtained from that. Wet prep revealed monilial forms. Viral culture obtained from the ulcerlike lesion on the right.

DIAGNOSIS: Primary herpes 1 infection; will R/O other infectious etiologies.

Analysis

Review the medical record *Primary Herpes 1 Infection* to answer the following questions.

1. Did the patient have any discharge? If so, describe it.

   _____

2. What type of discomfort was the patient experiencing around the vulvar area?

   _____

3. Has the patient been taking her oral contraceptive pills regularly?

   _____

4. Where was the viral culture obtained?

   _____

5. Even though the patient's partner used a condom, how do you think the patient became infected with herpes?

   _____

Medical Record Activity 12–2

Menometrorrhagia

Terminology

The terms listed in the chart come from the medical record *Menometrorrhagia* that follows. Use a medical dictionary such as *Taber's Cyclopedic Medical Dictionary*, the appendices of this book, or other resources to define each term. Then review the pronunciations for each term and practice by reading the medical record aloud.

Term	Definition
ablation ăb-LĀ-shŭn	
benign bē-NĪN	
Cesarean section sē-SĂR-ē-ăn	
cholecystectomy kō-lē-sĭs-TĔK-tō-mē	
dysmenorrhea dĭs-mĕn-ō-RĒ-ă	
endometrial biopsy ĕn-dō-MĒ-trē-ăl BĪ-ŏp-sē	
fibroids FĪ-broyds	
gravida 2 GRĂV-ĭ-dă	
hysterectomy hĭs-tĕr-ĔK-tō-mē	
laparoscopic lăp-ă-rō-SKŎP-ik	
mammogram MĂM-ō-grăm	
menometrorrhagia mĕn-ō-mĕt-rō-RĀ-jē-ă	
palliative PĂL-ē-ā-tĭv	
para I PĂR-ă	
postoperative pōst-ŎP-ĕr-ă-tĭv	

Term	Definition
Premarin PRĔM-ă-rĭn	
salpingo-oophorectomy săl-pĭng-gō-ō-ŏf-ō-RĔK-tō-mē	
therapeutic abortion thĕr-ă-PŪ-tĭk ă-BOR-shŭn	
thyroid function test THĪ-royd FŬNG-shŭn	

MENOMETRORRHAGIA

CHIEF COMPLAINT: Dysmenorrhea and night sweats

HISTORY OF PRESENT ILLNESS: The patient is a 43-year-old gravida 2, para 1 with multiple small uterine fibroids, irregular menses twice a month, family history of ovarian cancer, benign endometrial biopsy, normal Pap, normal mammogram, and normal thyroid function tests. Negative cervical cultures. She has completed childbearing and desires definitive treatment on endometrial ablation, hormonal regulation.

SURGICAL HISTORY: Cesarean section, therapeutic abortion, and cholecystectomy

ASSESSMENT: This is a patient with menometrorrhagia who declines palliative treatment and desires definitive treatment in the form of a hysterectomy.

PLAN: The plan is to perform a laparoscopic assisted vaginal hysterectomy as the patient has essentially no uterine prolapse and desires her ovaries taken out. She desires to be started on Premarin in the postoperative period. She has been counseled concerning the risks of surgery, including injury to bowel or bladder, infection, and bleeding.

She voices understanding and agrees to the plan to perform a laparoscopic assisted vaginal hysterectomy bilateral salpingo-oophorectomy.

Analysis

Review the medical record *Menometrorrhagia* to answer the following questions.

1. How many pregnancies did this patient have? How many viable infants did she deliver?

   _____

2. What is a therapeutic abortion?

   _____

3. Why did the physician propose to perform a hysterectomy?

   _____

4. What is a vaginal hysterectomy?

   _____

5. Does the surgeon plan to remove one or both ovaries and fallopian tubes?

   _____

6. Why do you think the physician will use the laparoscope to perform the hysterectomy?

   _____

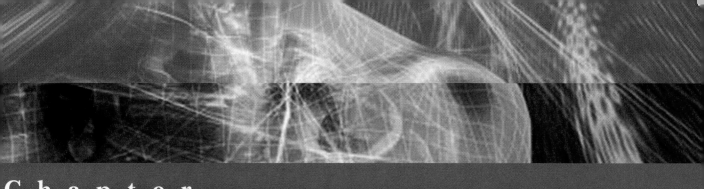

Chapter

13

Endocrine System

CHAPTER OUTLINE

OBJECTIVES

Upon completion of this chapter, you will be able to:

- Locate and describe the structures of the endocrine system.
- Recognize, pronounce, spell, and build words related to the endocrine system.
- Describe pathological conditions, diagnostic and therapeutic procedures, and other terms related to the endocrine system.
- Explain pharmacology related to the treatment of endocrine disorders.
- Demonstrate your knowledge of this chapter by completing the learning and medical record activities.

387

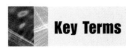

Key Terms

This section introduces important endocrine system terms and their definitions. Word analyses are also provided.

Term	Definition
diabetes insipidus di-ă-BĒ-tēz in-SĬ-pĭ-dŭs	Disorder of insufficient secretion of antidiuretic hormone (ADH) by the posterior portion of the pituitary gland *Diabetes insipidus is characterized by polyuria and polydipsia.*
diabetes mellitus di-ă-BĒ-tēz MĚ-lĭ-tŭs	Chronic metabolic disorder of impaired carbohydrate, protein, and fat metabolism due to insufficient secretion of insulin or insulin resistance of target tissues *When body cells are deprived of glucose, their principal energy fuel, they begin to metabolize fats and proteins, depositing unusually high levels of wastes in the blood, causing a condition called ketosis. Hyperglycemia and ketosis are responsible for the host of troubling and commonly life-threatening symptoms of diabetes mellitus.*
electrolytes ē-LĚK-trō-lits	Mineral salts (sodium, potassium, and calcium) that carry an electrical charge in solution *A proper balance of electrolytes is essential to the normal functioning of the entire body.*
glucagon GLOO-kă-gŏn	Hormone produced by pancreatic alpha cells that increases the blood glucose level by stimulating the liver to change stored glycogen (a starch form of sugar) to glucose *Glucagon opposes the action of insulin and is used to reverse hypoglycemic reactions in insulin shock.*
glucose GLOO-kōs	Simple sugar that is the end product of carbohydrate digestion *Glucose is the primary source of energy for living organisms.*

homeostasis
hō-mē-ō-STĀ-sĭs
 	
   homeo-: same, alike
   -stasis: standing still
	The body's internal state of equilibrium that is maintained by the every-changing processes of feedback and regulation in response to external or internal changes

hormone HOR-mōn	Chemical substances produced by specialized cells of the body that are released slowly in minute amounts directly into the bloodstream *Hormones are produced primarily by endocrine glands and are carried through the bloodstream to the target organ.*

hyperglycemia
hi-pĕr-gli-SĒ-mē-ă
 	
   hyper-: excessive, above normal
   glyc: sugar, sweetness
   -emia: blood condition
	Greater than normal amount of glucose in the blood; commonly associated with diabetes mellitus

Term	Definition
idiopathic ĭd-ē-ō-PĂTH-ĭk *idi/o:* unknown, peculiar *path:* disease *-ic:* pertaining to, relating to	Pertaining to conditions without clear pathogenesis or disease without recognizable cause
insulin ĬN-sŭ-lĭn	Hormone produced by pancreatic beta cells that acts to clear sugar (glucose) from the blood by promoting its storage in tissues as carbohydrates (glycogen)
mimetic mĭm-ĔT-ĭk	Imitation or simulation of a certain effect
sympathomimetic sĭm-pă-thō-mĭm-ĔT-ĭk	Agent that mimics the effects of the sympathetic nervous system *Epinephrine and norepinephrine are sympathomimetic hormones because they produce effects that mimic those brought about by the sympathetic nervous system.*
target	A structure, organ, or tissue to which something is directed *In the endocrine system, a target is the structure, organ, or tissue on which a hormone exerts its specific effect.*

Anatomy and Physiology

The endocrine system comprises a network of ductless glands that produce specific effects on body functions by slowly discharging **hormones** directly into the bloodstream. The ductless glands of the endocrine system are not to be confused with exocrine glands such as the sweat and oil glands of the skin, which release their secretions externally through ducts. Although the general effects of most hormones are well known, the manner in which specific hormones affect different organs or tissues of the body is just now becoming clear. The organs or tissues that respond to the effects of a hormone are called **target organs** or **target tissues.** The release of a hormone by an endocrine gland to a target organ is determined by the body's need for the hormone at any given time and is regulated to avoid overproduction **(hypersecretion)** or underproduction **(hyposecretion).** Unfortunately, there are times when the body's regulating mechanism does not operate properly and hormonal levels become excessive or deficient, causing various disorders.

This chapter discusses the structure, hormones, and functions of the *pituitary, thyroid, parathyroid, adrenal, pancreatic,* and *pineal glands.* The function of the *thymus* is covered in Chapter 9, the *testes* in Chapter 11, and the *ovaries* in Chapter 12. (See Figure 13–1.)

Pituitary Gland

The (1) **pituitary gland,** or **hypophysis,** is no larger than a pea and is located at the base of the brain. It is known as the "master gland" because it regulates many body activities and stimu-

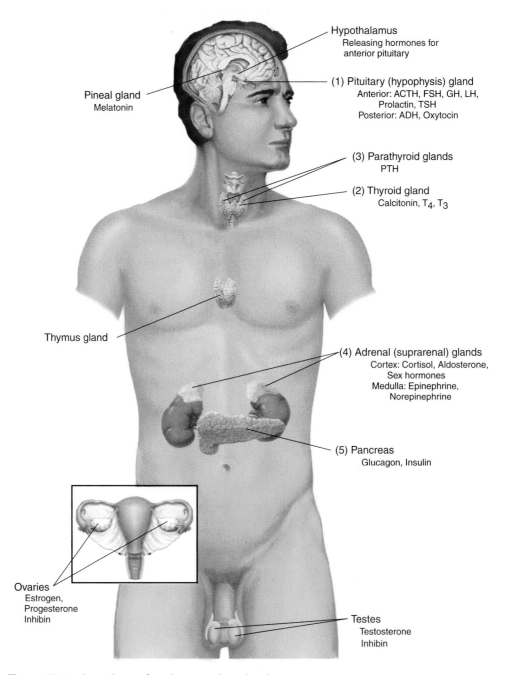

Hypothalamus
Releasing hormones for
anterior pituitary

(1) Pituitary (hypophysis) gland
Anterior: ACTH, FSH, GH, LH,
Prolactin, TSH
Posterior: ADH, Oxytocin

Pineal gland
Melatonin

(3) Parathyroid glands
PTH

(2) Thyroid gland
Calcitonin, T$_4$, T$_3$

Thymus gland

(4) Adrenal (suprarenal) glands
Cortex: Cortisol, Aldosterone,
Sex hormones
Medulla: Epinephrine,
Norepinephrine

(5) Pancreas
Glucagon, Insulin

Ovaries
Estrogen,
Progesterone
Inhibin

Testes
Testosterone
Inhibin

Figure 13–1   Locations of major exocrine glands.

lates other glands to secrete their own specific hormones. (See Figure 13–2.) The pituitary gland consists of two distinct portions, an anterior lobe (adenohypophysis) and a posterior lobe (neurohypophysis). The anterior lobe, triggered by the action of the hypothalamus, produces at least six hormones. The hypothalamus also produces and secretes two hormones directly to the posterior lobe, where they are stored and released into the bloodstream as needed. (See Table 13–1.)

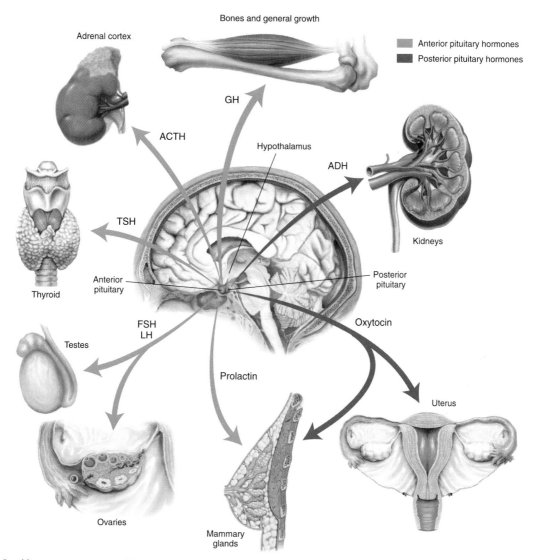

Figure 13–2   Hormones secreted by anterior and posterior pituitary gland along with target organs.

Table 13–1	PITUITARY HORMONES	

This table outlines pituitary hormones, along with their target organs and functions and selected associated disorders.

Hormone	Target Organ and Functions	Disorders
Posterior Pituitary Hormones (Neurohypophysis)		
Antidiuretic hormone (ADH)	• Kidney—increases water reab-sorption (water returns to the blood)	• Hyposecretion causes diabetes insipidus. • Hypersecretion causes syndrome of inappro-priate antidiuretic hormone (SIADH).
Oxytocin	• Uterus—stimulates uterine contractions; initiates labor • Breast—promotes milk secre-tion from the mammary glands	• Unknown

(Continued)

Table 13–1   PITUITARY HORMONES *(Continued)*

Hormone	Target Organ and Functions	Disorders
Anterior Pituitary Hormones (Adenohypophysis)		
Adrenocorticotropic hormone (ACTH)	• Adrenal cortex—promotes secretions of some hormones by adrenal cortex, especially cortisol	• Hyposecretion is rare. • Hypersecretion causes Cushing disease.
Follicle-stimulating hormone (FSH)	• Ovaries—in females, stimulates egg production; increases secretion of estrogen • Testes—in males, stimulates sperm production	• Hyposecretion causes failure of sexual maturation. • Hypersecretion has no known significant effects.
Growth hormone (GH) or somatotropin	• Bone, cartilage, liver, muscle, and other tissues—stimulates somatic growth; increases use of fats for energy	• Hyposecretion in children causes pituitary dwarfism. • Hypersecretion in children causes gigantism; hypersecretion in adults causes acromegaly.
Luteinizing hormone (LH)	• Ovaries—in females, promotes ovulation; stimulates production of estrogen and progesterone • Testes—in males, promotes secretion of testosterone	• Hyposecretion causes failure of sexual maturation. • Hypersecretion has no known significant effects.
Prolactin	• Breast—in conjunction with other hormones, promotes lactation	• Hyposecretion in nursing mothers causes poor lactation. • Hypersecretion in nursing mothers causes galactorrhea.
Thyroid-stimulating hormone (TSH)	• Thyroid gland—stimulates secretion of thyroid hormone	• Hyposecretion in infants causes cretinism; hyposecretion in adults causes myxedema. • Hypersecretion causes Graves disease, exophthalmos. (See Figure 13–3.)

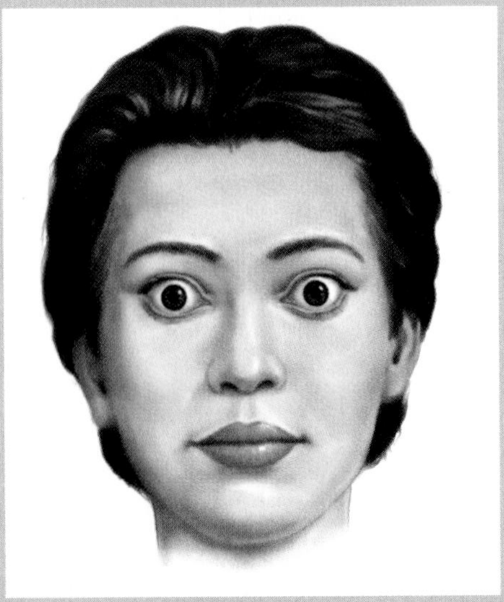

Figure 13–3   Exophthalmos caused by Graves disease.

Thyroid Gland

The (2) **thyroid gland** is the largest gland of the endocrine system. An H-shaped organ located in the neck just below the larynx, this gland is composed of two large lobes that are separated by a strip of tissue called an **isthmus.** Thyroid hormone (TH) is the body's major metabolic hormone, which increases the rate of oxygen consumption and thus the rate at which carbohydrates, proteins, and fats are metabolized. TH is actually two active iodine-containing hormones, **thyroxine (T_4)** and **triiodothyronine (T_3).** Thyroxine is the major hormone secreted by the thyroid; most triiodothyronine is formed at the target tissues by conversion of T_4 to T_3. Except for the adult brain, spleen, testes, uterus, and the thyroid gland itself, thyroid hormone affects virtually every cell in the body. TH also influences growth hormone and plays an important role in maintaining blood pressure. (See Table 13–2.)

Table 13–2   THYROID HORMONES

This table outlines thyroid hormones, along with their functions and selected associated disorders.

Hormone	Functions	Disorders
Calcitonin	• Regulates calcium levels in the blood in conjunction with parathyroid hormone • Secreted when calcium levels in the blood are high in order to maintain homeostasis	• Exerts its most significant effects in childhood when bones are growing and changing dramatically in mass, size, and shape • At best, a weak hypocalcemic agent in adults
Thyroxine (T_4) and triiodothyronine (T_3)	• Increases energy production from all food types • Increases rate of protein synthesis	• Hyposecretion in infants causes cretinism; hyposecretion in adults causes myxedema. • Hypersecretion causes Graves disease, exophthalmos. (See Figure 13–3.)

Parathyroid Glands

The (3) **parathyroid glands** consist of at least four separate glands located on the posterior surface of the lobes of the thyroid gland. The only hormone known to be secreted by the parathyroid glands is parathyroid hormone (PTH). PTH helps to regulate calcium balance by stimulating three target organs: bones, kidneys, and intestines. (See Table 13–3.) Because of PTH stimulation, calcium and phosphates are released from bones, increasing concentration of these substances in blood. Thus, calcium that is necessary for the proper functioning of body tissues is available in the bloodstream. At the same time, PTH enhances the absorption of calcium and phosphates from foods in the intestine, causing a rise in the blood levels of calcium and phosphates. PTH causes the kidneys to conserve blood calcium and to increase the excretion of phosphates in the urine.

Adrenal Glands

The (4) **adrenal glands** are paired organs covering the superior surface of the kidneys. Because of their location, the adrenal glands are also known as *suprarenal glands.* Each adrenal gland is divided into two sections, each of which has its own structure and function. The outer adrenal cortex makes up the bulk of the gland and the adrenal medulla makes up the inner portion. Although these regions are not sharply divided, they represent distinct glands that secrete different hormones.

Table 13–3	PARATHYROID HORMONES	

This table outlines parathyroid hormones, along with their target organs and functions and selected associated disorders.

Hormone	Target Organ and Functions	Disorders
Parathyroid hormone (PTH)	• Bones—increases the reabsorption of calcium and phosphate from bone to blood • Kidneys—increases calcium absorption and phosphate excretion • Small intestine—increases absorption of calcium and phosphate	• Hyposecretion causes tetany. • Hypersecretion causes osteitis fibrosa cystica.

Adrenal Cortex

The adrenal cortex secretes three types of steroid hormones:

1. **Mineralocorticoids,** mainly aldosterone, are essential to life. These hormones act mainly through the kidneys to maintain the balance of sodium and potassium **(electrolytes)** in the body. More specifically, aldosterone causes the kidneys to conserve sodium and excrete potassium. At the same time, it promotes water conservation and reduces urine output.
2. **Glucocorticoids,** mainly cortisol, influence the metabolism of carbohydrates, fats, and proteins. The glucocorticoid with the greatest activity is *cortisol.* It helps to regulate the concentration of glucose in the blood, protecting against low blood sugar levels between meals. Cortisol also stimulates the breakdown of fats in adipose tissue and releases fatty acids into the blood. The increase in fatty acids causes many cells to use relatively less glucose.
3. **Sex hormones,** including androgens, estrogens, progestins, help maintain secondary sex characteristics, such as development of the breasts and adult distribution of hair. (See Table 13–4.)

Adrenal Medulla

The adrenal medulla cells secrete two closely related hormones, **epinephrine** (adrenaline) and **norepinephrine** (noradrenaline). Both of these hormones are activated when the body responds to crisis situations, and are considered sympathomimetic agents because they produce effects that mimic those brought about by the sympathetic nervous system. Because hormones of the adrenal medulla merely intensify activities set into motion by the sympathetic nervous system, their deficiency is not a problem.

Of the two hormones, epinephrine is secreted in larger amounts. In the physiological response to stress, epinephrine is responsible for maintaining blood pressure and cardiac output, keeping airways open wide, and raising blood glucose levels. All these functions are useful for frightened, traumatized, injured, or sick persons. Norepinephrine reduces the diameter of blood vessels in the periphery (vasoconstriction), thereby raising blood pressure. (See Table 13–4.)

Pancreas (Islets of Langerhans)

The (5) **pancreas** lies inferior to the stomach in a bend of the duodenum. It functions both as an exocrine and endocrine gland. A large pancreatic duct runs through the gland, carrying enzymes and other exocrine digestive secretions from the pancreas to the small intestine. The endocrine portion of the pancreas consists of groups of cells called islets of Langerhans that produce two distinct types of hormones: alpha cells that produce glucagon and beta cells that produce insulin. Both hormones play important roles in the proper metabolism of sugars and starches in the body.

When blood glucose levels are low **(hypoglycemia),** glucagon stimulates the release of glucose from storage sites in the liver. Because the liver converts stored glycogen to glucose **(glycogenolysis),** the blood glucose level rises. The overall effect, therefore, is a rise in the

Table 13-4   ADRENAL HORMONES

This table outlines adrenal hormones, along with their target organs and functions and selected associated disorders.

Hormone	Target Organ and Functions	Disorders
Adrenal Cortex Hormones		
Glucocorticoids (mainly cortisol)	• Body cells—promote gluconeogenesis; regulate metabolism of carbohydrates, proteins, and fats; help depress inflammatory and immune responses	• Hyposecretion causes Addison disease. • Hypersecretion causes Cushing syndrome. (See Figure 13–4.)
Mineralocorticoids (mainly aldosterone)	• Kidneys—increase blood levels of sodium and decrease blood levels of potassium in the kidneys	• Hyposecretion causes Addison disease. • Hypersecretion causes aldosteronism.
Sex hormones (any of the androgens, estrogens, or related steroid hormones) produced by the ovaries, testes, and adrenal cortices	• In females, possibly responsible for female libido and source of estrogen after menopause; otherwise, effects in adults are insignificant.	• Hypersecretion of adrenal androgen in females leads to virilism (development of male characteristics). • Hypersecretion of adrenal estrogen and progestin secretion in males leads to feminization (development of feminine characteristics). • Hyposecretion has no known significant effects.
Adrenal Medullary Hormones		
Epinephrine and norepinephrine	• Sympathetic nervous system target organs—hormone effects mimic sympathetic nervous system activation (sympathomimetic); increase metabolic rate and heart rate; raise blood pressure by promoting vasoconstriction	• Hyposecretion has no known significant effects. • Hypersecretion causes prolonged "fight-or-flight" reaction and hypertension.

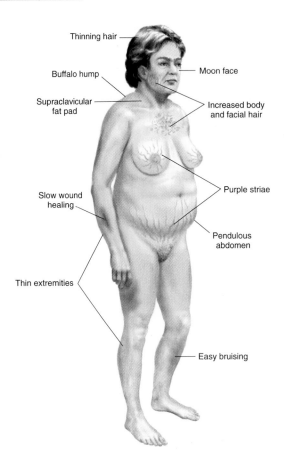

Thinning hair

Moon face

Buffalo hump

Supraclavicular
fat pad

Increased body
and facial hair

Purple striae

Slow wound
healing

Pendulous
abdomen

Thin extremities

Easy bruising

Figure 13–4   Physical manifestations of Cushing syndrome.

blood glucose level. When blood glucose levels are high **(hyperglycemia),** the pancreatic beta cells are stimulated to produce insulin, which causes glucose to enter body cells to be used for energy and acts to clear glucose from the blood by promoting its storage as glycogen. Insulin and glucagon function as opposites—normal secretion of both hormones ensures a blood glucose level that fluctuates within normal limits. (See Table 13–5.)

Table 13–5	PANCREATIC HORMONES	

This table outlines pancreatic hormones, along with their target organs and functions and selected associated disorders.

Hormone	Target Organ and Functions	Disorders
Glucagon	• Liver and blood—raises blood glucose level by accelerating conversion of glycogen into glucose in the liver (glycogenolysis) and other nutrients into glucose in the liver (gluconeogenesis) and releasing glucose into blood (glycogen to glucose)	• Persistently low blood glucose levels (hypoglycemia) may be caused by deficiency in glucagon.
Insulin	• Tissue cells—lowers blood glucose level by accelerating glucose transport into cells and the use of that glucose for energy production (glucose to glycogen)	• Hyposecretion of insulin causes diabetes mellitus. • Hypersecretion of insulin causes hyperinsulinism.

Pineal Gland

The (6) **pineal gland,** which is shaped like a pinecone, is attached to the posterior part of the third ventricle of the brain. Although the exact functions of this gland have not been established, there is evidence that it secretes the hormone melatonin. It is believed that melatonin may inhibit the activities of the ovaries. When melatonin production is high, ovulation is blocked, and there may be a delay in puberty development.

 It is time to review anatomy by completing Learning Activity 13–1.

 Medical Word Elements

This section introduces combining forms, suffixes, and prefixes related to the endocrine system. Word analyses are also provided.

Element	Meaning	Word Analysis
COMBINING FORMS		
adren/o	adrenal glands	adren/o/megaly (ăd-rēn-ō-MĔG-ă-lē): enlargement of the adrenal glands
		-megaly: enlargement
adrenal/o		adrenal/ectomy (ăd-rē-năl-ĔK-tō-mē): excision of one or both adrenal glands
		-ectomy: excision, removal
calc/o	calcium	hyper/calc/emia (hī-pĕr-kăl-SĒ-mē-ă): abnormally high level of calcium in the blood
		hyper-: excessive, above normal
		-emia: blood condition
crin/o	secrete	endo/crin/o/logy (ĕn-dō-krĭn-ŎL-ō-jē): study of the endocrine glands and their functions
		endo-: in, within
		-logy: study of
gluc/o	sugar, sweetness	gluc/o/genesis (gloo-kō-JĔN-ĕ-sĭs): forming or producing glucose
		-genesis: forming, producing, origin
glycos/o		glycos/uria (glī-kō-SŪ-rē-ă): abnormal amount of sugar, especially glucose, in the urine
		-uria: urine
glyc/o		hypo/glyc/emia (hī-pō-glī-SĒ-mē-ă): abnormally low level of glucose in the blood
		hypo-: under, below
		-emia: blood condition
		Hypoglycemia is usually caused by administration of too much insulin, excessive secretion of insulin by the islet cells of the pancreas, or dietary deficiency.

(Continued)

Element	Meaning	Word Analysis	*(Continued)*
home/o	same, alike	home/o/stasis (hō-mē-ō-STĀ-sĭs): state of equilibrium in the internal environment of the body *-stasis:* standing still	
kal/i*	potassium (an electrolyte)	kal/emia (kă-LĒ-mē-ă): presence of potassium in the blood *-emia:* blood condition	
pancreat/o	pancreas	pancreat/o/tomy (păn-krē-ă-TŎT-ō-mē): incision in the pancreas *-tomy:* incision	
parathyroid/o	parathyroid glands	parathyroid/ectomy (păr-ă-thī-royd-ĔK-tō-mē): excision of one or more of the parathyroid glands *-ectomy:* excision, removal	
thym/o	thymus gland	thym/oma (thī-MŌ-mă): rare neoplasm of the thymus gland *-oma:* tumor *Treatment for thymoma may include surgical removal, radiation therapy, or chemotherapy.*	
thyr/o **thyroid/o**	thyroid gland	thyr/o/megaly (thī-rō-MĔG-ă-lē): enlargement of the thyroid gland *-megaly:* enlargement hyper/thyroid/ism (hī-pĕr-THĪ-royd-ĭzm): condition characterized by hyperactivity of the thyroid gland *hyper-:* excessive, above normal *-ism:* condition	
toxic/o	poison	toxic/o/logist (tŏks-ĭ-KŎL-ō-jĭst): specialist in poisons, their effects, and antidotes *-logist:* specialist in study of	

SUFFIXES

Element	Meaning	Word Analysis	
-crine	secrete	endo/crine (ĔN-dō-krĭn): secrete internally or within *endo-:* in, within	
-dipsia	thirst	poly/dipsia (pŏl-ē-DĬP-sē-ă): excessive thirst *-poly-:* many, much	
-gen	forming, producing, origin	andr/o/gen (ĂN-drō-jĕn): any steroid hormone that increases masculinization *andr/o:* male	
-toxic	poison	thyr/o/toxic (thī-rō-TŎKS-ĭk): pertaining to, affected by, or marked by toxic activity of the thyroid gland *thyr/o:* thyroid gland	
-uria	urine	glycos/uria (glī-kō-SŪ-rē-ă): abnormal amount of glucose in the urine *glycos:* sugar, sweetness	

Element	Meaning	Word Analysis
PREFIXES		
eu-	good, normal	eu/thyr/oid (ū-THĪ-royd): pertains to a normal thyroid gland *thyr/o:* thyroid gland *-oid:* resembling
exo-	outside, outward	exo/crine (ĔKS-ō-krĭn): secrete outwardly *-crine:* secrete *Exocrine denotes a gland that secretes outwardly through excretory ducts*
hyper-	excessive, above normal	hyper/glyc/emia (hī-pĕr-glĭ-SĒ-mē-ă): increased blood glucose, as occurs in diabetes *glyc:* sugar, sweetness *-emia:* blood condition
hypo-	under, below	hypo/insulin/ism (hī-pō-ĬN-sŭ-lĭn-ĭzm): deficiency of insulin secretion by cells of the pancreas *-ism:* condition
poly-	many, much	poly/uria (pŏl-ē-Ū-rē-ă): excessive secretion and discharge of urine *-uria:* urine *Some causes of polyuria are diabetes, use of diuretics, excessive fluid intake, and hypercalcemia.*

*The combining vowel *i* is used instead of *o*. This is an exception to the rule.

It is time to review medical word elements by completing Learning Activity 13–2.

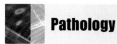

Pathology

Disorders of the endocrine system are caused by underproduction **(hyposecretion)** or overproduction **(hypersecretion)** of hormones. In general, hyposecretion is treated with drug therapy in the form of hormone replacement. Hypersecretion is generally treated by surgery. Most hormone deficiencies result from genetic defects in the glands, surgical removal of the glands, or production of poor-quality hormones.

Pituitary Disorders

Hypersecretion or hyposecretion of growth hormone leads to body-size abnormalities. Abnormal variations of ADH secretion lead to disorders in the composition of blood and marked electrolyte imbalance. (See Table 13–1.)

Thyroid Disorders

Thyroid gland disorders are common and may develop at any time during life. They may be the result of a developmental problem, injury, disease, or dietary deficiency. One form of hypothyroidism that develops in infants is called *cretinism*. If not treated, this disorder leads to mental retardation, impaired growth, low body temperatures, and abnormal bone formation. Usually these symptoms do not appear at birth because the infant has received thyroid hormones from the mother's blood during fetal development. When hypothyroidism develops during adulthood, it is known as **myxedema.** The characteristics of this disease are edema, low blood levels of T_3 and T_4, mental retardation, weight gain, and sluggishness.

Hyperthyroidism results from excessive secretions of T_3, T_4, or both. Two of the most common disorders of hyperthyroidism are **Graves disease** and **toxic goiter.** Graves disease is considerably more prevalent and is characterized by an elevated metabolic rate, abnormal weight loss, excessive perspiration, muscular weakness, and emotional instability. Also, the eyes are likely to protrude **(exophthalmos)** because of edematous swelling in the tissues behind them. (See Figure 13–3.) At the same time, the thyroid gland is likely to enlarge, producing *goiter*. (See Figure 13–5.)

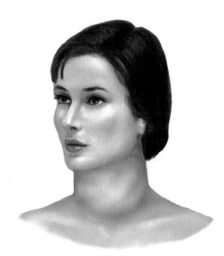

Figure 13–5   Enlargement of the thyroid gland in goiter.

It is believed that toxic goiter may occur because of excessive release of thyroid-stimulating hormone (TSH) from the anterior lobe of the pituitary gland. Overstimulation by TSH causes thyroid cells to enlarge and secrete extra amounts of hormones. Treatment for this condition may involve drug therapy to block the production of thyroid hormones or surgical removal of all or part of the thyroid gland. Another method for treating this disorder is to administer a sufficient amount of radioactive iodine to destroy the thyroid secretory cells. (See Table 13–2.)

Parathyroid Disorders

As with the thyroid gland, dysfunction of the parathyroids is usually characterized by inadequate hormone secretion **(hypoparathyroidism),** or excessive hormone secretion **(hyperparathyroidism).**

Insufficient production of parathyroid hormone (PTH), called *hypoparathyroidism*, can be caused by primary parathyroid dysfunction or by elevated blood calcium levels. This condition can result from an injury or from surgical removal of the glands, sometimes in conjunction with thyroid surgery. The primary effect of hypoparathyroidism is a decreased blood calcium level (**hypocalcemia**). Decreased calcium lowers the electrical threshold, causing neurons to depolarize more easily, and increases the number of nerve impulses, resulting in muscle twitches and spasms (**tetany**).

Excessive production of PTH, called *hyperparathyroidism,* is commonly caused by a benign tumor. The increase in PTH secretion leads to demineralization of bones (**osteitis fibrosa cystica**), making them porous (**osteoporosis**) and highly susceptible to fracture and deformity. When this condition is the result of a benign glandular tumor (**adenoma**) of the parathyroid, the tumor is removed. Treatment may also include orthopedic surgery to correct severe bone deformities. Excess PTH also causes calcium to be deposited in the kidneys. When the disease is generalized and all bones are affected, this disorder is known as *von Recklinghausen disease.* Renal symptoms and kidney stones (**nephrolithiasis**) may also develop. (See Table 13–3.)

Disorders of the Adrenal Glands

As outlined before, the adrenal glands consist of the adrenal cortex and adrenal medulla. Each has its own structure and function as well as its own set of associated disorders.

Adrenal Cortex

The adrenal cortex is mainly associated with Addison disease and Cushing syndrome.

Addison disease. Addison disease, a relatively uncommon chronic disorder caused by a deficiency of cortical hormones, results when the adrenal cortex is damaged or atrophied. Atrophy of the adrenal glands is probably the result of an autoimmune process in which circulating adrenal antibodies slowly destroy the gland. The gland usually suffers 90% destruction before clinical signs of adrenal insufficiency appear. Hypofunction of the adrenal cortex interferes with the body's ability to handle internal and external stress. In severe cases, the disturbance of sodium and potassium metabolism may be marked by depletion of sodium and water through urination, resulting in severe chronic dehydration. Other clinical manifestations include muscular weakness, anorexia, gastrointestinal symptoms, fatigue, hypoglycemia, hypotension, low blood sodium (**hyponatremia**), and high serum potassium (**hyperkalemia**). If treatment for this condition begins early, usually with adrenocortical hormone therapy, the prognosis is excellent. If untreated, the disease will continue a chronic course with progressive but relatively slow deterioration. In some patients, the deterioration may be rapid.

Cushing syndrome. Cushing syndrome is a cluster of symptoms caused by excessive amounts of cortisol, adrenocorticotropin hormone (ACTH), or both circulating in the blood. (See Figure 13–4.) Causes of this excess secretion include:

- long-term administration of steroid drugs (glucocorticoids) in treating such diseases as rheumatoid arthritis, lupus erythematosus, and asthma
- adrenal tumor resulting in excessive production of cortisol
- Cushing disease, a pituitary disorder that results in increased secretion of ACTH.

Regardless of the cause, Cushing syndrome alters carbohydrate and protein metabolism and electrolyte balance. The overproduction of mineralocorticoids and glucocorticoids causes blood glucose concentration to remain high, depleting tissue protein. In addition, sodium retention causes increased fluid in tissue that leads to edema. These metabolic changes produce weight gain and may cause structural changes, such as a moon-shaped face, grossly exaggerated head and trunk, and pencil-thin arms and legs. Other symptoms include fatigue, high blood pressure, and excessive hair growth in unusual places (**hirsutism**), especially in women. The treatment goal for this disease is to restore serum cortisol to normal levels. Nevertheless, treatment varies with the cause and may necessitate radiation, drug therapy, surgery, or a combination of these methods.

Adrenal Medulla

No specific diseases can be traced directly to a deficiency of hormones from the adrenal medulla. However, medullary tumors sometimes cause excess secretions. The most common disorder is a neoplasm known as *pheochromocytoma*, which produces excessive amounts of epinephrine and norepinephrine. Most of these tumors are encapsulated and benign. These hypersecretions produce stress, fear, palpitations, headaches, visual blurring, muscle spasms, and sweating. Typical treatment consists of antihypertensive drugs and surgery.

Pancreatic Disorders

Diabetes is a general term that when used alone refers to diabetes mellitus (DM). It is by far the most common pancreatic disorder. DM is a disease in which the body does not produce sufficient insulin or does not utilize it properly. Insulin is an essential hormone for conversion of sugar, starches, and other food into energy required for daily life.

Although genetics and environmental factors, such as obesity and lack of exercise, seem significant in the development of this disease, the cause of diabetes is not always clear. It is characterized by an upset in carbohydrate metabolism and disturbance in protein and fat metabolism with a subsequent rise in the concentration of blood glucose **(hyperglycemia)**. Glucose is excreted in the urine **(glycosuria)** along with electrolytes, particularly sodium. Sodium and potassium losses result in muscle weakness and fatigue. Because glucose cannot enter the cells, cellular starvation results and leads to hunger and an increased appetite **(polyphagia)**. (See Table 13–5.) Diabetes mellitus occurs in two primary forms:

- *Type 1 diabetes*, also known as *insulin-dependent diabetes mellitus (IDDM)*, is usually diagnosed in children and young adults and was previously called *juvenile diabetes*. In type 1 diabetes, the body does not produce insulin. Treatment includes injection of insulin to maintain a normal level of glucose in the blood. (See Table 13–6.)
- *Type 2 diabetes*, also known as *non-insulin-dependent diabetes mellitus (NIDDM)*, is the most common form and is distinctively different from type 1. Its onset is usually later in life (maturity onset), and risk factors include a family history of diabetes and obesity. In type 2 diabetes, the body is deficient in producing enough insulin or the body's cells are resistant to insulin action in target tissues. The hyperglycemia that results may cause cell starvation and, over time, may damage the kidneys, eyes, nerves, or heart. Treatment for type 2 diabetes includes exercise, diet, weight loss and, if needed, insulin or oral antidiabetic agents. Oral antidiabetic agents activate the release of pancreatic insulin and improve the body's sensitivity to insulin. (See Table 13–6.)

Complications

Diabetes is associated with a number of primary and secondary complications. Patients with type 1 diabetes usually report rapidly developing symptoms. With type 2 diabetes, the patient's symptoms are usually vague, long-standing, and develop gradually.

Primary complications of type 1 include diabetic ketoacidosis (DKA). DKA, also referred to as *diabetic acidosis* or *diabetic coma*, may develop over several days or weeks. It can be caused by too little insulin, failure to follow a prescribed diet, physical or emotional stress, or undiagnosed diabetes.

Secondary complications due to long-standing diabetes emerge years after the initial

Table 13-6	CLINICAL MANIFESTATIONS OF DIABETES

According to the American Diabetes Association, the following signs and symptoms are manifestations of type 1 and type 2 diabetes.

Type 1 Diabetes

Type 1 diabetes may be suspected if any one of the associated signs and symptoms appears. Children usually exhibit dramatic, sudden symptoms and must receive prompt treatment. Signs and symptoms that signal type 1 diabetes can be remembered using the acronym *CAUTION*. Type 1 diabetes is characterized by the sudden appearance of:
- **C**onstant urination (polyuria) and glycosuria
- **A**bnormal thirst (polydipsia)
- **U**nusual hunger (polyphagia)
- **T**he rapid loss of weight
- **I**rritability
- **O**bvious weakness and fatigue
- **N**ausea and vomiting.

Type 2 Diabetes

Many adults may have type 2 diabetes with none of the associated signs or symptoms. The disease is commonly discovered during a routine physical examination. In addition to any of the signs and symptoms associated with type 1 diabetes, those for type 2 diabetes can be remembered using the acronym *DIABETES*:
- **D**rowsiness
- **I**tching
- **A** family history of diabetes
- **B**lurred vision
- **E**xcessive weight
- **T**ingling, numbness, and pain in the extremities
- **E**asily fatigued
- **S**kin infections and slow healing of cuts and scratches, especially of the feet.

diagnosis. Common chronic complications include diabetic retinopathy and diabetic nephropathy. In diabetic retinopathy, the retina's blood vessels are destroyed, causing visual loss and, eventually, blindness. In diabetic nephropathy, destruction of the kidneys causes renal insufficiency and commonly requires hemodialysis or renal transplantation. Another secondary complication known as *gestational diabetes* may occur in pregnant women because of the body's hormonal changes during pregnancy. Gestational diabetes usually subsides after the child is born **(parturition).** However, mothers with type 1 or type 2 diabetes mellitus have a two to three times greater risk of giving birth to infants who suffer fetal distress and congenital malformations.

Oncology

Pancreatic Cancer

Most carcinomas of the pancreas arise as epithelial tumors **(adenocarcinomas)** and make their presence known by obstruction and local invasion. Because the pancreas is richly supplied with nerves, pain is a prominent feature of pancreatic cancer, whether it arises in the head, body, or tail of the organ.

The prognosis in pancreatic cancer is poor, with only a 2% survival rate in 5 years. Pancreatic cancer is the fourth leading cause of cancer death in the United States. The highest incidence is among people ages 60 to 70. The etiology is unknown, but cigarette smoking, exposure to occupational chemicals, a diet high in fats, and heavy coffee intake are associated with an increased incidence of pancreatic cancer.

Pituitary Tumors

Pituitary tumors are generally not malignant, however because their growth is invasive, they are considered neoplastic and are usually treated as such. Initial signs and symptoms include headache, blurred vision, and, commonly, personality changes, dementia, and seizures. Tomography, skull radiographs, pneumoencephalography, angiography, and computed tomography scans assist in diagnosis. Depending on the size of the tumor and its location, different treatment modalities are employed. Treatments include surgical removal, radiation, or both.

Thyroid Carcinoma

Cancer of the thyroid gland, or *thyroid carcinoma*, is classified according to the specific tissue that is affected. In general, however, all types share many predisposing factors, including radiation, prolonged TSH stimulation, familial disposition, and chronic goiter. The malignancy usually begins with a painless, commonly hard nodule or a nodule in the adjacent lymph nodes accompanied with an enlarged thyroid. When the tumor is large, it typically destroys thyroid tissue, which results in symptoms of hypothyroidism. Sometimes the tumor stimulates the production of thyroid hormone, resulting in symptoms of hyperthyroidism. Treatment includes surgical removal, radiation, or both.

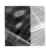

Diagnostic, Symptomatic, and Related Terms

This section introduces diagnostic, symptomatic, and related terms and their meanings. Word analyses for selected terms are also provided.

Term	Definition

acromegaly
ăk-rō-MĔG-ă-lē
 	
  acr/o: extremity
  -megaly: enlargement
	Chronic metabolic disorder characterized by a gradual, marked enlargement and thickening of the bones of the face and jaw
	
	Acromegaly afflicts middle-aged and older persons and is caused by overproduction of growth hormone (GH). Treatment includes radiation, pharmacological agents, or surgery, which commonly involves partial resection of the pituitary gland.

diuresis
dī-ū-RĒ-sĭs
 	
  di-: double
  ur: urine
  -esis: condition
	Abnormal secretion of large amounts of urine
	
	Diuresis occurs in such conditions as diabetes mellitus, diabetes insipidus, and acute renal failure.

glucagon GLOO-kă-gŏn	Hormone secreted by the pancreatic alpha cells *Glucagon increases the blood glucose level by stimulating the liver to change stored glycogen to glucose. Glucagon opposes the action of insulin and is used as an injection in diabetes to reverse hypoglycemic reactions and insulin shock.*

Term	Definition
glucose GLOO-kōs	Simple sugar that is the end product of carbohydrate digestion *Glucose is found in many foods, especially fruits, and is a major source of energy. The determination of blood glucose levels is an important diagnostic test in diabetes and other disorders.*
glycosuria glī-kō-SŪ-rē-ă *glycos:* sugar, sweetness *-uria:* urine	Presence of glucose in the urine, abnormal amount of sugar in the urine
Graves disease	Multisystem autoimmune disorder characterized by pronounced hyperthyroidism usually associated with enlarged thyroid gland and exophthalmos (abnormal protrusion of the eyeball) (See Figure 13–3.)
hirsutism HŬR-sūt-ĭzm	Excessive distribution of body hair, especially in women *Hirsutism in women is usually caused by abnormalities of androgen production or metabolism.*
hypercalcemia hī-pĕr-kăl-SĒ-mē-ă *hyper-:* excessive, above normal *calc:* calcium *-emia:* blood	Excessive amount of calcium in the blood
hyperkalemia hī-pĕr-kă-LĒ-mē-ă *hyper-:* excessive, above normal *kal:* potassium (an electrolyte) *-emia:* blood	Excessive amount of potassium in the blood *Hyperkalemia is most commonly a result of defective renal excretion of potassium.*
hypervolemia hī-pĕr-vŏl-Ē-mē-ă *hyper-:* excessive, above normal *vol:* volume *-emia:* blood	Abnormal increase in the volume of circulating fluid (plasma) in the body *Hypervolemia commonly results from retention of large amounts of sodium and water by the kidneys. Signs and symptoms of hypervolemia include weight gain, edema, dyspnea, tachycardia, and pulmonary congestion.*
hyponatremia hī-pō-nă-TRĒ-mē-ă *hypo-:* under, below, deficient *natr:* sodium (an electrolyte) *-emia:* blood	Abnormal condition of low sodium in the blood
insulinoma ĭn-sū-lĭn-Ō-mă *insulin:* insulin *-oma:* tumor	Tumor of the islets of Langerhans of the pancreas

(Continued)

Term	Definition	(Continued)
obesity ō-BĒ-sĭ-tē	Abnormal increase in the proportion of fat cells, mainly in the viscera and subcutaneous tissues of the body *Obesity may be due to an excessive intake of food (exogenous) or metabolic or endocrine abnormalities (endogenous).*	

panhypopituitarism
păn-hī-pō-pĭ-TŪ-ĭ-tăr-ĭzm
 	
  pan-: all
  hypo: under, below, deficient
  pituitar: pituitary gland
  -ism: condition
	Total pituitary impairment that brings about a progressive and general loss of hormonal activity	

pheochromocytoma fē-ō-krō-mō-sī-TŌ-mă	Small chromaffin cell tumor, usually located in the adrenal medulla	

thyroid storm
THĪ-royd
 	
  thyr: thyroid gland
  -oid: resembling
	Crisis of uncontrolled hyperthyroidism caused by the release into the bloodstream of increased amount of thyroid hormone; also called *thyroid crisis* or *thyrotoxic crisis*
	Thyroid storm may occur spontaneously or be precipitated by infection, stress, or thyroidectomy performed on a patient who is inadequately prepared with antithyroid drugs. If left untreated, it may be fatal.	

virile VĬR-ĭl	Masculine or having characteristics of a man, especially copulative powers	
virilism VĬR-ĭl-ĭzm	Masculinization in a woman or development of male secondary sex characteristics in the woman	

 It is time to review pathological, diagnostic, symptomatic, and related terms by completing Learning Activity 13–3.

Diagnostic and Therapeutic Procedures

This section introduces procedures used to diagnose and treat endocrine disorders. Descriptions are provided as well as pronunciations and word analyses for selected terms.

Procedure	Description
DIAGNOSTIC PROCEDURES	
Clinical	

exophthalmometry
ĕk-sŏf-thăl-MŎM-ĕ-trē
   ex-: out, out from
   ophthalm/o: eye
   -metry: act of measuring
	Test that measures the degree of forward displacement of the eyeball (exophthalmos) as seen in Graves disease (See Figure 13–3.)
	The test is administered with an instrument called an exophthalmometer, which allows measurement of the distance from the center of the cornea to the lateral orbital rim.

Laboratory	
fasting blood glucose (FBG)	Test that measures blood glucose level after a 12-hour fast
glucose tolerance test (GTT) GLOO-kōs	Test that measures the body's ability to metabolize carbohydrates by administering a standard dose of glucose and measuring glucose level in blood and urine at regular intervals *GTT is commonly used to help diagnose diabetes or other disorders that affect carbohydrate metabolism.*
insulin tolerance test	Test that determines insulin levels in serum (blood) by administering insulin and measuring blood glucose level in blood at regular intervals *In hypoglycemia, glucose levels may be lower and return to normal more slowly.*
protein-bound iodine (PBI)	Test that measures the concentration of thyroxine in a blood sample *Result of the PBI test provides an index of thyroid activity.*
thyroid function test (TFT)	Test that determines increase or decrease in thyroid function *The thyroid function test measures levels of thyroid-stimulating hormone (TSH), triiodothyronine (T_3), and thyroxine (T_4).*
total calcium	Test that measures calcium to detect bone and parathyroid disorders *Hypercalcemia can indicate primary hyperparathyroidism; hypocalcemia can indicate hypoparathyroidism.*

Procedure	Description	*(Continued)*

Radiographic

computed tomography (CT) scan
kŏm-PŪ-tĕd tō-MŎG-ră-fē

tom/o: to cut
-graphy: process of recording

Imaging technique achieved by rotating an x-ray emitter around the area to be scanned and measuring the intensity of transmitted rays from different angles

In a CT scan, the computer generates a detailed cross-sectional image that appears as a slice. (See Figure 4–4D.) CT scan is used to detect disease and tumors in soft body tissues, such as the pancreas, thyroid, and adrenal glands, and may be used with or without a contrast medium.

---

magnetic resonance imaging (MRI)
măg-NĔT-ĭc RĔZ-ĕn-ăns
ĬM-ĭj-ĭng

Noninvasive imaging technique that uses radio waves and a strong magnetic field rather than an x-ray beam to produce multiplanar cross-sectional images

MRI is the method of choice for diagnosing a growing number of diseases because it provides superior soft-tissue contrast, allows multiple plane views, and avoids the hazards of ionizing radiation. MRI is used to identify abnormalities of pituitary, pancreatic, adrenal, and thyroid glands.

---

radioactive iodine uptake (RAIU)

Administration of radioactive iodine (RAI) orally as a tracer to test how quickly the thyroid gland takes up (uptake) iodine from the blood

Results of RAIU test are used to determine thyroid function.

---

thyroid scan
thyr: thyroid gland
-oid: resembling

Test that involves administration of a radioactive substance that is localized in the thyroid gland and use of a scanner to visualize the gland

Thyroid scanning is used to detect pathological formations such as tumors. It is useful in evaluating neck or substernal masses, thyroid nodules, hyperthyroidism, and metastatic tumors.

THERAPEUTIC PROCEDURES

Surgical

microneurosurgery of pituitary gland
mī-krō-nū-rō-SĔR-jĕr-ē,
pĭ-TŪ-ĭ-tār-ē

Microdissection of a tumor using a binocular surgical microscope for magnification

---

parathyroidectomy
păr-ă-thī-royd-ĔK-tō-mē

para-: near, beside; beyond
thyroid: thyroid gland
-ectomy: excision, removal

Excision of one or more of the parathyroid glands, usually to control hyperparathyroidism

---

pinealectomy
pĭn-ē-ăl-ĔK-tō-mē

Removal of the pineal body

---

thymectomy
thī-MĔK-tō-mē

thym: thymus gland
-ectomy: excision, removal

Excision of the thymus gland

Procedure	Description
thyroidectomy thi-royd-ĔK-tō-mē *thyroid:* thyroid gland *-ectomy:* excision, removal	Excision of the thyroid gland *Thyroidectomy is performed for goiter, tumors, or hyperthyroidism* *that does not respond to iodine therapy and antithyroid drugs.*
partial	Method of choice for removing a fibrous, nodular thyroid
subtotal	Removal of most of the thyroid to relieve hyperthyroidism

Pharmacology

Common disorders associated with endocrine glands include hyposecretion and hypersecretion of hormones. When deficiencies of this type occur, natural and synthetic hormones, such as insulin and thyroid agents, are prescribed. These agents normalize hormone levels to maintain proper functioning and homeostasis. Therapeutic agents are also available to regulate various substances in the body, such as glucose levels in diabetic patients. Hormone replacement therapy (HRT), such as synthetic thyroid and estrogen, treat these hormonal deficiencies. Although specific drugs are not covered in this section, hormonal chemotherapy drugs are used to treat certain cancers, such as testicular, ovarian, breast, and endometrial cancer. (See Table 13–7.)

Table 13–7   DRUGS USED TO TREAT ENDOCRINE DISORDERS

This table lists common drug classifications used to treat endocrine disorders, their therapeutic actions, and selected generic and trade names.

Classification	Therapeutic Action	Generic and Trade Names

insulins	Treat type 1 diabetes
	
	 Insulins are classified according to how quickly they act and the duration of their therapeutic action. They are administered by intermittent subcutaneous injection, implanted infusion pump, or directly into the bloodstream by I.V. injection or continuous I.V. infusion through a controlled infusion device. Currently, nasal sprays and oral capsules are being tested as a method of administration. Although type 2 diabetes may be treated with insulin, it is more commonly treated with oral antidiabetics.
		regular insulin
		 ĬN-sū-lĭn
		   Humulin R*, Novolin R
		 NPH insulin
		 ĬN-sū-lĭn
		   Humulin N, Novolin N
		 NPH/regular insulin mixtures
		 ĬN-sū-lĭn
		   Humulin 50/50, Humulin 70/30,
		   Novolin 70/30

(Continued)

Table 13-7   DRUGS USED TO TREAT ENDOCRINE DISORDERS
(Continued)

Classification	Therapeutic Action	Generic and Trade Names
oral antidiabetics	Stimulate the pancreas to produce more insulin and increase the number of insulin receptors *Contrary to popular opinion, oral antidiabetic drugs are not insulin and are not effective in treating type I diabetes mellitus.*	**glimepiride** GLĪ-mĕ-pī-rĭd *Amaryl* **glipizide** GLĬP-ĭ-zĭd *Glucotrol, Glucotrol XL* **glyburide** GLĪ-bū-rĭd *DiaBeta, Glynase, Micronase* **metformin** mĕt-FOR-mĭn *Glucophage*
antithyroids	Treat hyperthyroidism by impeding the formation of T_3 and T_4 hormone *Antithyroids are administered in preparation for a thyroidectomy and in thyrotoxic crisis.*	**methimazole** mĕth-ĬM-ă-zōl *Tapazole* **strong iodine solution** Ī-ō-dĭn *Lugol's solution*
corticosteroids	Replace hormones lost in adrenal insufficiency (Addison disease) *Corticosteroids are also widely used to suppress inflammation, control allergic reactions, reduce rejection in transplantation, and treat some cancer.*	**cortisone** KOR-tĭ-sōn *Cortone, Acetate* **hydrocortisone** hi-drō-KOR-tĭ-sōn *A-Hydrocort, Cortef, Hydrocortone, Solu-Cortef*
growth hormone replacements	Increase skeletal growth in children and growth hormone deficiencies in adults *Growth hormones increase spinal bone density and help manage growth failure in children.*	**somatropin (recombinant)** sō-mă-TRŌ-pĭn *Humatrope, Norditropin, Nutropin, Serostim* **somatrem (recombinant)** SŌ-mă-trĕm *Protropin*
thyroid supplements	Replace or supplement thyroid hormones *Each thyroid supplement contains T_3, T_4, or a combination of both. Thyroid supplements are also used to treat some types of thyroid cancer.*	**levothyroxine** lē-vō-thi-RŌK-sēn *Levo-T, Levoxyl, Synthroid, T_4 Unithroid* **liothyronine** lī-ō-THĪ-rō-nēn *Cytomel, I-triiodothyronine, T_3, Triostat* **thyroid** THĪ-royd *T_3/T_4, Thyrolar*

*The trade name for all human genetically produced insulins is *Humulin*. Traditionally, insulin has been derived from beef or pork pancreas. Human insulin is genetically produced using recombinant DNA techniques to avoid the potential for allergic reaction.

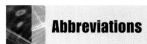

Abbreviations

This section introduces endocrine-related abbreviations and their meanings.

Abbreviation	Meaning
ACTH	adrenocorticotropic hormone
ADH	antidiuretic hormone (vasopressin)
BMR	basal metabolic rate
DI	diabetes insipidus; diagnostic imaging
DKA	diabetic ketoacidosis
DM	diabetes mellitus
FSH	follicle-stimulating hormone
GH	growth hormone
IDDM	insulin-dependent diabetes mellitus
K	potassium (an electrolyte)
LH	luteinizing hormone
MSH	melanocyte-stimulating hormone
NIDDM	non-insulin-dependent diabetes mellitus
NPH	neutral protamine Hagedorn (insulin)
PRL	prolactin
PGH	pituitary growth hormone
PTH	parathyroid hormone; also called *parathormone*
RAI	radioactive iodine
RAIU	radioactive iodine uptake
T_3	triiodothyronine (thyroid hormone)
T_4	thyroxine (thyroid hormone)
TFT	thyroid function test
TSH	thyroid-stimulating hormone

It is time to review procedures, pharmacology, and abbreviations by completing Learning Activity 13–4.

LEARNING ACTIVITIES

The activities that follow provide review of the endocrine system terms introduced in this chapter. Complete each activity and review your answers to evaluate your understanding of the chapter.

Learning Activity 13–1

Identifying endocrine structures

Label the following illustration using the terms listed below.

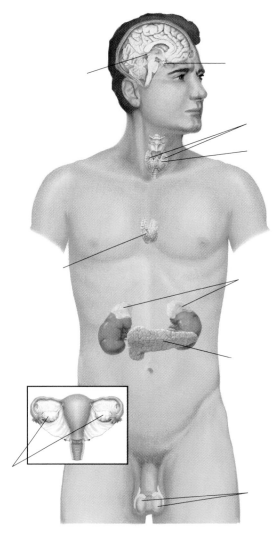

adrenal (suprarenal) glands   parathyroid glands   testes

ovaries   pineal gland   thymus gland

pancreas   pituitary (hypophysis) gland   thyroid gland

 Check your answers by referring to Figure 13–1 on page 390. Review material that you did not answer correctly.

Learning Activity 13–2

Building medical words

Use **glyc/o** *(sugar) to build words that mean:*

1. blood condition of excessive glucose _____
2. blood condition of deficiency of glucose _____
3. formation of glycogen _____

Use **pancreat/o** *(pancreas) to build words that mean:*

4. inflammation of the pancreas _____
5. destruction of the pancreas _____
6. disease of the pancreas _____

Use **thyr/o** *or* **thyroid/o** *(thyroid gland) to build words that mean:*

7. inflammation of the thyroid gland _____
8. enlargement of the thyroid _____

Build surgical words that mean:

9. excision of a parathyroid gland _____
10. removal of the adrenal gland _____

Check your answers in Appendix A. Review material that you did not answer correctly.

CORRECT ANSWERS _____ × 10 = _____ **% SCORE**

Learning Activity 13–3

Matching pathological, diagnostic, symptomatic, and related terms

Match the following terms with the definitions in the numbered list.

Addison disease	glycosuria	myxedema
cretinism	hirsutism	pheochromocytoma
Cushing syndrome	hyperkalemia	type 1 diabetes
diuresis	hyponatremia	type 2 diabetes
exophthalmic goiter	insulin	virile

1. _____ having characteristics of a man; masculine

2. _____ hypothyroidism acquired in adulthood

3. _____ increased excretion of urine

4. _____ excessive growth of hair or the presence of hair in unusual places, especially in women

5. _____ hypothyroidism that appears as a congenital condition and is commonly associated with other endocrine abnormalities

6. _____ hormone produced by beta cells of the pancreas

7. _____ caused by deficiency in the secretion of adrenocortical hormones

8. _____ characterized by protrusion of the eyeballs, increased heart action, enlargement of the thyroid gland, weight loss, and nervousness

9. _____ excessive amount of potassium in the blood

10. _____ small chromaffin cell tumor, usually located in the adrenal medulla

11. _____ insulin-dependent diabetes mellitus that occurs most commonly in children and adolescents (juvenile onset)

12. _____ decreased concentration of sodium in the blood

13. _____ abnormal presence of glucose in the urine

14. _____ metabolic disorder caused by hypersecretion of the adrenal cortex resulting in excessive production of glucocorticoids, mainly cortisol

15. _____ non-insulin-dependent diabetes mellitus that usually occurs later in life (maturity onset)

✓ Check your answers in Appendix A. Review material that you did not answer correctly.

CORRECT ANSWERS _____ × **6.67** = _____ **% SCORE**

Learning Activity 13–4

Matching procedures, pharmacology, and abbreviations

Match the following terms with the definitions in the numbered list.

antithyroids	growth hormone	protein-bound iodine
computed tomography (CT) scan	GTT	RAIU
corticosteroids	Humulin	T_3
exophthalmometry	magnetic resonance imaging (MRI)	T_4
FBS	oral antidiabetics	thyroid scan

1. _____ measures circulating glucose level after a 12-hour fast

2. _____ measures thyroid function and monitors how quickly ingested iodine is taken into the thyroid gland

3. _____ replacement hormones for adrenal insufficiency (Addison disease)

4. _____ increases skeletal growth in children

5. _____ radioactive compound is administered and localizes in the thyroid gland; used to detect thyroid abnormalities

6. _____ thyroxine

7. _____ used to treat type 1 diabetes

8. _____ diagnostic test used to determine hypoglycemia, hyperglycemia, and adjustments in insulin dosage

9. _____ used to treat hyperthyroidism by impeding the formation of T_3 and T_4 hormone

10. _____ test to measure the concentration of thyroxine in a blood sample

11. _____ triiodothyronine

12. _____ noninvasive imaging technique that uses radio waves and a strong magnetic field to produce multiplanar cross-sectional images

13. _____ test that measures the degree of forward displacement of the eyeball as seen in Graves disease

14. _____ imaging technique achieved by rotating an x-ray emitter around the area to be scanned and measuring the intensity of transmitted rays from different angles; used to detect disease in soft body tissues, such as the pancreas, thyroid, and adrenal glands

15. _____ trade name for all human genetically produced insulins

Check your answers in Appendix A. Review any material that you did not answer correctly.

CORRECT ANSWERS _____ $\times$ **6.67** = _____ **% SCORE**

MEDICAL RECORD ACTIVITIES

The two medical records included in the activities that follow use common clinical scenarios to show how medical terminology is used to document patient care. Complete the terminology and analysis sections for each activity to help you recognize and understand terms related to the endocrine system.

Medical Record Activity 13–1

Hyperparathyroidism

Terminology

The terms listed in the chart come from the medical record *Hyperparathyroidism* that follows. Use a medical dictionary such as *Taber's Cyclopedic Medical Dictionary,* the appendices of this book, or other resources to define each term. Then review the pronunciations for each term and practice by reading the medical record aloud.

Term	Definition
adenoma ăd-ĕ-NŌ-mă	
claudication klăw-dĭ-KĀ-shŭn	
diabetes mellitus dī-ă-BĒ-tēz MĔ-lĭ-tŭs	
endocrinologist ĕn-dō-krĭn-ŎL-ō-jĭst	
hypercalciuria hī-pĕr-kăl-sē-Ū-rē-ă	
hyperparathyroidism hī-pĕr-păr-ă-THĪ-roy-dĭzm	
impression ĭm-PRĔSH-ŭn	
osteoarthritis ŏs-tē-ō-ăr-THRĪ-tĭs	
parathyroid păr-ă-THĪ-royd	
peripheral vascular disease pĕr-ĬF-ĕr-ăl VĂS-kū-lăr dĭ-ZĒZ	

HYPERPARATHYROIDISM

HISTORY OF PRESENT ILLNESS: This 66-year-old former blackjack dealer is under evaluation for hyperparathyroidism. Surgery evidently has been recommended, but there is confusion as to how urgent this is. She has a 13-year history of type 1 diabetes mellitus, a history of shoulder pain, osteoarthritis of the spine, and peripheral vascular disease with claudication. She states her 548-pack-per-year smoking history ended 3.5 years ago. Her first knowledge of parathyroid disease was about 3 years ago when laboratory findings revealed an elevated calcium level. This subsequently led to the diagnosis of hyperparathyroidism. She was further evaluated by an endocrinologist in the Lake Tahoe area, who determined that she also had hypercalciuria, although there is nothing to suggest a history of kidney stones.

IMPRESSION: Hyperparathyroidism and hypercalciuria, probably a parathyroid adenoma

Analysis

Review the medical record *Hyperparathyroidism* to answer the following questions.

1. What is an adenoma?

   _____

2. What does the physician suspect caused the patient's hyperparathyroidism?

   _____

3. What type of laboratory findings revealed parathyroid disease?

   _____

4. What is hypercalciuria?

   _____

5. If the patient smoked 548 packs of cigarettes per year, how many packs did she smoke in an average day?

   _____

Medical Record Activity 13–2

Diabetes mellitus

Terminology

The terms listed in the chart come from the medical record *Diabetes Mellitus* that follows. Use a medical dictionary such as *Taber's Cyclopedic Medical Dictionary*, the appendices of this book, or other resources to define each term. Then review the pronunciations for each term and practice by reading the medical record aloud.

Term	Definition
Accu-chek ĂK-ū-chĕk	
morbid obesity MOR-bĭd ō-BĒ-sĭ-tē	

(Continued)

Term	Definition	(Continued)
obesity, exogenous ō-BĒ-sĭ-tē, ĕks-ŎJ-ĕ-nŭs		
polydipsia pŏl-ē-DĬP-sē-ă		
polyphagia pŏl-ē-FĀ-jē-ă		
polyuria pŏl-ē-Ū-rē-ă		

DIABETES MELLITUS

Chart Notes

This 200-pound patient was admitted to the hospital because of a 10-day history of polyuria, polydipsia, and polyphagia. She has been very nervous, irritable, and very sensitive emotionally and cries easily. During this period, she has had headaches and has become very sleepy and tired after eating. On admission, her Accu-Chek was 540.

Family history is significant in that both parents and two sisters have type 1 diabetes.

Physical examination was essentially negative. The abdomen was difficult to evaluate because of morbid obesity.

DIAGNOSIS: Diabetes mellitus; obesity, exogenous

Analysis

Review the medical record *Diabetes Mellitus* to answer the following questions.

1. How long has this patient been experiencing voracious eating?

   _____

2. Was the patient's obesity due to overeating or metabolic imbalance?

   _____

3. Why did the doctor experience difficulty in examining the patient's abdomen?

   _____

4. Was the patient's blood glucose above or below normal on admission?

   _____

5. What is the reference range for fasting blood glucose?

   _____

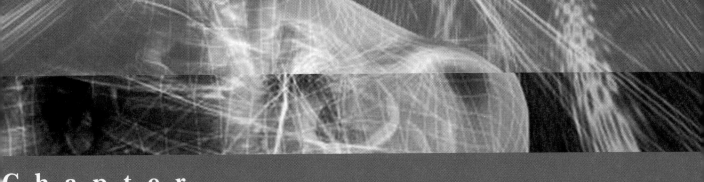

Chapter

14

Nervous System

OBJECTIVES

Upon completion of this chapter, you will be able to:

- Locate and describe the structures of the nervous system.
- Recognize, pronounce, spell, and build words related to the nervous system.
- Describe pathological conditions, diagnostic and therapeutic procedures, and other terms related to the nervous system.
- Explain pharmacology related to the treatment of nervous disorders.
- Demonstrate your knowledge of this chapter by completing the learning and medical record activities.

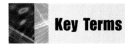

Key Terms

This section introduces important nervous system terms and their definitions. Word analyses are also provided.

Term	Definition
blood-brain barrier	Mechanism that blocks specific substances found in the bloodstream from entering the brain
cell body	Division of a neuron that includes the nucleus, cell organelles, and surrounding cytoplasm, but does not include the axon or dendrites
motor neuron	Neuron that transmits impulses from the central nervous system (brain or spinal cord) to a muscle or gland; also called *efferent neuron*
nervous impulse	Physiological change transmitted through certain tissues, especially nerve fibers and muscles, resulting in activity or inhibition
neurology nū-RŎL-ō-jē *neur/o:* nerve *-logy:* study of	Branch of medicine concerned with diagnosis and treatment of disorders of the nervous system
neurotransmitter nū-rō-TRĂNS-mĭt-ĕr	Chemical substance that transmits or inhibits nerve impulses at a synapse *Chemical substances that are neurotransmitters include acetylcholine, adrenaline, and dopamine.*
organelle or-găn-ĔL	Cytoplasm structure that provides specialized function for the cell
psychiatry sī-KĪ-ă-trē *psych:* mind *-iatry:* medicine; treatment	Branch of medicine concerned with the diagnosis and treatment of mental disorders
sensory neuron SĔN-sō-rē	Neuron that transmits impulses from receptors in the skin, sense organs, and internal organs to the central nervous system (brain or spinal cord); also called *afferent neuron*
synapse SĬN-ăps	Junction where a nerve impulse passes from an axon terminal to a neuron, muscle cell, or gland cell

Anatomy and Physiology

The nervous system is one of the most complicated systems of the body in both structure and function. It senses physical and chemical changes in the internal and external environments, processes them, and then responds to maintain homeostasis. Voluntary activities, such as walking and talking, and involuntary activities, such as digestion and circulation, are coordinated, regulated, and integrated by the nervous system. The entire neural network of the body relies on the transmission of electrochemical impulses. Impulses travel from cell to cell as they convey information from one area of the body to another. The speed at which this occurs is almost instantaneous, thus providing an immediate response to change.

Cellular Structure of the Nervous System

Despite its complexity, the nervous system is composed of only two principal types of cells: **neurons** and **neuroglia.** Neurons are cells that transmit impulses. They are commonly identified by the direction the impulse travels. **Sensory neurons,** also called *afferent nerves,* transmit stimuli to the brain and spinal cord; **motor neurons,** also called *efferent nerves,* transmit impulses from the brain or spinal cord to muscles and glands. Most nerves are composed of both afferent and efferent fibers and, thus, are called *mixed nerves.* Neuroglia are cells that support neurons and bind them to other tissues. They also play an important role when the nervous system suffers an injury or infection.

Neurons

The three major structures of the neuron are the *cell body,* the *axon,* and the *dendrites.* (See Figure 14–1.) The (1) **cell body** is the enlarged structure of the neuron that contains the (2) **nucleus** of the cell and various **organelles.** Its branching cytoplasmic projections are (3) **dendrites** that carry impulses to the cell body and (4) **axons** that carry impulses from the cell body. Dendrites resemble tiny branches on a tree, providing additional surface area for receiving impulses from other neurons. Axons are long, single projections ranging from a few millimeters to more than a meter in length. Axons transmit impulses to muscles, glands, and other dendrites.

Many axons in both the peripheral nervous system and the autonomic nervous system possess a white, lipoid covering called a (5) **myelin sheath.** This covering acts as an electrical insulator that reduces the possibility of an impulse stimulating adjacent nerves. It also accelerates impulse transmission through the axon. The myelin that covers axons in the brain and spinal cord gives these structures a white appearance and constitutes the white matter of the central nervous system. Unmyelinated fibers, dendrites, and nerve cell bodies make up the gray matter of the brain and spinal cord.

On peripheral nerves, the myelin sheath is formed by a neuroglial cell called a (6) **Schwann cell** that wraps tightly around the axon. It forms a thin cellular membrane called (7) **neurilemma,** or *neurolemma.* The space between adjacent Schwann cells is called the (8) **node of Ranvier.** This space helps maintain the electrical potentials needed for impulse conduction.

Neurons are not continuous with one another. Instead, a small space, known as a (9) **synapse,** is found between the (10) **axon terminal** of one neuron and the dendrite of another. For an impulse to travel from neuron to neuron, it must cross the synapse. The impulse within the neuron causes a chemical substance called a (11) **neurotransmitter** to be released at the end of the axon. The neurotransmitter diffuses across the synapse to receptor sites on the dendrite of the next neuron. Here it generates the next electrical stimulus. The receiving neuron immediately inactivates the neurotransmitter, thereby preventing an unwanted continued stimulation, and prepares the site for another stimulus by a neurotransmitter. Thus, impulses travel through neural pathways.

Neuroglia

The term **neuroglia** literally means "nerve glue." Scientists once believed that neuroglia served only a supporting role for neurons; however, we now know that neuroglia cells perform many functions. There are four types of neuroglia and each serves a distinct function:

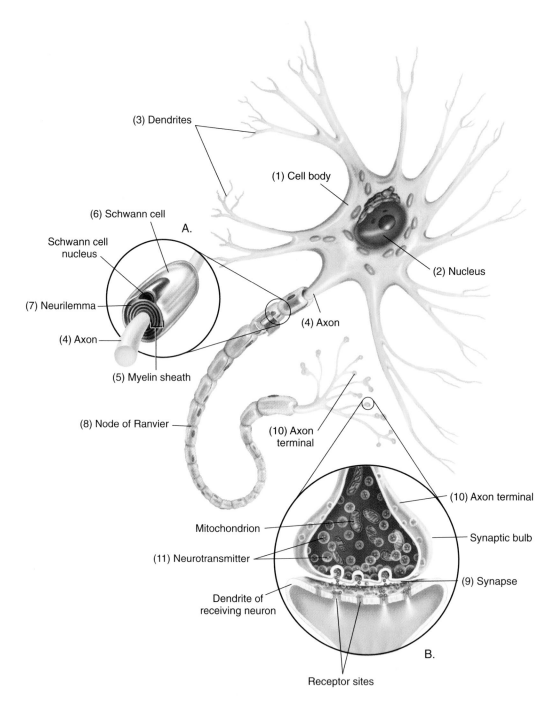

(3) Dendrites

(1) Cell body

(6) Schwann cell

Schwann cell nucleus

A.

(7) Neurilemma

(4) Axon

(5) Myelin sheath

(2) Nucleus

(4) Axon

(8) Node of Ranvier

(10) Axon terminal

(10) Axon terminal

Synaptic bulb

Mitochondrion

(11) Neurotransmitter

(9) Synapse

Dendrite of receiving neuron

B.

Receptor sites

Figure 14–1   Neuron. (A) Schwann cell. (B) Axon terminal synapse.

- *Astrocytes,* as their name suggests, are star-shaped neuroglia. They provide three-dimensional mechanical support for neurons and form tight sheaths around the capillaries of the brain. These sheaths provide an obstruction, called the *blood-brain barrier,* that keeps large molecular substances from entering the delicate tissue of the brain. Even so, small molecules, such as water, carbon dioxide, oxygen, and alcohol, readily pass from blood vessels through the barrier and enter the interstitial spaces of the brain. Researchers must take the blood-brain barrier into consideration when developing drugs for treatment of brain disorders.

- *Oligodendrocytes,* also called *oligodendroglia,* help in the development of myelin on neurons of the central nervous system.
- *Microglia,* the smallest of the neuroglia, possess phagocytic properties and may become very active during times of infection.
- *Ependyma* are ciliated cells that line fluid-filled cavities of the central nervous system, especially the ventricles of the brain. They assist in cerebrospinal fluid (CSF) circulation.

Nervous System Divisions

The nervous system consists of two main divisions, the central nervous system (CNS) and the peripheral nervous system (PNS). The CNS consists of the brain and spinal cord. The PNS consists of 12 pairs of cranial nerves, which emerge from the base of the skull, and 31 pairs of spinal nerves, which emerge from the spinal cord. (See Table 14–1.)

Central Nervous System

The CNS consists of the brain and spinal cord, which are enclosed within three protective membranes called the *meninges.*

Brain. In addition to being one of the largest organs of the body, the brain is highly complex in structure and function. (See Figure 14–2.) It integrates almost every physical and mental activity of the body and is the center for memory, emotion, thought, judgment, reasoning, and consciousness. The brain is composed of four major structures:

Table 14–1   NERVOUS SYSTEM DIVISIONS AND FUNCTIONS

This table lists the divisions of the nervous system along with their functions.

Division	Function
Central	
Brain	Center for thought and emotion, interpretation of sensory stimuli, and coordination of body functions
Spinal cord	Main pathway for transmission of information between the brain and body
Peripheral	
Cranial nerves	Includes 12 pairs of nerves that emerge from the base of the skull and may act in a motor or sensory capacity
Spinal nerves	Includes 31 pairs of nerves that emerge from the spine and act in motor and sensory capacities
Somatic	Transmits sensory impulses to the central nervous system and motor impulses to voluntary (skeletal) muscles
Autonomic • Sympathetic • Parasympathetic	Regulates involuntary (visceral) muscles and glands • Division of the autonomic nervous system that prepares the body for "fight or flight" • Division of the autonomic nervous system that moderates or reverses the action of the sympathetic nervous system

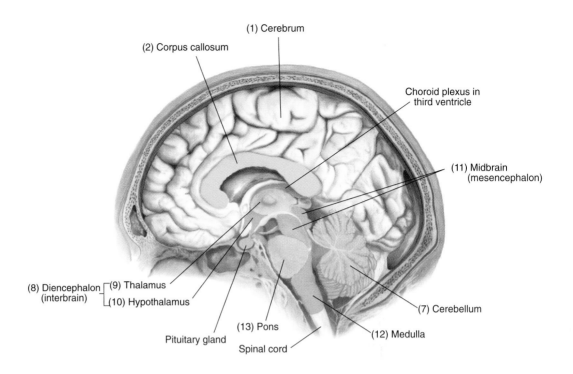

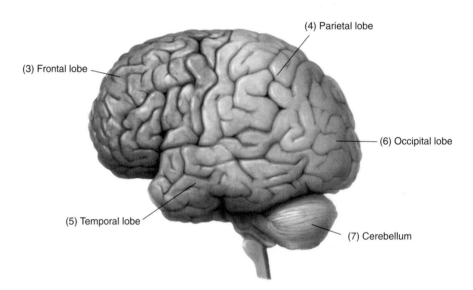

Figure 14–2 Brain structures.

- cerebrum
- cerebellum
- diencephalon
- brainstem

Cerebrum. The (1) **cerebrum** is the largest and uppermost portion of the brain. It consists of two hemispheres divided by a deep longitudinal fissure, or groove. The fissure does not completely separate the hemispheres. A structure called the (2) **corpus callosum** joins these hemispheres, permitting communication between the right and left sides of the brain. Each hemisphere is divided into five lobes. Four of these lobes are named for the bones that lie directly above them: (3) **frontal,** (4) **parietal,** (5) **temporal,** and (6) **occipital.** The fifth lobe, the **insula** (not shown in the figure), is hidden from view and can be seen only upon dissection.

The cerebral surface consists of numerous folds, or convolutions, called *gyri.* The gyri are separated by furrows or fissures called *sulci.* A thin gray layer called the *cerebral cortex* covers the entire cerebrum and is composed of millions of cell bodies, which give it its gray color.

The remainder of the cerebrum is primarily composed of white matter (myelinated axons). Major functions of the cerebrum include sensory perception and interpretation, language, voluntary movement, and the emotional aspects of behavior and memory.

Cerebellum. The second largest part of the brain, the (7) **cerebellum,** occupies the posterior portion of the brain. All functions of the cerebellum involve movement. When the cerebrum initiates muscular movement, the cerebellum coordinates and refines it. The cerebellum also aids in maintaining equilibrium and balance.

Diencephalon. The (8) **diencephalon (interbrain)** is composed of many smaller structures, two of which are the (9) **thalamus** and the (10) **hypothalamus.** The thalamus receives all sensory stimuli except olfactory stimuli and processes and transmits them to the cerebral cortex. In addition, the thalamus receives impulses from the cerebrum and relays them to efferent nerves. The hypothalamus integrates autonomic nerve impulses, regulates body temperature, and controls endocrine functions.

Brainstem. The brainstem completes the last major section of the brain. It is composed of three structures: the (11) **midbrain (mesencephalon),** separating the cerebrum from the brainstem; the (12) **medulla,** which attaches to the spinal cord; and (13) the **pons,** or "bridge," connecting the midbrain to the medulla. In general, the brainstem is a pathway for impulse conduction between the brain and spinal cord. The brainstem is the origin of 10 of the 12 pairs of cranial nerves and controls respiration, blood pressure, and heart rate. Because the brainstem is the site that controls the beginning of life (the initiation of the beating heart in a fetus) and the end of life (the cessation of respiration and heart activity) it is sometimes called the *primary brain.*

Spinal cord. The spinal cord transmits sensory impulses from the body to the brain and motor impulses from the brain to muscles and organs of the body. The sensory nerve tracts are called *ascending tracts* because the direction of the impulse is upward. Conversely, motor nerve tracts are called *descending tracts* because they carry impulses in a downward direction to muscles and organs. A cross-section of the spinal cord reveals an inner gray area composed of cell bodies and dendrites and a white outer area composed of myelinated tissue of the ascending and descending tracts.

The entire spinal cord is located within the spinal cavity of the vertebral column, with spinal nerves exiting between the intervertebral spaces throughout almost the entire length of the spinal column. Unlike the cranial nerves, which have specific names, the spinal nerves are identified by the region of the vertebral column from which they exit.

Meninges. The brain and the spinal cord receive limited protection from three coverings called *meninges* (singular, *meninx*). These coverings include:

- The *dura mater,* the outermost covering, is tough, fibrous, and composed primarily of connective tissue. Beneath the dura mater is a cavity called the **subdural space** filled with serous fluid.
- The *arachnoid,* the middle covering, has (as its name suggests) a spider-web appearance. A **subarachnoid space** contains cerebrospinal fluid (CSF) that provides additional protection for the brain and spinal cord by acting as a shock absorber.

- The *pia mater,* the innermost covering of the meninges, contains numerous blood vessels and lymphatics that nourish the underlying tissues.

Cerebrospinal fluid (CSF) is a colorless fluid that contains proteins, glucose, urea, salts, and some white blood cells. It circulates around the spinal cord and brain and through spaces called *ventricles* located within the inner portion of the brain, and provides nutritive substances to the CNS. Normally, CSF is absorbed as rapidly as it is formed, maintaining a constant fluid volume. Any interference with absorption results in a collection of fluid in the brain, a condition called **hydrocephalus.**

Peripheral Nervous System

The peripheral nervous system is composed of all nervous tissue located outside of the spinal column and skull. It includes 12 pairs of cranial nerves that carry impulses to and from the brain and 31 pairs of spinal nerves that carry impulses to and from the spinal cord.

Functionally, the PNS is subdivided into two specialized systems: the somatic nervous system (SNS) and the autonomic nervous system (ANS).

Cranial nerves. The cranial nerves are designated by name or number. (See Figure 14–3.) Cranial nerves consist of fibers that may serve a sensory or motor function, or a mixture of both. Sensory nerves receive impulses from the sense organs, including the eyes, ears, nose, tongue, and skin, and transmit them to the CNS. Because sensory nerves conduct impulses toward the CNS, they are also known as afferent nerves. Motor nerves, in contrast, conduct impulses away from the CNS, so they are called efferent nerves. They conduct impulses to muscles, causing them to contract, or to glands, causing them to secrete. Nerves composed of both sensory and motor fibers are called mixed nerves. An example of a mixed nerve is the facial nerve. It acts in a motor capacity by transmitting impulses for smiling or frowning. However, it also acts in a sensory capacity by transmitting taste impulses from the tongue to the brain.

Spinal nerves. All spinal nerves are mixed nerves. (See Figure 14–4.) They have two points of attachment to the spinal cord: an *anterior root* and a *posterior root.* The anterior root contains motor fibers and the posterior root contains sensory fibers. These two roots unite to form the spinal nerve.

Somatic nervous system. The SNS primarily innervates (supplies with nerves) skeletal muscles and is associated with voluntary movement. Examples of voluntary movement include walking and talking.

Autonomic nervous system. In contrast, the ANS innervates glands, smooth muscles, and cardiac muscles. This system is considered involuntary, because it operates without conscious control. Examples of autonomic activities include digestion, heart contraction, and vasoconstriction.

The ANS is further subdivided into the *sympathetic* and *parasympathetic* systems. To a large extent, these subdivisions oppose the action of the other, although in certain instances, they may exhibit independent action. In general, sympathetic nerve fibers produce vasoconstriction, increased heart rate, elevated blood pressure, and slowing of gastrointestinal activity. Sympathetic functions are evident in "fight-or-flight" situations. Blood flow increases in skeletal muscles to prepare an individual to either fight or retreat from a threatening situation. The parasympathetic system generally transmits impulses that bring about vasodilation, a slower heart rate, a decrease in blood pressure, and a return to normal gastrointestinal activity.

It is time to review nervous system structures by completing Learning Activity 14–1.

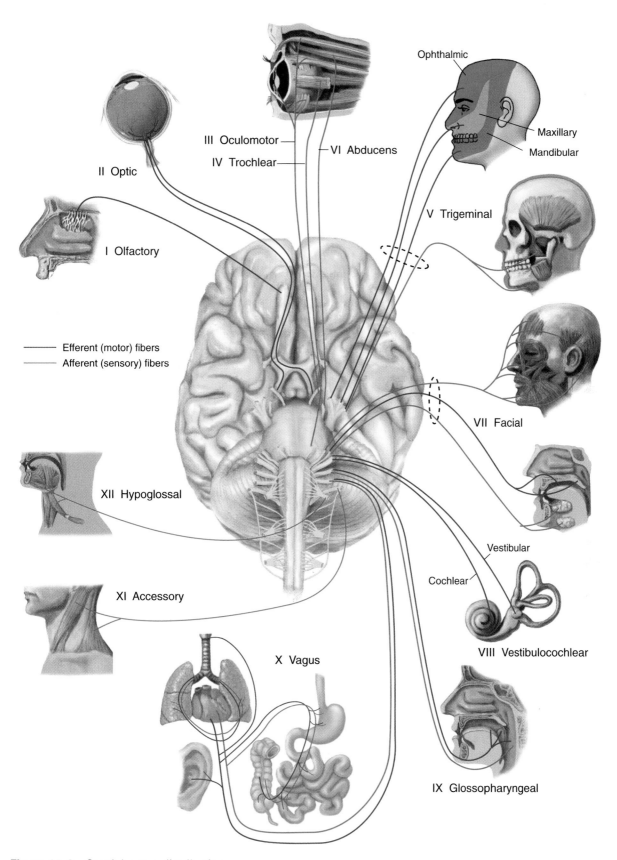

Figure 14–3 Cranial nerve distribution.

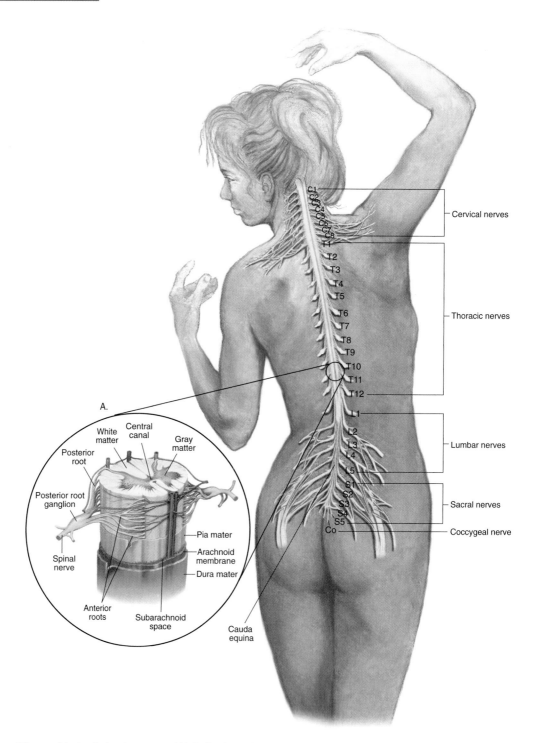

Cervical nerves

Thoracic nerves

Lumbar nerves

Sacral nerves

Coccygeal nerve

Cauda
equina

A.

White
matter

Central
canal

Gray
matter

Posterior
root

Posterior root
ganglion

Spinal
nerve

Anterior
roots

Subarachnoid
space

Pia mater

Arachnoid
membrane

Dura mater

Figure 14–4   Spinal nerves. (A) Spinal cord enlargement

Medical Word Elements

This section introduces combining forms, suffixes, and prefixes related to the nervous system. Word analyses are also provided.

Element	Meaning	Word Analysis
COMBINING FORMS		
cerebr/o	cerebrum	cerebr/o/tomy (sĕr-ĕ-BRŎT-ō-mē): incision of the cerebrum *-tomy:* incision
crani/o	cranium (skull)	crani/o/malacia (krā-nē-ō-mă-LĀ-shē-ă): softening of the cranial bones *-malacia:* softening
dendr/o	tree	dendr/oid (DĔN-droyd): resembling a branching tree such as cytoplasmic branches of a neuron *-oid:* resembling *Dendrons conduct nerve impulses to the cell body.*
encephal/o	brain	encephal/o/cele (ĕn-SĔF-ă-lō-sēl): herniation of the brain *-cele:* hernia, swelling *Encephalocele is a condition in which portions of the brain and meninges protrude through a bony midline defect in the skull. It is usually associated with a neural tube defect.*
gangli/o	ganglion (knot or knotlike mass)	gangli/ectomy (găng-glē-ĔK-tō-mē): excision of a ganglion *-ectomy:* excision, removal *A ganglion is a mass of nerve cell bodies (gray matter) in the peripheral nervous system.*
gli/o	glue; neuroglial tissue	gli/oma (glĭ-Ō-mă): tumor composed of neuroglial or supporting tissue of the nervous system *-oma:* tumor
lex/o	word, phrase	dys/lex/ia (dĭs-LĔK-sē-ă): difficulty using and interpreting written forms of communication *dys-:* bad; painful; difficult *-ia:* condition *In dyslexia, disability is not associated with vision or intelligence.*
kinesi/o	movement	brady/kinesia (brăd-ē-kĭ-NĒ-sē-ă): slow movement *brady-:* slow

(Continued)

Element	Meaning	Word Analysis	(Continued)
lept/o	thin, slender	lept/o/mening/o/pathy (lĕp-tō-mĕn-ĭn-GŎP-ă-thē): disease of the leptomeninges *mening/o:* meninges (membranes covering brain and spinal cord) *-pathy:* disease *The leptomeninges include the pia mater and arachnoid, both of which are thin and delicate in structure, as opposed to the dura mater.*	
mening/o **meningi/o**	meninges (membranes covering brain and spinal cord)	mening/o/cele (mĕn-ĬN-gō-sēl): herniation of the meninges through the skull or spinal column *-cele:* hernia, swelling meningi/oma (mĕn-in-jē-Ō-mă): slow-growing tumor that originates in the meninges *-oma:* tumor	
myel/o	bone marrow; spinal cord	poli/o/myel/itis (pōl-ē-ō-mi-ĕl-Ī-tĭs): inflammation of the gray matter of the spinal cord *poli/o:* gray; gray matter (of brain or spinal cord) *-itis:* inflammation	
narc/o	stupor; numbness; sleep	narc/o/tic (năr-KŎT-ĭk): relating to or producing stupor or sleep *-tic:* pertaining to, relating to *Narcotics depress the central nervous system, thus relieving pain and producing sleep.*	
neur/o	nerve	neur/o/lysis (nū-RŎL-ĭs-ĭs): loosening of adhesions surrounding a nerve *-lysis:* separation; destruction; loosening	
sthen/o	strength	hyper/sthen/ia (hī-pĕr-STHĒ-nē-ă): abnormal strength with excessive tension in all parts of the body *hyper-:* excessive, above normal *-ia:* condition	
radicul/o	nerve root	radicul/algia (ră-dĭk-ū-LĂL-jē-ă): pain in the nerve roots *-algia:* pain	
thec/o	sheath (usually refers to meninges)	intra/thec/al (ĭn-tră-THĒ-kăl): pertaining to the space within a sheath, especially the meninges *intra-:* in, within *-al:* pertaining to, relating to	
thalam/o	thalamus	thalam/o/tomy (thăl-ă-MŎT-ō-mē): incision of the thalamus to treat intractable pain or psychoses *-tomy:* incision	
ton/o	tension	dys/ton/ia (dĭs-TŌ-nē-ă): any abnormality in muscle tone *dys-:* bad; painful; difficult *-ia:* condition *Dystonia usually refers to a movement disorder characterized by sustained muscle contractions resulting in a persistently abnormal posture.*	

Element	Meaning	Word Analysis
ventricul/o	ventricle (of heart or brain)	ventricul/o/metry (věn-trĭk-ū-LŎM-ĕ-trē): measurement of intraventricular cerebral pressure *-metry:* act of measuring

SUFFIXES

Element	Meaning	Word Analysis
-algesia	pain	an/algesia (ăn-ăl-JĒ-zē-ă): absence of a normal sense of pain *an-:* without, not
-algia		syn/algia (sĭn-ĂL-jē-ă): referred pain *syn-:* union, together, joined
-asthenia	weakness, debility	my/asthenia (mī-ăs-THĒ-nē-ă): muscular weakness and abnormal fatigue *my:* muscle
-esthesia	feeling	hyper/esthesia (hī-pěr-ěs-THĒ-zē-ă): increased sensitivity to sensory stimuli, such as pain and touch *hyper-:* excessive, above normal
-kinesia	movement	hyper/kinesia (hī-pěr-kĭ-NĒ-zē-ă): increased muscular movement and physical activity *hyper-:* excessive, above normal
-lepsy	seizure	epi/lepsy (ĔP-ĭ-lěp-sē): any disorder characterized by recurrent seizures *epi-:* above, upon
-paresis	partial paralysis	hemi/paresis (hěm-ē-PĂR-ě-sĭs): paralysis of one side of the body; also called *hemiplegia* *hemi-:* one-half *When used alone, the term* paresis *means partial paralysis or motor weakness.*
-phasia	speech	a/phasia (ă-FĀ-zē-ă): impairment in the ability to communicate through speech, writing, or signs because of brain dysfunction *a-:* without, not
-plegia	paralysis	quadri/plegia (kwŏd-rĭ-PLĒ-jē-ă): paralysis of all four extremities *quadri-:* four
-plexy	stroke	cata/plexy (KĂT-ă-plěks-ē): sudden, brief loss of muscle control that commonly results in collapse *cata-:* down *Cataplexy is commonly brought on by extreme emotion, such as surprise, anger, and excitement.*
-taxia	order, coordination	a/taxia (ă-TĂK-sē-ă): defective muscle coordination, especially when voluntary movements are attempted *a-:* without, not

(Continued)

Element	Meaning	Word Analysis	(Continued)
-trophy	development, nourishment	dys/trophy (DĬS-trō-fē): disorder caused by defective nutrition or metabolism *dys-:* bad; painful; difficult	

PREFIXES

Element	Meaning	Word Analysis	
contra-	against	contra/later/al (kŏn-tră-LĂT-ĕr-ăl): pertaining to opposite sides *later:* side, to one side *-al:* pertaining to, relating to	
pachy-	thick	pachy/mening/itis (păk-ē-mĕn-ĭn-JĪ-tĭs): inflammation of the dura mater *mening:* meninges (membranes covering brain and spinal cord) *-itis:* inflammation *The dura mater is a thick membrane that provides protection for the brain and spinal cord.*	
para-	near, beside; beyond	para/plegia (păr-ă-PLĒ-jē-ă): paralysis of the lower part of the body and both legs *-plegia:* paralysis	
syn-	union, together, joined	syn/esthesia (sĭn-ĕs-THĒ-zē-ă): stimulation of one sense that causes a perception in one or more different senses *-esthesia:* feeling *An example of synesthesia is hearing a sound that may also produce a sensation of smell.*	
uni-	one	uni/later/al (ū-nĭ-LĂT-ĕr-ăl): pertaining to or affecting only one side *later:* side, to one side *-al:* pertaining to, relating to	

 It is time to review medical word elements by completing Learning Activity 14–2.

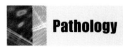 **Pathology**

Damage to the brain and spinal cord invariably causes signs and symptoms in other parts of the body. Therefore, it is always essential to identify the neurological deficit as involving a muscle, a nerve, the spinal cord, or the brain. Common symptoms for many neurological disorders include headache, insomnia, back or neck pain, weakness, and involuntary movement **(dyskinesia).** Careful observation of the patient during the patient history and physical examination may provide valuable clues about mental status and cognitive and motor ability. Muscle strength, coordination, gait, balance, and reflexes provide additional diagnostic clues. Lumbar punctures provide a sample of CSF for analysis and help identify various types of meningitis and encephalitis. Radiology—especially CT and MRI scans—provide detailed images that can locate cerebrovascular irregularities, lesions, and tumors.

Bell Palsy

Bell palsy is a facial paralysis caused by a functional disorder of the seventh cranial nerve and any or all of its branches and is associated with herpes virus. It may be unilateral, bilateral, transient, or permanent. Symptoms include weakness **(asthenia)** and numbness of the face, distortion of taste perception, facial disfigurement, and facial spasms. The cornea becomes dry because of an absent blink reflex and commonly leads to corneal infection **(keratitis)**. Speech difficulties **(dysphasia)** and pain behind the ear or in the face are also symptoms of this disease. Anti-inflammatory drugs and the application of heat promote circulation and ease pain. Spontaneous recovery can be expected in about 3 to 5 weeks.

Cerebrovascular Disease

Cerebrovascular disease (CVD) refers to any functional abnormality of the cerebrum caused by disorders of the blood vessels of the brain. CVD is most commonly associated with a stroke, also called *cerebrovascular accident (CVA)*. The three major types of strokes are *ischemic stroke, intracerebral hemorrhage*, and *subarachnoid hemorrhage*. The most common type, which accounts for about 80% of all strokes, is ischemic stroke. It is caused by a narrowing of the arteries of the brain or neck **(carotid)**, generally due to arteriosclerosis. This narrowing causes insufficient oxygen delivery to the brain tissue and, within a few minutes, the tissue begins to die. An intracerebral hemorrhage is a type of stroke caused by the sudden rupture of an artery within the brain. After the rupture, released blood compresses brain structures and destroys them. In a subarachnoid hemorrhage, blood is released into the space surrounding the brain. This condition is commonly caused by a ruptured aneurysm and is usually fatal.

Signs and symptoms of stroke include weakness in one half of the body **(hemiparesis),** paralysis in one half of the body **(hemiplegia),** inability to speak **(aphasia),** lack of muscular coordination **(ataxia),** stupor, coma, or even death. If the CVA is mild, the patient may experience a brief "blackout," blurred vision, or dizziness and may be unaware of the "minor stroke." Stroke symptoms that resolve within 24 hours are known as a *transient ischemic attack (TIA)*. About one-third of all strokes are preceded by a TIA. A family history of cerebrovascular disease and high blood pressure appears to be a contributing factor to stroke. Treatment involves speech, physical, and occupational therapy and various medications, depending on the type of stroke.

Seizure Disorders

Chronic or recurring seizure disorders are called *epilepsies*. These disorders involve electrical disturbances **(dysrhythmias)** in the brain that result in abnormal, recurrent, and uncontrolled electrical discharges. Causes of epilepsy include brain injury, congenital anomalies, metabolic disorders, brain tumors, vascular disturbances, and genetic disorders.

Seizures are characterized by sudden bursts of abnormal electrical activity in neurons, resulting in temporary changes in brain function. Two major types of seizures are *partial* and *generalized*. In partial seizures there is a short alteration of consciousness of about 10 to 30 seconds, characterized by repetitive, unusual movements and confusion. In generalized seizures there is a temporary lapse in consciousness, accompanied by rhythmic movement of the eyes, head, or hands, without convulsions.

Status epilepticus is a life-threatening emergency that involves the whole cortex. It is diagnosed when a continuous seizure occurs without a pause; that is, without an intervening period of normal brain function. It is characterized by tonic-clonic convulsions that may cause irreversible brain damage or even death. Diagnosis and evaluation commonly rely on *electroencephalography* and *magnetoencephalography* to locate the affected area of the brain. Epilepsy is controlled by antiepileptic medications.

Parkinson Disease

Parkinson disease, also called "shaking palsy," is a progressive neurological disorder affecting the portion of the brain responsible for controlling movement. As neurons degenerate, the patient develops uncontrollable nodding of the head, decreased speed of movement (**bradykinesia, hypokinesia),** tremors, large joint stiffness, and a shuffling gait. Muscle rigidity causes facial expressions to appear fixed and masklike with unblinking eyes. Sometimes the patient exhibits "pill rolling," in which he or she inadvertently rubs the thumb against the index finger.

In patients with Parkinson disease, dopamine, a neurotransmitter that facilitates the transmission of impulses at synapses, is lacking in the brain. Management involves the administration of L-dopa, which can cross the blood-brain barrier. L-dopa is converted in the brain to dopamine. Even so, this treatment only reduces symptoms; it is not a cure for Parkinson disease.

Multiple Sclerosis

Multiple sclerosis (MS) is a progressive, degenerative disease of the CNS. MS is characterized by inflammation, hardening and, finally, loss of myelin (**demyelination)** throughout the spinal cord and brain. As myelin deteriorates, the transmission of electrical impulses from one neuron to another is impeded. In effect, the conduction pathway develops "short circuits."

Signs and symptoms of MS include tremors, muscle weakness, and bradykinesia. Occasionally, visual disturbances exist. During remissions, symptoms temporarily disappear, but progressive hardening of myelin areas leads to other attacks. Ultimately, most voluntary motor control is lost and the patient becomes bedridden. Death occurs anywhere from 7 to 30 years after the onset of the disease. Young adults, usually women, between ages 20 and 40 are the most common victims of MS. The etiology of the disease is unclear, but autoimmune disease or a slow viral infection is believed to be the most probable cause.

Alzheimer Disease

Alzheimer disease is a progressive neurological disorder that causes memory loss and serious mental deterioration. Small lesions called *plaques* develop in the cerebral cortex and disrupt the passage of electrochemical signals between cells. The clinical manifestations of Alzheimer disease include memory loss and cognitive decline. There is also a decline in social skills and ability to carry out activities of daily living. Most patients undergo personality, emotional, and behavioral changes. As the disease progresses, loss of concentration and increased fatigue, restlessness, and anxiety are common. Alzheimer disease was once considered rare but is now identified as a leading cause of senile dementia. Although there is no specific treatment, moderate relief has been associated with medications that prevent a breakdown of brain chemicals required for neurotransmission.

Mental Illness

Mental illness includes an array of psychological disorders, syndromes, and behavioral patterns that cause alterations in mood, behavior, and thinking. (See Table 14–2.) Its forms range from mild to profound. For example, anxiety may manifest as a slight apprehension or uneasiness lasting a few days to a more severe form, involving intense fears lasting for months and even years.

Psychosis refers to a serious mental disorder commonly characterized by false beliefs despite overwhelming evidence to the contrary **(delusions).** The psychotic patient typically "hears voices" and "sees visions" in the absence of an actual stimulus **(hallucinations).** The patient's speech is usually incoherent and disorganized and behavior is erratic.

Neurosis is a mental disorder caused by an emotion experienced in the past that overwhelmingly interferes or affects a present emotion. For example, a child bitten by a dog may show irrational fear of animals as an adult. Many mental disorders are forms of neuroses, including irrational fears **(phobias),** exaggerated emotional and reflexive behaviors **(hysterias),** or irrational, uncontrolled performance of ritualistic actions for fear of a dire consequence **(obsessive compulsive disorders).**

Research and education have removed much of the stigma attached to mental illness. Today, mental illness is becoming a more recognizable and treatable disorder. Many psychological disorders can be effectively treated or managed by family physicians, school psychologists, marriage counselors, family counselors, and even support groups such as grief support groups and Alcoholics Anonymous.

Diagnosis and treatment of serious mental disorders usually require the skills of a medical specialist called a *psychiatrist*. In the capacity of a physician, the psychiatrist is licensed to prescribe medications and perform medical procedures not available to those who do not hold a medical license. Psychiatrists commonly work in association with *clinical psychologists*, who are individuals trained in evaluating human behavior, intelligence, and personality.

Table 14–2   COMMON TERMS ASSOCIATED WITH MENTAL ILLNESS

This table lists common terms or disorders associated with mental illness along with their definitions.

Term	Definition
affective disorder	Psychological disorder in which the major characteristic is an abnormal mood, usually mania or depression
anorexia nervosa	Eating disorder characterized by a refusal to maintain adequate weight for age and height and an all-consuming desire to remain thin
anxiety	Psychological "worry" disorder characterized by excessive pondering or thinking "what if..." *Feelings of worry, dread, lack of energy, and a loss of interest in life are common signs associated with anxiety.*
attention-deficit hyperactivity disorder (ADHD)	Disorder affecting children and adults characterized by impulsiveness, overactivity, and the inability to remain focused on a task
bipolar disorder	Mental disorder that causes unusual shifts in mood, emotion, energy, and ability to function; also called *manic-depressive illness*
bulimia nervosa	Eating disorder characterized by binging (overeating) and purging (vomiting or use of laxatives)
depression	Mood disorder associated with sadness, despair, discouragement, and, commonly, feelings of low self-esteem, guilt, and withdrawal
mania	Mood disorder characterized by mental and physical hyperactivity, disorganized behavior, and hyper-elevated mood
panic attack	Sudden, profound, overwhelming feeling of fear that comes without warning and is not attributable to any immediate danger *A key symptom of a panic attack is the fear of its recurrence.*

Oncology

Intracranial tumors can arise from any structure within the cranial cavity, including the pituitary and pineal glands, cranial nerves, and the arachnoid and pia mater **(leptomeninges).** However, most intracranial tumors originate directly in brain tissue. In addition, all of these tissues may be the site of metastatic spread from primary malignancies that occur outside of the nervous system. Metastatic tumors of the cranial cavity tend to exhibit growth characteristics similar to those of the primary malignancy but tend to grow more slowly than the parent tumor. Metastatic tumors of the cranial cavity are usually easier to remove than primary intracranial tumors.

Primary intracranial tumors are commonly classified according to histological type and include those that originate in neurons and those that develop in glial tissue. Signs and symptoms of intracranial tumors include headaches, especially upon arising in the morning, during coughing episodes, and upon bending or sudden movement. Occasionally, the optic disc in the back of the eyeball swells **(papilledema)** because of increased intracranial pressure. Personality changes are common and include depression, anxiety, and irritability.

Computed tomography (CT) scans and magnetic resonance imaging (MRI) help establish a diagnosis but are not definitive. Surgical removal relieves pressure and confirms or rules out malignancy. Even after surgery, most intracranial tumors require radiation therapy (RT) as a second line of treatment. Chemotherapy, when added to RT, provides the best chance for survival and quality of life.

 ## Diagnostic, Symptomatic, and Related Terms

This section introduces diagnostic, symptomatic, and related terms and their meanings. Word analyses for selected terms are also provided.

Term	Definition
agnosia ăg-NŌ-zē-ă *a-:* without, not *gnos:* knowing *-ia:* condition	Inability to comprehend auditory, visual, spacial, olfactory, or other sensations even though the sensory sphere is intact *The type of agnosia is usually identified by the sense or senses affected, such as* visual agnosia. *Agnosia is common in parietal lobe tumors.*
asthenia ăs-THĒ-nē-ă *a-:* without, not *sthen:* strength *-ia:* condition	Weakness, debility, or loss of strength *Asthenia is a characteristic of multiple sclerosis.*
ataxia ă-TĂK-sē-ă *a-:* without, not *tax:* order, coordination *-ia:* condition	Lack of muscle coordination in the execution of voluntary movement *Ataxia may be the result of head injury, stroke, MS, alcoholism, or a variety of hereditary disorders.*
aura AW-ră	Premonitory awareness of an approaching physical or mental disorder; peculiar sensation that precedes seizures

Term	Definition
autism AW-tĭzm	Mental disorder chracterized by extreme withdrawal and an abnormal absorption in fantasy, usually accompanied by an inability to communicate even on a basic level *A person with autism may engage in repetitive behavior, such as rocking or repeating words.*
cerebral palsy sĕ-RĒ-brăl PAWL-zē *cerebr:* cerebrum *-al:* pertaining to, relating to	Self-limiting paralysis due to developmental defects in the brain or trauma during the birth process
clonic spasm KLŎN-ĭk SPĂZM	Alternate contraction and relaxation of muscles
closed head trauma TRAW-mă	Injury to the head in which the dura mater remains intact and brain tissue is not exposed *In closed head trauma, the injury site may occur at the impact site where the brain hits the inside of the skull (coup), or at the rebound site where the opposite side of the brain strikes the skull (contrecoup).*
coma KŌ-mă	Abnormally deep unconsciousness with absence of voluntary response to stimuli
concussion kŏn-KŬSH-ŭn	Transient loss of consciousness as a result of trauma to the head *Delayed symptoms of concussion may include headache, nausea, vomiting, and blurred vision.*
dementia dĭ-MĔN-shē-ă *de-:* cessation *ment:* mind *-ia:* condition	Broad term that refers to cognitive deficit, including memory impairment
dyslexia dĭs-LĔK-sē-ă *dys-:* bad; painful; difficult *lex:* word, phrase *-ia:* condition	Inability to learn and process written language despite adequate intelligence, sensory ability, and exposure
Guillain-Barré syndrome gē-YĂ băr-RĀ SĬN-drōm	Condition of acute polyneuritis with progressive muscle weakness in extremities *Guillain-Barré syndrome occurs most commonly in people ages 30 to 50 with spontaneous and complete recovery in about 95% of cases.*
herpes zoster HĔR-pēz ZŎS-tĕr	Painful, acute infectious disease of the posterior root ganglia of only a few segments of the spinal or cranial nerves; also called *shingles* *Herpes zoster is caused by the same organism (varicella-zoster) that causes chickenpox in children. The disease is self-limiting and usually resolves in 10 days to 5 weeks.*

(Continued)

Term	Definition	(Continued)
Huntington chorea HŬNT-ing-tŭn kō-RĒ-ă	Inherited disease of the CNS that usually has its onset in people between ages 30 and 50 *Huntington chorea is characterized by quick, involuntary movements; speech disturbances; and mental deterioration.*	
hydrocephalus hi-drō-SĔF-ă-lŭs	Accumulation of fluid in the ventricles of the brain, causing thinning of brain tissue and separation of cranial bones	
lethargy LĔTH-ăr-jē	Abnormal activity or lack of response to normal stimuli; also called *sluggishness*	
neurosis nū-RŌ-sĭs *neur:* nerve *-osis:* abnormal condition; increase (used primarily with blood cells)	Unconscious conflict that produces anxiety and other symptoms and leads to maladaptive use of defense mechanisms	
psychosis sī-KŌ-sĭs *psych:* mind *-osis:* abnormal condition; increase (used primarily with blood cells)	Major emotional disorder where contact with reality is lost to the point that the individual is incapable of meeting challenges of daily life	
spina bifida SPĪ-nă BĬ-fĭ-dă	Defect in which the neural tube (tissue that forms the brain and spinal cord in the fetus) fails to close during embryogenesis *Spina bifida is a serious birth defect. Forms of spina bifida include meningomyelocele, meningocele, and occulta. (See Figure 14–5.)*	
meningocele mĕn-ĬN-gō-sēl *mening/o:* meninges (membranes covering brain and spinal cord) *-cele:* hernia, swelling	Form of spina bifida in which the spinal cord develops properly but the meninges protrude through the spine	
myelomeningocele mī-ĕ-lō-mĕn-ĬN-gō-sēl *myel/o:* bone marrow; spinal cord *mening/o:* meninges (membranes covering brain and spinal cord) *-cele:* hernia, swelling	Most severe form of spina bifida where the spinal cord and meninges protrude through the spine	

Term	Definition
occulta ŏ-KŬL-tă	Form of spina bifida where one or more vertebrae are malformed and the spinal cord is covered with a layer of skin

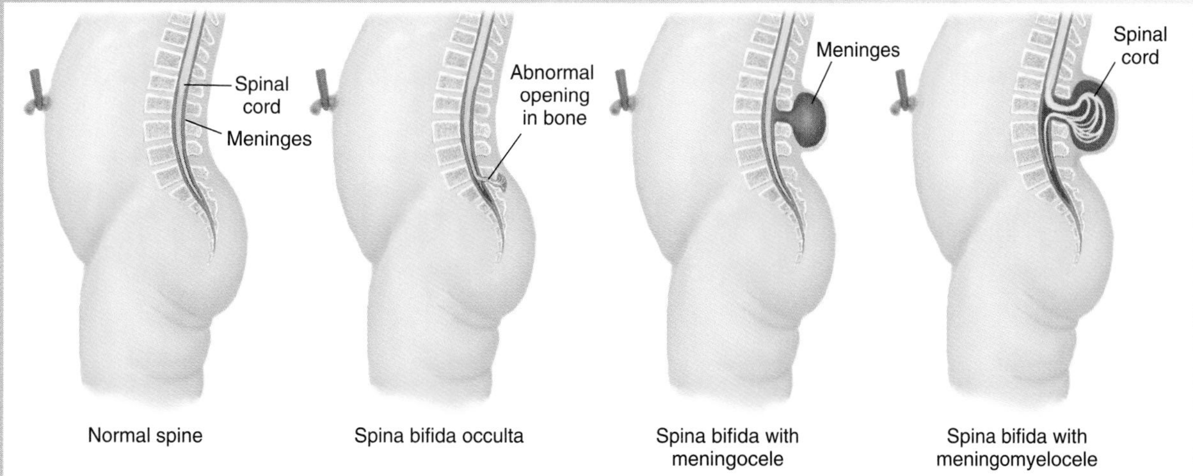

Figure 14–5 Spina bifida.

Term	Definition
paraplegia păr-ă-PLĒ-jē-ă *para-:* near, beside; beyond *-plegia:* paralysis	Paralysis of the lower portion of the trunk and both legs usually as a result of injury or disease of the spine
paresthesia păr-ĕs-THĒ-zē-ă	Sensation of numbness, prickling, tingling, or heightened sensitivity *Paresthesia can be caused by disorders affecting the central nervous system, such as stroke, transient ischemic attack, multiple sclerosis, transverse myelitis, and encephalitis.*
poliomyelitis pōl-ē-ō-mi-ĕl-Ī-tĭs *poli/o:* gray; gray matter (of brain or spinal cord) *myel:* bone marrow; spinal cord *-itis:* inflammation	Inflammation of the gray matter of the spinal cord caused by a virus, commonly resulting in spinal and muscle deformity and paralysis *Through the Global Polio Eradication Initiative of 1988, the incidence of polio has decreased worldwide by 99%.*
quadriplegia kwŏd-rĭ-PLĒ-jē-ă *quadri-:* four *-plegia:* paralysis	Paralysis of all four extremities and usually the trunk
Reye syndrome RĪ SĬN-drōm	Acute encephalopathy and fatty infiltration of the brain, liver and, possibly, the pancreas, heart, kidney, spleen, and lymph nodes; usually seen in children younger than age 15 who had an acute viral infection *Mortality in Reye syndrome may be as high as 80%. The use of aspirin by children experiencing chickenpox or influenza may induce Reye syndrome.*

(Continued)

Term	Definition	(Continued)
sciatica sĭ-ĂT-ĭ-kă	Severe pain in the leg along the course of the sciatic nerve felt at the base of the spine, down the thigh, and radiating down the leg due to a compressed nerve	
syncope SĬN-kō-pē	Temporary loss of consciousness due to the sudden decline of blood flow to the brain; also called *fainting*	
vasovagal văs-ō-VA-găl	Syncope due to a drop in blood pressure brought on by the response of the nervous system to abrupt emotional stress, pain, or trauma	
transient ischemic attack (TIA) TRĂN-zē-ĕnt ĭs-KĒ-mĭk	Temporary interference with blood supply to the brain lasting from a few minutes to a few hours *Symptoms of TIA may include numbness or weakness in the extremities, especially on one side of the body; confusion or difficulty in talking or understanding speech; visual impairment; dizziness; loss of balance; and difficulty walking.*	

 It is time to review pathological, diagnostic, symptomatic, and related terms by completing Learning Activity 14–3.

Diagnostic and Therapeutic Procedures

This section introduces procedures used to diagnose and treat nervous disorders. Descriptions are provided as well as pronunciations and word analyses for selected terms.

Procedure	Description
DIAGNOSTIC PROCEDURES	
Clinical	
electroencephalography (EEG) ē-lĕk-trō-ĕn-sĕf-ă-LŎG-ră-fē *electr/o:* electricity *encephal/o:* brain *-graphy:* process of recording	Recording of electrical activity in the brain, whose cells emit distinct patterns of rhythmic electrical impulses *Different wave patterns on the EEG are associated with normal and abnormal waking and sleeping states and help diagnose such conditions as tumors, infections, and seizure disorders.*
electromyography (EMG) ē-lĕk-trō-mi-ŎG-ră-fē *electr/o:* electricity *my/o:* muscle *-graphy:* process of recording	Recording of electrical signals (action potentials) that occur in a muscle when it is at rest and during contraction to assess nerve damage *In EMG, an electrode inserted into a muscle records the impulses and displays them on a monitor called an* oscilloscope.

Procedure	Description
lumbar puncture LŬM-băr PŬNK-chūr	Needle puncture of the spinal cavity to extract spinal fluid for diagnostic purposes, introduce anesthetic agents into the spinal canal, or remove fluid to allow other fluids (such as radiopaque substances) to be injected; also called *spinal puncture* and *spinal tap*
magnetoencephalography (MEG) măg-nĕt-ō-ĕn-cĕf-ă-LŎG-ră-fē	Noninvasive test that records electromagnetic activity produced as neurons discharge and maps their pathway through the brain *MEG is performed in seizure disorders because it can pinpoint active regions in the brain and trace their movement from region to region. A helmet that contains magnetic sensors tracks the impulses and records them.*
nerve conduction velocity (NCV) NĔRV kŏn-DŬK-shŭn vĕ-LŎ-sĭ-tē	Test that measures the speed at which impulses travel through a nerve *In NCV, one electrode stimulates a nerve while other electrodes, placed over different areas of the nerve, record an electrical signal (action potential) as it travels through the nerve. This test is used for diagnosing muscular dystrophy and neurological disorders that destroy myelin.*

Laboratory

cerebrospinal fluid (CSF) analysis sĕr-ē-brō-SPĪ-năl, ă-NĂL-ĭ-sĭs *cerebr/o:* cerebrum *spin:* spine *-al:* pertaining to, relating to	Series of chemical, microscopic, and microbial tests used to diagnose disorders of the central nervous system, including viral and bacterial infections, tumors, and hemorrhage

Radiographic

angiography ăn-jē-ŎG-ră-fē *angi/o:* vessel (usually blood or lymph) *-graphy:* process of recording	Radiography of the blood vessels after introduction of a contrast medium *Angiography is used to visualize vascular abnormalities. The contrast medium may be injected into an artery or vein or administered through a catheter inserted in a peripheral artery, run through the vessel, and positioned at a visceral site.*
cerebral sĕr-Ē-brăl *cerebr/o:* cerebrum *-al:* pertaining to, relating to	Angiography of blood vessels of the brain after injection of a contrast medium; also called *cerebral arteriography* *Vascular tumors, aneurysms, and occlusions are identified using cerebral angiography. In addition, abscesses, nonvascular tumors, and hematomas are commonly identified because they distort the normal vascular image.*
myelography mi-ĕ-LŎG-ră-fē *myel/o:* bone marrow; spinal cord *-graphy:* process of recording	Diagnostic radiological examination of the spinal canal, nerve roots, and spinal cord after injection of contrast medium into the spinal canal *Myelography is usually performed in conjunction with a CT scan and when an MRI is not possible because the patient has a pacemaker or other implantable device.*

(Continued)

Procedure	Description	*(Continued)*
scan	Term used to describe a computerized image by modality (such as *computed tomography, magnetic resonance,* and *nuclear*) or by structure (such as *thyroid, bone,* or *brain*)	
brain	Diagnostic procedure using radioisotope imaging to localize and identify intracranial masses, lesions, tumors, or infarcts *Because radioactive material concentrates in rapidly growing cells, a brain scan is used to identify brain tumors and evaluate the progress of treatment.*	
computed tomography (CT) kŏm-PŪ-tĕd tō-MŎG-ră-fē *tom/o:* to cut *-graphy:* process of recording	Imaging technique that rotates an x-ray emitter around the area to be scanned and measures the intensity of transmitted rays from different angles	
positron emission tomography (PET) PŎZ-ĭ-trŏn ē-MĬSH-ŭn tō-MŎG-ră-fē	Scan using computed tomography to record the positrons (positively charged particles) emitted from a radiopharmaceutical and produce a cross-sectional image of metabolic activity in body tissues to determine the presence of disease *PET is especially useful in scanning the brain and nervous system to diagnose disorders that involve abnormal tissue metabolism, such as schizophrenia, brain tumors, epilepsy, stroke, and Alzheimer disease. The images are produced using colors that indicate degrees of metabolism or blood flow. The highest rates appear red; lower rates appear yellow, then green; and the lowest rates appear blue. (See Figure 4–4F.)*	
ultrasonography ŭl-tră-sŏn-ŎG-ră-fē *ultra-:* excess, beyond *son/o:* sound *-graphy:* process of recording	Image produced by using high-frequency sound waves (ultrasound) and displaying the reflected "echoes" on a monitor; also called *ultrasound, sonography, echo,* and *echogram*	
echoencephalography ĕk-ō-ĕn-sĕf-ă-LŎG-ră-fē *echo-:* repeated sound *encephal/o:* brain *-graphy:* process of recording	Ultrasound technique used to study the intracranial structures of the brain and, especially, diagnose conditions that cause a shift in the midline structures of the brain	

THERAPEUTIC PROCEDURES

Surgical

cryosurgery krī-ō-SĔR-jĕr-ē	Technique that exposes abnormal tissue to extreme cold to destroy it *Cryosurgery is sometimes used to destroy malignant tumors of the brain.*	

Procedure	Description
stereotaxic radiosurgery stĕr-ē-ō-TĂK-sĭk rā-dē-ō-SŬR-jĕr-ē	Precise method of locating and destroying sharply circumscribed lesions on specific, tiny areas of pathological tissue in deep-seated structures of the central nervous system; also called *stereotaxy* or *stereotactic surgery* *Stereotaxic radiosurgery is used in the treatment of seizure disorders, aneurysms, brain tumors, and many other neuropathological conditions and is performed without a surgical incision. The site to be worked on is localized with three-dimensional coordinates, and methods of destroying lesions include heat, cold, and radiation.*
thalamotomy thăl-ă-MŎT-ō-mē *thalam/o:* thalamus *-tomy:* incision	Partial destruction of the thalamus to treat intractable pain, involuntary movements, or emotional disturbances *Thalamotomy produces few neurological deficits or changes in personality.*
tractotomy trăk-TŎT-ō-mē	Transection of a nerve tract in the brainstem or spinal cord *Tractotomy is sometimes used to relieve intractable pain.*
trephination trĕf-ĭn-Ā-shŭn	Technique that cuts a circular opening into the skull to reveal brain tissue and decrease intracranial pressure
vagotomy vā-GŎT-ō-mē	Interruption of the function of the vagus nerve to relieve peptic ulcer *Vagotomy is performed when ulcers in the stomach and duodenum do not respond to medication or changes in diet.*

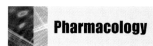

Pharmacology

Neurological agents are used to relieve or eliminate pain, suppress seizures, control tremors, and reduce muscle rigidity. Hypnotics, a class of drugs used as sedatives, depress central nervous system (CNS) function to relieve agitation and induce sleep. Anesthetics are capable of producing a complete or partial loss of feeling and are used for surgery. Psychotherapeutic agents alter brain chemistry to treat mental illness. These drugs are used as mood stabilizers in various mental disorders. They also reduce symptoms of depression and treat attention deficit hyperactivity disorder and narcolepsy. (See Table 14–3.)

Table 14-3   DRUGS USED TO TREAT NEUROLOGICAL AND PSYCHIATRIC DISORDERS

This table lists common drug classifications used to treat neurological and psychiatric disorders, their therapeutic actions, and selected generic and trade names.

Classification	Therapeutic Action	Generic and Trade Names
Neurological		

analgesics	Relieve or eliminate pain
	
	Nonnarcotic and nonsteroidal anti-inflammatory drugs (NSAIDs), such as Bayer and Vioxx, are used to treat mild aches and pain. Moderate to severe pain is commonly treated with narcotic analgesics, such as Demerol. Because they are addictive in nature, narcotic analgesics require a prescription.
		aspirin
		ĂS-pĕr-ĭn
		   Bayer, Bufferin, Ecotrin
		acetaminophen
		ă-sē-tă-MĬN-ō-fĕn
		   Tylenol, Panadol, Tempra
		rofecoxib
		rō-fĕ-CŌKS-ĭb
		   Vioxx
		meperidine
		mĕ-PĔR-ĭ-dēn
		   Demerol

anesthetics	Produce partial or complete loss of sensation, with or without loss of consciousness
	
	Anesthetics may be classified as general or local.
		lidocaine
		LĪ-dō-kān
		   Xylocaine
		nitrous oxide
		NĪ-trŭs ŎK-sĭd
		   N₂O

general	Act upon the brain to produce complete loss of feeling with loss of consciousness *General anesthetics are commonly used for surgical procedures and include Nembutal, Diprivan, and Versed.*	**pentobarbital** pĕn-tō-BĂR-bĭ-tăl *Nembutal* **propofol** PRŌ-pō-fŏl
local	Act upon nerves or nerve tracts and affect a local area only *Local anesthetics include Xylocaine and Novocain.*	*Diprivan* **procaine** PRŌ-kān *Novocain*

anticonvulsants	Suppress or control seizures by stabilizing the neuron membrane and reducing its excitability
	
	Anticonvulsants are used to prevent or control partial and generalized epileptic seizures.
		carbamazepine
		kăr-bă-MĂZ-ĕ-pēn
		   Tegretol
		valproate
		văl-PRŌ-āt
		   Depakote
		lamotrigine
		lă-MŌ-trĭ-jēn
		   Lamictal

antiparkinsonian agents	Reduce the signs and symptoms associated with Parkinson disease by increasing dopamine in the brain
	
	Antiparkinsonian agents control tremors and muscle rigidity.
		levodopa
		lē-vō-DŌ-pă
		   L-dopa, Larodopa, Dopar
		levodopa/carbidopa
		kăr-bĭ-DŌ-pă
		   Sinemet, Sinemet CR

Table 14-3 · DRUGS USED TO TREAT NEUROLOGICAL AND PSYCHIATRIC DISORDERS

Classification	Therapeutic Action	Generic and Trade Names
hypnotics	Depress central nervous system (CNS) functions and promote sedation and sleep *Hypnotics may be nonbarbiturates or barbiturates. Nonbarbiturate hypnotics (such as Restoril) carry a low risk of addiction; barbiturate hypnotics (such as Seconal) carry a higher risk of addiction.*	**secobarbital** sē-kō-BĂR-bĭ-tŏl *Seconal* **temazepam** tĕ-MĂZ-ĕ-păm *Restoril*
Psychiatric		
antipsychotics	Treat hallucinations, delusions, agitation, and paranoia and symptoms associated with schizophrenia *The first antipsychotics, known as* neuroleptics *(such as Thorazine and Haldol), caused numerous adverse effects. Newer medications called* atypical antipsychotics *(such as Zyprexa and Risperdal) have fewer adverse effects. In addition to psychotic disorders, antipsychotics are used to treat agitation associated with post-traumatic stress disorder and dementia.*	**clozapine** CLŌ-ză-pēn *Clozaril* **haloperidol** hă-lō-PĔR-ĭ-dŏl *Haldol* **olanzapine** ō-LĂN-ză-pēn *Zyprexa* **risperidone** rĭs-PĔR-ĭ-dōn *Risperdal*
antidepressants	Treat multiple symptoms of depression *Antidepressants fall under different classifications and some are also used to treat anxiety and pain.*	**paroxetine** pă-RŎK-sĕ-tēn *Paxil* **fluoxetine** floo-ŎK-sĕ-tēn *Prozac* **amitriptyline** ăm-ĭ-TRĬP-tĭ-lēn *Elavil*
psychostimulants	Treat narcolepsy and attention-deficit hyperactivity disorder (ADHD) in children and adults *Psychostimulants used to treat ADHD are mainly amphetamines. Amphetamines reduce the symptoms of restlessness, emotional lability, and impulsive behavior and may increase attention span without overstimulation.*	**dextroamphetamine** dĕks-trō-ăm-FĔT-ă-mēn *Dexedrine* **methylphenidate** mĕth-ĭl-FĔN-ĭ-dāt *Ritalin*

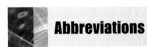

Abbreviations

This section introduces nervous system-related abbreviations and their meanings.

Abbreviation	Meaning
AD	Alzheimer disease
ALS	amyotrophic lateral sclerosis; also called *Lou Gehrig disease*
ANS	autonomic nervous system
BEAM	brain electrical activity mapping
CNS	central nervous system
CP	cerebral palsy
CSF	cerebrospinal fluid
CT scan, CAT scan	computed tomography scan
CVA	cerebrovascular accident
EEG	electroencephalogram; electroencephalography
ICP	intracranial pressure
LOC	loss of consciousness
LP	lumbar puncture
MEG	magnetoencephalography
MRA	magnetic resonance angiogram; magnetic resonance angiography
MRI	magnetic resonance imaging
MS	musculoskeletal; multiple sclerosis; mental status; mitral stenosis
NCV	nerve conduction velocity
PET	positron emission tomography
SNS	sympathetic nervous system
TIA	transient ischemic attack

It is time to review procedures, pharmacology, and abbreviations by completing Learning Activity 14–4.

LEARNING ACTIVITIES

The activities that follow provide a review of the nervous system terms introduced in this chapter. Complete each activity and review your answers to evaluate your understanding of the chapter.

Learning Activity 14–1

Identifying structures of the brain

Label the following illustration using the terms listed below.

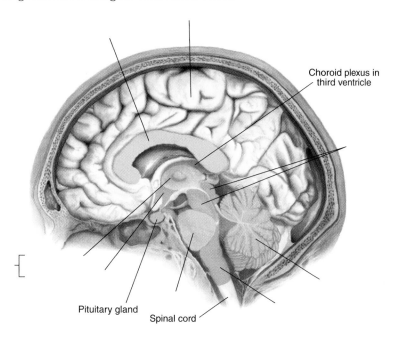

Choroid plexus in third ventricle

Pituitary gland

Spinal cord

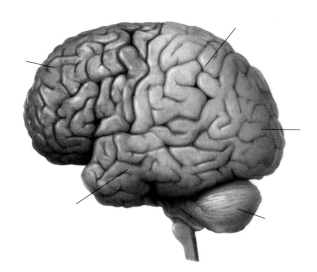

cerebellum	*hypothalamus*	*parietal lobe*
cerebrum	*medulla*	*pons*
corpus callosum	*midbrain (mesencephalon)*	*temporal lobe*
diencephalon (interbrain)	*occipital lobe*	*thalamus*
frontal lobe		

Check your answers by referring to Figure 14–2 on page 424. Review material that you did not answer correctly.

Building medical words

Use **encephal/o** *(brain) to build words that mean:*

1. disease of the brain _____
2. herniation of the brain _____
3. radiography of the brain _____

Use **cerebr/o** *(cerebrum) to build words that mean:*

4. disease of the cerebrum _____
5. inflammation of the cerebrum

Use **crani/o** *(cranium [skull]) to build words that mean:*

6. herniation (through the) cranium _____
7. instrument for measuring the skull _____

Use **neur/o** *(nerve) to build words that mean:*

8. pain in a nerve _____
9. specialist in the study of the nervous system _____
10. crushing a nerve _____

Use **myel/o** *(bone marrow; spinal cord) to build words that mean:*

11. herniation of the spinal cord _____
12. paralysis of the spinal cord _____

Use **psych/o** *(mind) to build words that mean:*

13. pertaining to the mind _____
14. abnormal condition of the mind _____

Use the suffix **-kinesia** *(movement) to build words that mean:*

15. movement that is slow _____
16. movement that is painful or difficult _____

Use the suffix **-plegia** *(paralysis) to build words that mean:*

17. paralysis of one half (of the body) _____
18. paralysis of four (limbs) _____

Use the suffix **-phasia** *(speech) to build words that mean:*

19. difficult speech _____
20. lacking or without speech _____

Build surgical terms that mean:

21. destruction of a nerve _____

22. incision of the skull _____

23. surgical repair of the skull _____

24. suture of a nerve _____

25. incision of the brain _____

✓ Check your answers in Appendix A. Review material that you did not answer correctly.

CORRECT ANSWERS _____ × 4 = _____ **% SCORE**

Learning Activity 14–3

Matching pathological, diagnostic, symptomatic, and related terms

Match the following terms with the definitions in the numbered list.

Alzheimer disease	dysrhythmias	paraplegia
asthenia	hemiparesis	Parkinson disease
autism	Guillain-Barré syndrome	poliomyelitis
bipolar disorder	leptomeningitis	shingles
bulimia nervosa	lethargy	stroke
clonic spasm	multiple sclerosis	transient ischemic attack (TIA)
concussion	phobias	

1. _____ weakness in one half of the body

2. _____ electrical disturbances in the brain

3. _____ pathological condition associated with the formation of small plaques in the cerebral cortex

4. _____ eating disorder characterized by binging and purging

5. _____ alternate contraction and relaxation of muscles

6. _____ acute polyneuritis with progressive muscle weakness in extremities

7. _____ type of neurosis characterized by irrational fears

8. _____ mental disorder that causes unusual shifts in mood, emotion, and energy

9. _____ inflammation of the arachnoid and pia mater

10. _____ weakness, debility, or loss of strength

11. _____ disease caused by the same organism that causes chickenpox in children

12. _____ abnormal activity or lack of response to normal stimuli; sluggishness

13. _____ paralysis of the lower portion of the trunk and both legs

14. _____ disease that causes inflammation of the gray matter of the spinal cord

15. _____ disease in which the brain fails to receive an adequate supply of oxygen

16. _____ denoting stroke symptoms that resolve within 24 hours

17. _____ mental disorder characterized by extreme withdrawal and abnormal absorption in fantasy

18. _____ disease characterized by head nodding, bradykinesia, tremors, and shuffling gait

19. _____ disease characterized by demyelination in the spinal cord and brain

20. _____ loss of consciousness caused by trauma to the head

✓ Check your answers in Appendix A. Review any material that you did not answer correctly.

CORRECT ANSWERS _____ × 5 = _____ **% SCORE**

Learning Activity 14–4

Matching procedures, pharmacology, and abbreviations

Match the following terms with the definitions in the numbered list.

analgesics	*electromyography*	*PET*
antipsychotics	*encephalography*	*psychostimulants*
cerebral angiography	*general anesthetics*	*tractotomy*
cryosurgery	*hypnotics*	*trephination*
CSF analysis	*myelography*	
echoencephalography	*NVC*	

1. _____ tests the speed at which impulses travel through a nerve

2. _____ treat narcolepsy and attention-deficit hyperactivity disorder (ADHD) in children and adults

3. _____ treat hallucinations, delusions, agitation, paranoia, and symptoms associated with schizophrenia

4. _____ act upon the brain to produce complete loss of feeling with loss of consciousness

5. _____ ultrasound technique used to study the intracranial structures of the brain

6. _____ technique that employs extreme cold to destroy tissue

7. _____ radiological examination of the spinal canal, nerve roots, and spinal cord

8. _____ visualization of the cerebrovascular system after injection of radiopaque dye

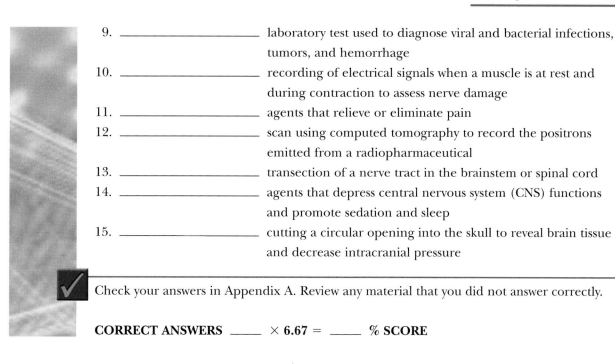

9. _____ laboratory test used to diagnose viral and bacterial infections, tumors, and hemorrhage

10. _____ recording of electrical signals when a muscle is at rest and during contraction to assess nerve damage

11. _____ agents that relieve or eliminate pain

12. _____ scan using computed tomography to record the positrons emitted from a radiopharmaceutical

13. _____ transection of a nerve tract in the brainstem or spinal cord

14. _____ agents that depress central nervous system (CNS) functions and promote sedation and sleep

15. _____ cutting a circular opening into the skull to reveal brain tissue and decrease intracranial pressure

Check your answers in Appendix A. Review any material that you did not answer correctly.

CORRECT ANSWERS _____ × **6.67** = _____ **% SCORE**

MEDICAL RECORD ACTIVITIES

The two medical records included in the activities that follow use common clinical scenarios to show how medical terminology is used to document patient care. Complete the terminology and analysis sections for each activity to help you recognize and understand terms related to the nervous system.

Medical Record Activity 14–1

Subarachnoid hemorrhage

Terminology

The terms listed in the chart come from the medical record *Subarachnoid Hemorrhage* that follows. Use a medical dictionary such as *Taber's Cyclopedic Medical Dictionary*, the appendices of this book, or other resources to define each term. Then review the pronunciations for each term and practice by reading the medical record aloud.

Term	Definition
aneurysm ĂN-ū-rĭzm	
cerebral MRI	
cisterna subarachnoidalis sĭs-TĔR-nă sŭb-ă-răk- NOYD-ă-lĭs	
CSF	
CT scan	
hydrocephalus hi-drō-SĔF-ă-lŭs	
lumbar puncture LŬM-băr PŬNK-chūr	
meningismus mĕn-ĭn-JĬS-mŭs	
occipital ŏk-SĬP-ĭ-tăl	
R/O	
subarachnoid sŭb-ă-RĂK-noyd	

SUBARACHNOID HEMORRHAGE

HISTORY OF PRESENT ILLNESS: The patient is a 61-year-old woman with a history of developing sudden onset of "extremely severe headaches" while swimming. She had associated neck pain, occipital pain, nausea, and vomiting.

A CT scan was obtained that showed blood in the cisterna subarachnoidalis consistent with subarachnoid hemorrhage. The patient also had mild acute hydrocephalus. Neurologically, the patient was found to be within normal limits. A cerebral MRI was performed and no aneurysm was noted. The patient was hospitalized on 7/5/xx. On 7/7/xx, she had sudden worsening of her headache associated with nausea and vomiting. Also, she was noted to have meningismus on examination. A lumbar puncture was performed to R/O possible rebleed. At the time of the lumbar puncture, CSF in four tubes was read as consistent with recurrent subarachnoid hemorrhage. A repeat MRI was performed without evidence of an aneurysm.

PROCEDURE: On 7/16/xx, the patient underwent repeat MRI, which again showed no aneurysm. The patient was deemed stable for discharge on 7/16/xx.

ACTIVITY: She was instructed to avoid any type of activity that could result in raised pressure in the head. The patient was advised that she should undergo no activity more vigorous than walking.

DISCHARGE DIAGNOSIS: Subarachnoid hemorrhage

Analysis

Review the medical record *Subarachnoid Hemorrhage* to answer the following questions.

1. In what part of the head did the patient feel pain?

   _____

2. What imaging tests were performed, and what was the finding in each test?

   _____

3. How does meningismus differ from meningitis?

   _____

4. Did the lumbar puncture rule out or confirm a second subarachnoid hemorrhage?

   _____

Medical Record Activity 14–2

Consultation report: Acute onset paraplegia

Terminology

The terms listed in the chart come from the medical record *Consultation Report: Acute Onset Paraplegia* that follows. Use a medical dictionary such as *Taber's Cyclopedic Medical Dictionary*, the appendices of this book, or other resources to define each term. Then review the pronunciations for each term and practice by reading the medical record aloud.

Term	Definition
abscess ĂB-sĕs	
acute ă-KŪT	
clonidine KLŌ-nĭ-dēn	
epidural ĕp-ĭ-DOO-răl	
fluoroscopy floo-ŏr-ŎS-kō-pē	
infarct ĬN-fărkt	
L2-3	
lumbar LŬM-băr	
methadone MĔTH-ă-dōn	
myelitis mī-ĕ-LĪ-tĭs	
paraplegia păr-ă-PLĒ-jē-ă	
paresthesia păr-ĕs-THĒ-zē-ă	
subarachnoid sŭb-ă-RĂK-noyd	
T10-11	
transverse trăns-VĔRS	

CONSULTATION REPORT: ACUTE ONSET PARAPLEGIA

DATE OF CONSULTATION: 4/14/xx

HISTORY OF PRESENT ILLNESS: This is a 41-year-old, right-handed, white female with a history of low back pain for the past 15 to 20 years after falling at work. She has had four subsequent lumbar surgeries, with the most recent in July 20xx. She was admitted to the hospital for pain management. The patient had a subarachnoid catheter placement for pain control and management, placed 4/10/xx, at the L2–3 level with the catheter placed at the T10–11 level. This was followed by trials of clonidine for hypertension and methadone for pain control, with bladder retention noted after clonidine administration. Upon catheter removal the patient noted the subacute onset of paresis, paresthesias, and pain in the legs approximately $2\frac{1}{2}$ to 3 hours later. We were consulted neurologically for assessment of the lower extremity weakness.

IMPRESSION AND PLAN: The patient has symptoms of acute onset paraplegia. Differential diagnoses include a subarachnoid hemorrhage, epidural abscess, and transverse myelitis. The patient will be placed on I.V. steroids with compression stockings for lymphedema should physical therapy be cleared by cardiology for manipulation of that region. Documentation of spinal fluid will be obtained under fluoroscopy. Her glucose and blood pressures must be carefully monitored.

Analysis

Review the medical record *Consultation Report: Acute Onset Paraplegia* to answer the following questions.

1. What was the original cause of the patient's current problems and what treatments were provided?

   _____

2. Why was the patient admitted to the hospital?

   _____

3. What intravenous medications did the patient receive and why was each given?

   _____

4. What was the cause of bladder retention?

   _____

5. What occurred after the catheter was removed?

   _____

6. What three disorders were listed in the differential diagnosis?

   _____

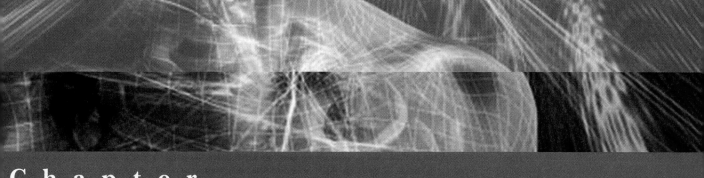

Chapter

15

Special Senses

OBJECTIVES

Upon completion of this chapter, you will be able to:

- Locate and describe the structures of the eye and ear.
- Recognize, pronounce, spell, and build words related to the special senses.
- Describe pathological conditions, diagnostic and therapeutic procedures, and other terms related to the special senses.

457

- Explain pharmacology related to the treatment of eye and ear disorders.
- Demonstrate your knowledge of this chapter by completing the learning and medical record activities.

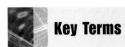

Key Terms

This section introduces important terms associated with the special senses and their definitions. Word analyses are also provided.

Term	Definition
accommodation ă-kŏm-ō-DĀ-shŭn	Adjustment of the eye for various distances so that the image falls on the retina of the eye
acuity ă-KŪ-ĭ-tē	Clearness or sharpness of a sensory function
adnexa ăd-NĔK-să	Tissues or structures in the body adjacent to or near a related structure *The adnexa of the eye include the extraocular muscles, orbits, eyelids, conjunctiva, and lacrimal apparatus.*
articulate ăr-TĬK-ū-lāt	To join or connect together loosely to allow motion between the parts
gustation gŭs-TĀ-shŭn	Sense and act of tasting foods, beverages, or other substances
humor HŪ-mor	Any fluid or semifluid of the body
labyrinth LĂB-ĭ-rĭnth	Series of intricate communicating passages *The labyrinth of the ear includes the cochlea, semicircular canals, and vestibule.*
olfaction ŏl-FĂK-shŭn	The act and sense of smelling *The sense of smell depends on airborne chemicals that stimulate receptors located in the deep nasal cavity. It not only warns of danger (such as from smoke or caustic chemicals) but may also influence mood, memory, emotions, and even the functioning of the immune and endocrine systems.*
ossicle ŎS-ĭ-kŭl	Any small bone, especially one of the three bones of the ear
photopigment fō-tō-PĬG-mĕnt	Light-sensitive pigment in the retinal cones and rods that absorbs light and initiates the visual process; also called *visual pigment*
slit lamp	Microscope with a specialized light that allows magnification of eye structures—especially the lens, cornea, and iris—and, with additional attachments, the vitreous humor and retina
tunic TŪ-nĭk	A layer or coat of tissue; also called *membrane layer* *The fibrous, vascular, and sensory tunics are the three tunics of the eyeball.*

Anatomy and Physiology

General sensations perceived by the body include touch, pressure, pain, and temperature. These sensations are not identified with any specific site of the body. Specific sensations include smell **(olfaction),** taste **(gustation),** vision, hearing **(audition),** and balance. Each sensation is connected to a specific organ or structure in the body. (For a discussion of olfaction, see Chapter 7, Respiratory System, and for a discussion of gustation, see Chapter 6, Digestive System.) This chapter presents information on the sense of vision provided by the eye and senses of hearing and equilibrium provided by the ear.

Eye

The eye is a globe-shaped organ composed of three distinct **tunics,** or layers: the fibrous tunic, the vascular tunic, and the sensory tunic. (See Figure 15–1.)

Fibrous Tunic

The outermost layer of the eyeball, the fibrous tunic, serves as a protective coat for the more sensitive structures beneath. It includes the (1) **sclera** and the (2) **cornea.** The sclera, or "white of the eye," provides strength, shape, and structure to the eye. As the sclera passes in front of the eye, it bulges forward to become the cornea. Rather than being opaque, the cornea is transparent, allowing light to enter the interior of the eye. The cornea is one of the few body

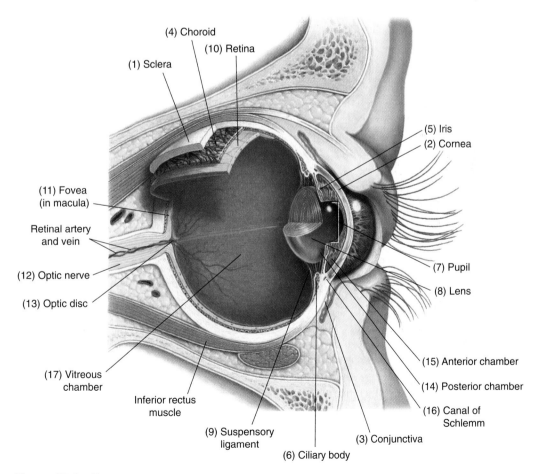

Figure 15–1   Eye structures.

structures that does not contain capillaries and must rely on eye fluids for nourishment. A thin membrane, the (3) **conjunctiva,** covers the outer surface of the eye and lines the eyelids.

Vascular Tunic

The middle layer of the eyeball, the vascular tunic, is also known as the *uvea.* The uvea consists of the choroid, iris, and ciliary body. The (4) **choroid** provides the blood supply for the entire eye. It contains pigmented cells that prevent extraneous light from entering the inside of the eye. An opening in the choroid allows the optic nerve to enter the inside of the eyeball. The anterior portion of the choroid contains two modified structures, the (5) **iris** and the (6) **ciliary body.** The iris is a colored, contractile membrane whose perforated center is called the (7) **pupil.** The iris regulates the amount of light passing through the pupil to the interior of the eye. As environmental light increases, the pupil constricts and as light decreases, the pupil dilates. The ciliary body is a circular muscle that produces aqueous humor. The ciliary body is attached to a capsular bag that holds the (8) **lens** by the (9) **suspensory ligaments.** As the ciliary muscle contracts and relaxes, it alters the shape of the lens making it thicker or thinner. These changes in shape allow the eye to focus on an image, a process called **accommodation.**

Sensory Tunic

The innermost sensory tunic is the delicate, double-layered (10) **retina.** It consists of a thin, outer *pigmented layer* lying over the choroid and a thick, inner *nervous layer,* or visual portion. The retina is responsible for the reception and transmission of visual impulses to the brain. It has two types of visual receptors called *rods* and *cones.* Rods function in dim light and produce black-and-white vision. Cones function in bright light and produce color vision. The (11) **fovea** is in the center of the macula. All of its receptors are cones that lie very close to each other. It provides the greatest **acuity** for color vision. When the eye focuses on an object, light rays from that object are directed to the fovea.

Other Structures

Rods and cones contain a chemical called **photopigment,** or *visual pigment.* As light strikes the photopigment, a chemical change occurs that stimulates rods and cones. The chemical changes produce impulses that are transmitted through the (12) **optic nerve** to the brain, where they are interpreted as vision. Both the optic nerve and blood vessels of the eye enter at the (13) **optic disc.** Its center is referred to as the *blind spot* because the area has neither rods nor cones for vision.

One of two major fluids **(humors)** of the eye is **aqueous humor.** It is found in the (14) **posterior chamber** and (15) **anterior chamber** and provides nourishment for the lens and the cornea. Aqueous humor is continually produced by the ciliary body and is drained from the eye through a small opening called the (16) **canal of Schlemm.** If aqueous humor fails to drain from the eye at the rate at which it is produced, a condition called *glaucoma* results. The second major humor of the eye is **vitreous humor,** a jellylike substance that fills the interior of eye, the (17) **vitreous chamber.** The vitreous humor, lens, and aqueous humor are the refractive structures of the eye. They bend light rays, focusing them sharply on the retina. If any one of these structures does not function properly, vision is impaired.

The **adnexa** of the eye include all supporting structures of the eye globe. Six muscles control the movement of the eye: the superior, inferior, lateral, and medial rectus muscles and the superior and inferior oblique muscles. These muscles coordinate the eyes so that they move in a synchronized manner.

Two movable folds of skin constitute the eyelids, each with eyelashes that protect the front of the eye. (See Figure 15–2.) The (1) **conjunctiva** lines the inner surface of the eyelids and the cornea. Lying superior and to the outer edge of each eye are the (2) **lacrimal glands,** which produce tears that bathe and lubricate the eyes. The tears collect at the inner edges of the eyes, the *canthi* (singular, *canthus*), and pass through pinpoint openings, the (3) **lacrimal canals,** to the mucous membranes that line the inside of the (4) **nasal cavity.**

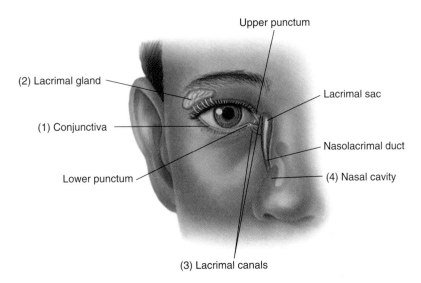

Upper punctum

(2) Lacrimal gland

Lacrimal sac

(1) Conjunctiva

Nasolacrimal duct

Lower punctum

(4) Nasal cavity

(3) Lacrimal canals

Figure 15–2   Lacrimal apparatus.

Ear

The ear is the sense receptor organ for hearing and equilibrium. Hearing is a function of the cochlea; the semicircular canals and vestibule control equilibrium.

Hearing

The ear consists of three major sections: the outer or **external ear,** the middle ear or **tympanic cavity,** and the inner ear or **labyrinth.** (See Figure 15–3.) Each of these sections transmits sound waves differently. The external ear conducts sound waves through air; the middle ear, through bone; and the inner ear, through fluid. This series of transmissions ultimately generates impulses that are sent to and interpreted by the brain as sound.

An (1) **auricle** (or **pinna**) collects waves traveling through air and channels them to the (2) **external auditory canal,** also called the *ear canal.* The ear canal is a slender tube lined with glands that produce a waxy secretion called **cerumen.** Its stickiness traps tiny foreign particles and prevents them from entering the deeper areas of the canal. The (3) **tympanic membrane** (also called the *tympanum* or *eardrum*) is a flat, membranous structure drawn over the end of the ear canal. Sound waves entering the ear canal strike against the tympanic membrane, causing it to vibrate. Its movement causes movement of the three smallest bones of the body, collectively called the *ossicles.* These tiny articulating bones, the (4) **malleus** (hammer), the (5) **incus** (anvil), and the (6) **stapes** (stirrups), are located within the tympanic cavity and form a coupling between the tympanic membrane and the (7) **cochlea,** the first structure of the inner ear. The malleus is attached to the eardrum and **articulates** with the incus. The stapes articulates with the incus and is attached to cochlea. The cochlea is a snail-shaped structure, filled with a fluid called perilymph. Its inner surfaces are lined with a highly sensitive hearing structure called the *organ of Corti,* which contains tiny nerve endings called the *hair cells.* A membrane-covered opening on the external surface of the cochlea called the (8) **oval window** provides a place for attachment of the stapes. The movement of the ossicles in the middle ear causes the stapes to exert a gentle pumping action against the oval window. The pumping action forces the perilymph to disturb the hair cells, generating impulses that are transmitted to the brain by way of the auditory nerve, where they are interpreted as sound. The (9) **eustachian tube** connects the middle ear to the pharynx. It equalizes pressure on the outer and inner surfaces of the eardrum. When sudden pressure changes occur, pressure can be equalized on either side of the tympanic membrane by deliberate swallowing.

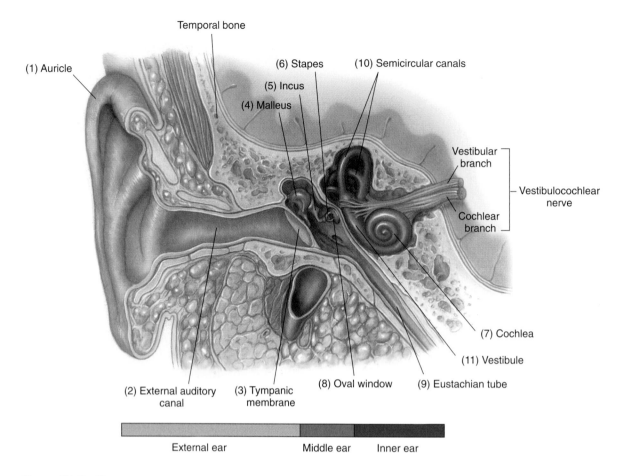

Figure 15–3   Ear structures.

Equilibrium

The inner ear consists of a system of fluid-filled tubes and sacs as well as the nerves that connect these structures to the brain. Because of its mazelike design, it is referred to as the *labyrinth.* The labyrinth, which rests inside the bone of the skull, includes not only the cochlea (the organ devoted to hearing) but also the vestibular system, which is devoted to the control of balance and eye movements. The vestibular system contains the (10) **semicircular canals** and the (11) **vestibule.** The vestibule joins the cochlea and the semicircular canals. Many complex structures located in this maze are responsible for maintaining both **static** and **dynamic equilibrium.** Static equilibrium refers to the orientation of the body relative to gravity. It allows an individual to maintain posture and orientation while at rest. Dynamic equilibrium refers to maintaining body position in response to movement.

 It is time to review eye and ear anatomy by completing Learning Activities 15–1 and 15–2.

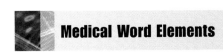

Medical Word Elements

This section introduces combining forms, suffixes, and prefixes related to the special senses. Word analyses are also provided.

Element	Meaning	Word Analysis
COMBINING FORMS		
Eye		
ambly/o	dull, dim	ambly/opia (ăm-blē-Ō-pē-ă): reduction or dimness of vision *-opia:* vision
aque/o	water	aque/ous (Ā-kwē-ŭs): pertaining to water *-ous:* pertaining to, relating to
blephar/o	eyelid	blephar/o/ptosis (blĕf-ă-rō-TŌ-sĭs): drooping of the upper eyelid *-ptosis:* prolapse, downward displacement
choroid/o	choroid	choroid/o/pathy (kō-roy-DŎP-ă-thē): any disease of the choroid *-pathy:* disease
core/o	pupil	core/o/meter (kō-rē-ŎM-ĕ-tĕr): instrument for measuring the pupil *-meter:* instrument for measuring
pupill/o		pupill/o/graphy (pū-pĭ-LŎG-ră-fē): process of recording movement of the pupil *-graphy:* process of recording
conjunctiv/o	conjunctiva	conjunctiv/al (kŏn-jŭnk-TĪ-văl): pertaining to the conjunctiva *-al:* pertaining to, relating to
corne/o	cornea	corne/al (KOR-nē-ăl): pertaining to the cornea *-al:* pertaining to, relating to
kerat/o	horny tissue; hard; cornea	kerat/o/tomy (kĕr-ă-TŎT-ō-mē): incision of the cornea *-tomy:* incision
cycl/o	ciliary body of eye; circular, cycle	cycl/o/plegia (sĭ-klō-PLĒ-jē-ă): paralysis of the ciliary body *-plegia:* paralysis

(Continued)

Element	Meaning	Word Analysis	(Continued)
dacry/o	tear; lacrimal apparatus (duct, sac, or gland)	dacry/oma (dăk-rē-Ō-mă): tumorlike swelling due to obstruction of the lacrimal duct *-oma:* tumor	
lacrim/o		lacrim/o/tome (LĂK-rĭ-mō-tōm): instrument used for incising the lacrimal sac or duct *-tome:* instrument to cut	
dacryocyst/o	lacrimal sac	dacryocyst/o/ptosis (dăk-rē-ō-sĭs-tŏp-TŌ-sĭs): prolapse of the lacrimal sac *-ptosis:* prolapse, downward displacement	
glauc/o	gray	glauc/oma (glaw-KŌ-mă): increased intraocular pressure that destroys the retina and optic nerve if not treated *-oma:* tumor *Poor blood flow to the back of the eye causes the optic nerve to appear pale gray, hence the name glaucoma.*	
goni/o	angle	goni/o/scopy (gŏ-nē-ŎS-kŏ-pē): examination of the angle and drainage area of the eye *-scopy:* visual examination *Gonioscopy is used to differentiate the two forms of glaucoma (open- and closed-angle).*	
irid/o	iris	irid/o/plegia (ĭr-ĭd-ō-PLĒ-jē-ă): paralysis of the sphincter of the iris *-plegia:* paralysis	
ocul/o	eye	ocul/o/myc/osis (ŏk-ū-lō-mĭ-KŌ-sĭs): fungal infection of the eye or its parts *myc:* fungus *-osis:* abnormal condition; increase (used primarily with blood cells)	
ophthalm/o		opthalm/o/logist (ŏf-thăl-MŎL-ō-jĭst): physician specializing in treating disorders of the eye *-logist:* specialist in study of	
opt/o	eye, vision	opt/o/kinet/ic (ŏp-tō-kĭ-NĔT-ĭk): pertaining to the twitching movement of the eyes, as in nystagmus *kinet:* movement *-ic:* pertaining to, relating to	
optic/o		optic/al (ŎP-tĭ-kăl): pertaining to the eye or vision *-al:* pertaining to, relating to	
phac/o	lens	phac/o/cele (FĀK-ō-sēl): displacement of the crystalline lens into the interior chamber of the eye *-cele:* hernia, swelling	

Element	Meaning	Word Analysis
phot/o	light	phot/o/phobia (fō-tō-FŌ-bē-ă): abnormal intolerance and sensitivity to light *-phobia:* fear
presby/o	old age	presby/opia (prĕz-bē-Ō-pē-ă): loss of accommodation of the crystalline lens associated with the aging process *-opia:* vision
retin/o	retina	retin/osis (rĕt-ĭ-NŌ-sĭs): any degenerative process of the retina not associated with inflammation *-osis:* abnormal condition; increase (used primarily with blood cells)
scler/o	hardening; sclera (white of eye)	scler/o/malacia (sklĕ-rō-mă-LĀ-shē-ă): softening of the sclera *-malacia:* softening
scot/o	darkness	scot/oma (skō-TŌ-mă): islandlike blind spot in the visual field *-oma:* tumor
vitr/o	vitreous body (of eye)	vitr/ectomy (vĭ-TRĔK-tō-mē): removal of the contents of the vitreous chamber and replacing with sterile saline *-ectomy:* excision, removal *The removal of the vitreous allows surgical procedures that would otherwise be impossible, including repair of macular holes and tears in the retina.*
Ear		
audi/o	hearing	audi/o/meter (aw-dē-ŎM-ĕ-tĕr): instrument used to measure hearing *-meter:* instrument for measuring
aur/o	ear	bi/aur/al (bī-AW-răl): pertaining to both ears *bi-:* two *-al:* pertaining to, relating to
ot/o		ot/o/py/o/rrhea (ō-tō-pī-ō-RĒ-ă): discharge of pus from the ear *py/o:* pus *-rrhea:* discharge, flow
labyrinth/o	labyrinth (inner ear)	labyrinth/o/tomy (lăb-ĭ-rĭn-THŎT-ō-mē): incision of the labyrinth *-tomy:* incision
mastoid/o	mastoid process	mastoid/ectomy (măs-toyd-ĔK-tō-mē): removal of the mastoid process *-ectomy:* excision, removal

(Continued)

Element	Meaning	Word Analysis	(Continued)
salping/o	tubes (usually fallopian or eustachian [auditory] tubes)	salping/o/scope (săl-PĬNG-gō-skōp): instrument to examine the eustachian tubes *-scope:* instrument to view or examine	
staped/o	stapes	staped/ectomy (stā-pĕ-DĔK-tō-mē): excision of the stapes to improve hearing, especially in cases of otosclerosis *-ectomy:* excision, removal	
myring/o	tympanic membrane (eardrum)	myring/o/myc/osis (mĭr-ĭn-gō-mi-KŌ-sĭs): inflammation of the tympanic membrane as a result of a fungal infection *myc:* fungus *-osis:* abnormal condition; increase (used primarily with blood cells)	
tympan/o		tympan/o/stomy (tĭm-pă-NŎS-tō-mē): forming an opening in the tympanic membrane, usually for tube insertion *-stomy:* forming an opening (mouth)	

SUFFIXES

-opia	vision	dipl/opia (dĭp-LŌ-pē-ă): double vision *dipl-:* double, twofold	
-opsia		heter/opsia (hĕt-ĕr-ŎP-sē-ă): inequality of vision in the two eyes *heter-:* different	
-tropia	turning	eso/tropia (ĕs-ō-TRŌ-pē-ă): marked turning inward of the eyes; also called *convergent strabismus* *eso-:* inward	
-acusia	hearing	an/acusia (ăn-ă-KŪ-sē-ă): deafness *an-:* without, not	
-cusis	hearing	presby/cusis (prĕz-bĭ-KŪ-sĭs): progressive hearing loss due to the aging process *presby:* old age	

PREFIXES

exo-	outside, outward	exo/tropia (ĕks-ō-TRŌ-pē-ă): abnormal turning outward of one or both eyes; also called *divergent strabismus* *-tropia:* turning	
hyper-	excessive, above normal	hyper/opia (hī-pĕr-Ō-pē-ă): farsightedness *-opia:* vision	

 It is time to review medical word elements by completing Learning Activity 15–3.

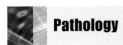

Pathology

For diagnosis, treatment, and management of visual disorders, the medical services of a specialist may be warranted. *Ophthalmology* is the medical specialty concerned with disorders of the eye. The physician who treats these disorders is called an *ophthalmologist.* *Optometrists* either work with ophthalmologists in a medical practice or practice independently. Optometrists are not medical doctors, but are doctors of optometry (OD). They diagnose vision problems and eye disease, prescribe eyeglasses and contact lenses, and prescribe drugs to treat eye disorders. Although they cannot perform surgery, they commonly provide preoperative and postoperative care.

For diagnosis, treatment, and management of hearing disorders, the medical services of a specialist may be warranted. *Otolaryngology* is the medical specialty concerned with disorders of the ear, nose, and throat. The physician who treats these disorders is called an *otolaryngologist.* Many otolaryngologists employ *audiologists.* Audiologists are allied health care professionals who work with patients that have hearing, balance, and related problems. They perform hearing examinations, evaluate hearing loss, clean and irrigate the ear canal, fit and dispense hearing aids or other assistive devices, and provide audiological rehabilitation, including auditory training and instruction in speech or lip reading.

Eye Disorders

Eye disorders include not only visual deficiencies associated with refractive errors, but also disorders of associated structures, such as the eye muscles, nerves, and blood vessels. A complete examination of the eye and its **adnexa** is necessary to identify the source of any disorder. Most ocular examinations begin by recording visual acuity and visual field. Then the eyelids, pupils, cornea, and lacrimal structures are examined and intraocular pressure is assessed as well. If infection is detected, it must be located and treated by testing eye and nasal discharge cultures and performing CT scans of the sinuses. Occasionally, the patient may be referred for dental examination to determine if abscesses in the mouth are the source of infection. Family history is important because many eye disorders have a genetic predisposition, including glaucoma. Common eye disorders include errors of refraction, cataracts, glaucoma, strabismus, and macular degeneration.

Errors of Refraction

An error of refraction (**ametropia**) exists when light rays fail to focus sharply on the retina. This may be due to a defect in the lens, cornea, or the shape of the eyeball. If the eyeball is too long, the image falls in front of the retina, causing nearsightedness (**myopia**). (See Figure 15–4.) In farsightedness (**hyperopia, hypermetropia**), the opposite of myopia, the eyeball is too short and the image falls behind the retina. A form of farsightedness is **presbyopia,** a defect associated with the aging process. The onset of presbyopia usually occurs between ages 40 and 45. Distant objects are seen clearly, but near objects are not in proper focus. In another form of ametropia called *astigmatism,* the cornea or lens has a defective curvature. This curvature causes light rays to diffuse over a large area of the retina, rather than being sharply focused.

Corrective lenses usually compensate for the various types of ametropia. An alternative to corrective lenses is laser-assisted *in situ* keratomileusis (LASIK) surgery. This procedure permanently changes the shape of the cornea. A small incision is made in the cornea to produce a flap. The flap is lifted to the side while a laser reshapes the underlying corneal tissue. At the completion of the procedure, the corneal flap is replaced. The procedure usually takes less than 15 minutes. However, not all people are candidates for this surgery. Some

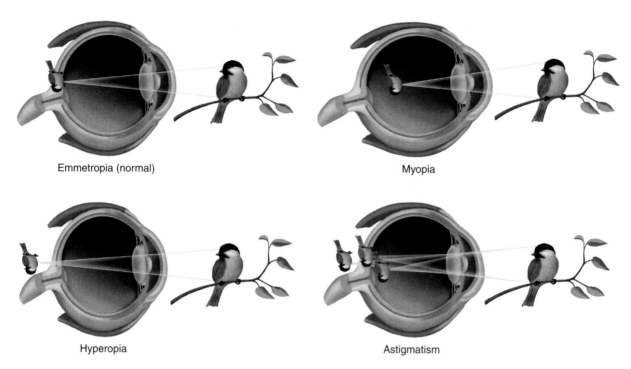

Emmetropia (normal)

Myopia

Hyperopia

Astigmatism

Figure 15–4   Refraction of eye.

medical conditions, certain medications, or the shape and structure of the eye may preclude this procedure as a viable alternative to corrective lenses.

Cataracts

Cataracts are opacities that form on the lens and impair vision. These opacities are commonly produced by protein that slowly builds up over time until vision is lost. The most common form of cataract is age related. More than one-half of Americans older than 65 are affected. Congenital cataracts found in children are usually a result of genetic defects or maternal rubella during the 1st trimester of pregnancy. This rare form of cataract is treated in the same manner as age-related cataract. The usual treatment is removal of the clouded lens by emulsifying it using ultrasound or a laser probe **(phacoemulsification).** (See Figure 15–5.) An artificial, bendable *intraocular lens* (IOL) is then inserted into the capsule. Once in position, the

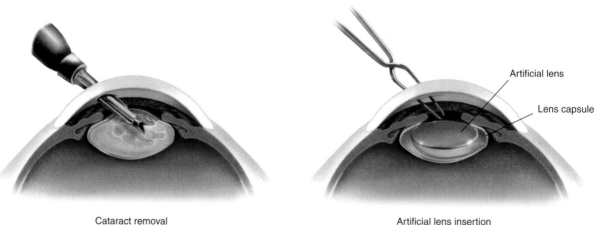

Cataract removal

Artificial lens

Lens capsule

Artificial lens insertion

Figure 15–5   Phacoemulsification.

lens unfolds. The surgery is usually performed using a topical anesthetic, and the incision normally does not require stitches. This is one of the safest and most effective surgical procedures performed in medicine.

Glaucoma

Glaucoma is characterized by increased intraocular pressure caused by the failure of aqueous humor to drain from the eye through a tiny duct called the *canal of Schlemm.* The increased pressure on the optic nerve destroys it, and vision is permanently lost.

Although there are various forms of glaucoma, all of them eventually lead to blindness unless the condition is detected and treated in its early stages. Glaucoma may occur as a primary or congenital disease or secondary to other causes, such as injury, infection, surgery, or prolonged topical corticosteroid use. Primary glaucoma can be chronic or acute. The chronic form is also called *open-angle, simple,* or *wide-angle glaucoma.* The acute form is called *angle-closure* or *narrow-angle glaucoma.* Chronic glaucoma may produce no symptoms except gradual loss of peripheral vision over a period of years. Headaches, blurred vision, and dull pain in the eye may also be present. Cupping of the optic discs may be noted on ophthalmoscopic examination. Acute glaucoma is accompanied by extreme ocular pain, blurred vision, redness of the eye, and dilation of the pupil. Nausea and vomiting may also occur. If untreated, acute glaucoma causes complete and permanent blindness within 2 to 5 days.

Glaucoma is diagnosed by **tonometry,** a screening test that measures intraocular pressure by determining the resistance of the eyeball to indentation by an applied force. A slit lamp with a high-intensity beam is used to examine the external surface and internal segments of the eye after administration of a local anesthetic. Devices such as a *tonometer,* which measures intraocular pressure, and a *gonioscope,* which visualizes the anterior chamber angle, expand the scope of the examination. (See Figure 15–6.) Several methods of tonometry are available, but the one that is considered most accurate is *applanation tonometry.* Numbing drops are used and the test is pain-free. Treatment for glaucoma includes medications that cause the pupils to constrict **(miotics),** which permits aqueous humor to escape from the eye, thereby relieving pressure. If miotics are ineffective, surgery may be necessary.

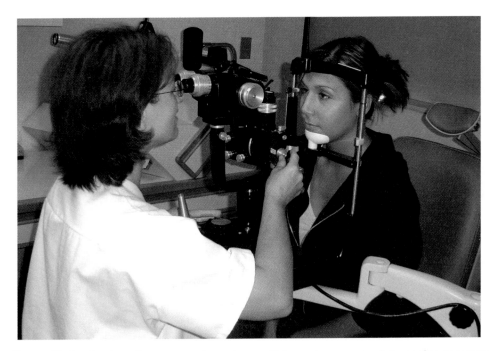

Figure 15–6 Applanation tonometry using a slit lamp to measure intraocular pressure (courtesy of Richard H. Koop, MD).

Strabismus

Strabismus, also called *heterotropia* or *tropia,* is a condition in which one eye is misaligned with the other and the eyes do not focus simultaneously when viewing an object. This misalignment may be in any direction—inward **(esotropia),** outward **(exotropia),** up, down, or any combination of these. The deviation may be a constant condition or may arise intermittently with stress, exhaustion, or illness. (See Figure 15–7.) In normal vision, each eye views an image from a somewhat different vantage point, thus transmitting a slightly different image to the brain. The result is binocular perception of depth or three-dimensional space, a phenomenon known as *stereopsis.* Strabismus commonly causes a loss of stereopsis. In children, strabismus is commonly but not always associated with "lazy-eye syndrome" **(amblyopia).** Vision is suppressed in the "lazy" eye so that the child uses only the "good" eye for vision. The vision pathway fails to develop in the "lazy" eye.

There is a critical period during which amblyopia must be corrected, usually before age 6. If not detected and treated early in life, amblyopia can cause a permanent loss of vision in the affected eye, with associated loss of stereopsis. Treatment for strabismus depends on the cause. It commonly consists of covering the normal eye, forcing the child to use the deviated one. Eye exercises and corrective lenses may be prescribed, or surgical correction may be necessary.

Macular Degeneration

Macular degeneration is the deterioration of the macula, the most sensitive portion of the retina. The macula is responsible for central, or "straight-ahead" vision required for reading, driving, detail work, and recognizing faces. (See Figure 15–8.) Although deterioration of the macula is associated with the toxic effects of some drugs, the most common type is age-related macular degeneration (ARMD, or AMD). ARMD is a leading cause of visual loss in the United States. The disease is unpredictable and progresses differently in each individual.

So far, two forms of ARMD have been identified: wet and dry. The less common but more severe form is wet, or *neovascular* ARMD. It affects about 10% of those afflicted with the disease. Small blood vessels form under the macula. Blood and other fluids leak from these vessels and destroy the visual cells, leading to severe loss of central vision and permanent visual impair-

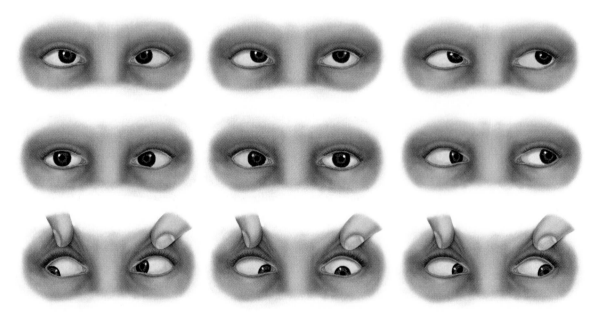

Figure 15–7   Types of strabismus.

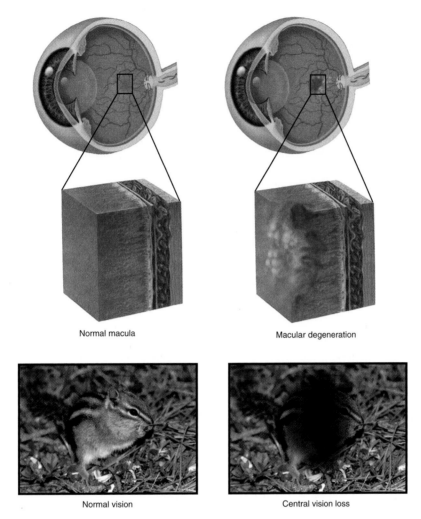

Normal macula

Macular degeneration

Normal vision

Central vision loss

Figure 15–8   Macular degeneration.

ment. If identified in its early stages, laser surgery can be employed to destroy the newly form-ing vessels. This treatment is called *laser photocoagulation*. It is successful in about one-half of the patients with wet ARMD. However, the effects of the procedure commonly do not last and new vessels begin to form.

The more common form of the disease is dry ARMD. Small yellowish deposits called *drusen* develop on the macula and interfere with central vision. Drusen are dried retinal pigment epithelial cells that form granules on the macula. Although some vision is lost, this form of the disease rarely leads to total blindness. Patients with dry ARMD are encour-aged to see their ophthalmologist frequently and perform a simple at-home test that iden-tifies visual changes that may indicate the development of the more serious neovascular ARMD.

Ear Disorders

Common signs and symptoms of ear disorders include hearing loss, earache, vertigo, and tinni-tus. Hearing tests are important in diagnosing hearing loss as well as aiding in localizing the source and nature of the hearing deficiency. In addition, many infections of the nose and throat refer pain to the ear. Therefore, an examination of the nose and throat is usually essential in identifying the cause of ear pain. Common ear disorders include otitis media and otosclerosis.

Otitis Media

Otitis media is an inflammation of the middle ear. This infection may be caused by a virus or bacterium. However, the most common culprit is *Streptococcus pneumoniae*. Otitis media is found most commonly in infants and young children, especially in the presence of an upper respiratory infection (URI). Symptoms may include earache and draining of pus from the ear **(otopyorrhea)**. In its most severe form, otitis media may lead to infection of the mastoid process **(mastoiditis)** or inflammation of brain tissue near the middle ear **(otoencephalitis)**. Recurrent episodes of otitis media may cause scarring of the tympanic membrane, leading to hearing loss. Treatment consists of bed rest, medications to relieve pain **(analgesics),** and antibiotics. Occasionally, an incision of the eardrum **(myringotomy, tympanotomy)** may be necessary to relieve pressure and promote drainage.

The main treatment for children with recurrent infection is the use of pressure-equalizing tubes (PE tubes) that are passed through the tympanic membrane. These tubes help drain fluid from the middle ear.

Otosclerosis

Otosclerosis is a disorder characterized by an abnormal hardening **(ankylosis)** of bones of the middle ear that causes hearing loss. The ossicle most commonly affected is the stapes, the bone that attaches to the oval window of the cochlea. The formation of a spongy growth at the footplate of the stapes decreases its ability to move the oval window, resulting in hearing loss. Occasionally, the patient perceives a ringing sound **(tinnitus)** within the ear, along with dizziness and a progressive loss of hearing, especially of low tones. Development of otosclerosis is typically closely tied to genetic factors; if one or both parents have the disorder, the child is at high risk for developing the disease. Surgical correction involves removing part of the stapes **(stapedectomy,** or more commonly **stapedotomy)** and implanting of a prosthetic device that allows sound waves to pass to the inner ear. The procedure requires only a local anesthetic and usually lasts only 45 minutes. Hearing is immediately restored.

Oncology

Two major neoplastic diseases account for more than 90% of all primary intraocular diseases: *retinoblastoma,* found primarily in children, and *melanoma,* found primarily in adults. Most retinoblastomas tend to be familial. The cell involved is the retinal neuron. Vision is impaired, and, in about 30% of patients, the disease is found in both eyes **(bilateral).** Melanoma may occur in the orbit, the bony cavity of the eyeball, the iris, or the ciliary body, but it arises most commonly in the pigmented cells of the choroid. The disease is usually asymptomatic until there is a hemorrhage into the anterior chamber. Any discrete, fleshy mass on the iris should be examined by an ophthalmologist. If malignancy occurs in the choroid, it usually appears as a brown or gray mushroom-shaped lesion.

Treatment for retinoblastoma usually involves the removal of the affected eye(s) **(enucleation),** followed by radiation. In melanoma where the lesion is on the iris, an iridectomy is performed. For melanoma of the choroid, enucleation is necessary. Many eye tumors are noninvasive and are not necessarily life threatening.

Diagnostic, Symptomatic, and Related Terms

This section introduces diagnostic, symptomatic, and related terms and their meanings. Word analyses for selected terms are also provided.

Term	Definition
EYE	
achromatopsia ă-krō-mă-TŎP-sē-ă *a-:* without, not *chromat:* color *-opsia:* vision	Severe congenital deficiency in color perception; also called *complete color blindness*
chalazion kă-LĀ-zē-ōn	Small, hard tumor developing on the eyelid, somewhat similar to a sebaceous cyst
conjunctivitis kŏn-jŭnk-tĭ-VĪ-tĭs *conjunctiv:* conjunctiva *-itis:* inflammation	Inflammation of the conjunctiva with vascular congestion, producing a red or pink eye; may be secondary to viral, chlamydial, bacterial, or fungal infections or allergy
convergence kŏn-VĔR-jĕnts	Medial movement of the two eyeballs so that they are both directed at the object being viewed
diopter dī-ŎP-tĕr	Measurement of refractive error *A negative diopter value signifies an eye with myopia and a positive diopter value signifies an eye with hyperopia.*
ectropion ĕk-TRŌ-pē-ŏn	Eversion, or outward turning, of the edge of the lower eyelid
emmetropia ĕm-ĕ-TRŌ-pē-ă	Normal condition of the eye in refraction in which, when the eye is at rest, parallel rays focus exactly on the retina
entropion ĕn-TRŌ-pē-ŏn	Inversion, or inward turning, of the edge of the lower eyelid
epiphora ĕ-PĬF-ō-ră	Abnormal overflow of tears *Epiphora is sometimes caused by obstruction of the tear ducts.*
exophthalmos ĕks-ŏf-THĂL-mŏs	Protrusion of one or both eyeballs *Common causes of exophthalmos include hyperactive thyroid, trauma, and tumor.*
hordeolum hor-DĒ-ō-lŭm	Localized, circumscribed, inflammatory swelling of one of the several sebaceous glands of the eyelid, generally caused by a bacterial infection; also called *sty*

(Continued)

Term	Definition	(Continued)
metamorphopsia mĕt-ă-mor-FOP-sē-ă *meta-:* change; beyond *morph:* form, shape, structure *-opsia:* vision	Visual distortion of objects *Metamorphopsia is commonly associated with errors of refraction, retinal disease, choroiditis, detachment of the retina, and tumors of the retina or choroid.*	
nyctalopia nĭk-tă-LO-pē-ă *nyctal:* night *-opia:* vision	Inability to see well in dim light; also called *night blindness* *Common causes of nyctalopia include cataracts, vitamin A deficiency, certain medications, and hereditary causes.*	
nystagmus nĭs-TĂG-mŭs	Involuntary eye movements that appear jerky and may reduce vision or be associated with other, more serious conditions that limit vision	
papilledema păp-ĭl-ĕ-DE-mă	Edema and hyperemia of the optic disc usually associated with increased ocular pressure resulting from intracranial pressure; also called *choked disc*	
photophobia fō-tō-FO-bē-ă *phot/o:* light *-phobia:* fear	Unusual intolerance and sensitivity to light *Photophobia commonly occurs in such diseases as meningitis, inflammation of the eyes, measles, and rubella.*	
presbyopia prĕz-bē-O-pē-ă *presby:* old age *-opia:* vision	Loss of accommodation of the crystalline lens associated with the aging process *During the aging process, proteins in the lens become harder and less elastic and muscle fibers surrounding the lens lose strength. These changes cause a decreased ability to focus, especially at close range.*	
retinopathy rĕt-ĭn-ŎP-ă-thē *retin/o:* retina *-pathy:* disease	Any disorder of retinal blood vessels	
diabetic dī-ă-BĔT-ĭk	Disorder that occurs in patients with diabetes and is manifested by small hemorrhages, edema, and formation of new vessels on the retina, leading to scarring and eventual loss of vision	
trachoma trā-KO-mă	Chronic, contagious form of conjunctivitis common in the southwestern United States that typically leads to blindness	
visual field VĬZH-ū-ăl	Area within which objects may be seen when the eye is in a fixed position	

EAR

anacusis ăn-ă-KU-sĭs *an-:* without, not *-acusis:* hearing	Deafness; also called *anacusia* *Anacusis may be unilateral or bilateral. Hearing loss should not be confused with anacusis, which refers to the complete inability to hear and is commonly congenital.*	

Term	Definition
conduction impairment kŏn-DŬK-shŭn	Blocking of sound waves as they are conducted through the external and middle ear (conduction pathway)
labyrinthitis lăb-i-rĭn-THĪ-tĭs *labyrinth:* labyrinth (inner ear) *-itis:* inflammation	Inflammation of the inner ear that usually results from an acute febrile process *Labyrinthitis may lead to progressive vertigo.*
Ménière disease mĕn-ē-ĀR	Disorder of the labyrinth that leads to progressive loss of hearing *Ménière disease is characterized by vertigo, sensorineural hearing loss, and tinnitus.*
otitis externa ō-TĪ-tĭs ĕks-TĔR-nă *ot:* ear *-itis:* inflammation	Infection of the external auditory canal *Common causes of otitis externa include exposure to swimming pool water (swimmer's ear), bacterial or fungal infections, seborrhea, eczema, and chronic conditions such as allergies.*
presbyacusis prĕz-bē-ă-KŪ-sĭs *presby:* old age *-acusis:* hearing	Impairment of hearing resulting from old age; also called *presbyacusia* *In presbyacusis, patients are generally able to hear low tones but ability to hear higher tones is lost. This condition usually affects speech perception, especially in the presence of background noise, as in a restaurant or a large crowd. This type of hearing loss is irreversible.*
pressure-equalizing (PE) tubes	Tubes that are inserted through the tympanic membrane, commonly to treat chronic otitis media; also called *tympanostomy tubes* or *ventilation tubes* *The average period that PE tubes remain in the ear is about 9 months, at which time they fall out on their own. If they do not fall out, they are removed surgically, usually by age 5 or 6.*
tinnitus tĭn-Ī-tŭs	Perception of ringing, hissing, or other sounds in the ears or head when no external sound is present *Tinnitus may be caused by a blow to the head, ingestion of large doses of aspirin, anemia, noise exposure, stress, impacted wax, hypertension, and certain types of medications and tumors.*
vertigo VĔR-tĭ-gō	Hallucination of movement, or a feeling of spinning or dizziness *Vertigo may be caused by a variety of disorders, including Ménière disease and labyrinthitis.*

 It is time to review pathological, diagnostic, symptomatic, and related terms by completing Learning Activity 15–4.

Diagnostic and Therapeutic Procedures

This section introduces procedures used to diagnose and treat eye and ear disorders. Descriptions are provided as well as pronunciations and word analyses for selected terms.

Procedure	Description
DIAGNOSTIC PROCEDURES	
Clinical	

audiometry
aw-dē-ŎM-ĕ-trē
 	
    audi/o: hearing
    -metry: act of measuring
	Measurement of hearing acuity at various sound wave frequencies
	
	In audiometry, pure tones of controlled intensity are delivered through earphones to one ear at a time while the patient indicates if the tone was heard. The minimum intensity (volume) required to hear each tone is graphed.

caloric stimulation test	Test that uses different temperatures to assess the vestibular portion of the nerve of the inner ear (acoustic nerve) to determine if nerve damage is the cause of vertigo *In the caloric stimulation test, cold and warm water are separately introduced into each ear while electrodes, placed around the eye, record nystagmus. Eyes move in a predictable pattern when the water is introduced, except with acoustic nerve damage.*
electronystagmography ē-lĕk-trō-nĭs-tăg-MŎG-ră-fē	Method of assessing and recording eye movements by measuring the electrical activity of the extraocular muscles *In electronystagmography, electrodes are placed above, below, and to the side of each eye. A ground electrode is placed on the forehead. The electrodes record eye movement relative to the position of the ground electrode.*
ophthalmodynamometry ŏf-thăl-mō-di-nă-MŎM-ĕ-trē	Measurement of the blood pressure of the retinal vessels *Ophthalmodynamometry is a screening test used to determine reduction of blood flow in the carotid artery.*

tonometry
tōn-ŎM-ĕ-trē
 	
    ton/o: tension
    -metry: act of measuring
	Evaluation of intraocular pressure by measuring the resistance of the eyeball to indentation by an applied force
	
	Tonometry is used to detect glaucoma. Several kinds of tonometers can be used. The applanation method of tonometry uses a sensor to depress the cornea and is considered the most accurate method of tonometry.

visual acuity test ă-KŪ-ĭ-tē	Part of an eye examination that determines the smallest letters that can be read on a standardized chart at a distance of 20′ *Visual acuity is expressed as a fraction. The top number refers to the distance from the chart (usually 20′) and the bottom number indicates the distance at which a person with normal eyesight could read the same line. For example 20/40 indicates that the patient correctly read letters at 20′ that could be read by a person with normal vision at 40′.*

Procedure	Description
Endoscopic	
gonioscopy gō-nē-ŎS-kō-pē *goni/o:* angle *-scopy:* visual examination	Examination of the angle of the anterior chamber of the eye to determine ocular motility and rotation and diagnose and manage glaucoma
ophthalmoscopy ŏf-thăl-MŎS-kō-pē *ophthalm/o:* eye *-scopy:* visual examination	Visual examination of the interior of the eye using a handheld instrument called an *ophthalmoscope,* which has various adjustable lenses for magnification and a light source to illuminate the interior of the eye *Ophthalmoscopy is used to detect eye disorders as well as disorders of other organs that cause changes in the eye.*
otoscopy ō-TŎS-kŏ-pē *ot/o:* ear *-scopy:* visual examination	Visual examination of the external auditory canal and the tympanic membrane using an otoscope
pneumatic nū-MĂT-ĭk	Procedure that assesses the ability of the tympanic membrane to move in response to a change in air pressure *In pneumatic otoscopy, a tight seal is created in the ear canal and then a very slight positive pressure and then a negative pressure is applied by squeezing and releasing a rubber bulb attached to the pneumatic otoscope. The fluctuation in air pressure causes movement of a normal tympanic membrane.*
retinoscopy rĕt-ĭn-ŎS-kō-pē *retin/o:* retina *-scopy:* visual examination	Evaluation of refractive errors of the eye by projecting a light into the eyes and determining the movement of reflected light rays *Retinoscopy is especially important in determining errors of refraction in babies and small children who cannot be refracted by traditional methods.*
Radiographic	
dacryocystography dăk-rē-ō-sĭs-TŎG-ră-fē *dacryocyst/o:* lacrimal sac *-graphy:* process of recording	Radiographic imaging procedures of the nasolacrimal (tear) glands and ducts *Dacryocystography is performed for excessive tearing (epiphora) to determine the cause of hypersecretion of the lacrimal gland or obstruction in the lacrimal passages.*
fluorescein angiography floo-RĔS-ēn ăn-jē-ŎG-ră-fē *angio:* vessel (usually blood or lymph) *-graphy:* process of recording	Assesses blood vessels and their leakage in and beneath the retina by injecting a colored dye (fluorescein) and allowing it to circulate while photographs of the intraocular circulation are recorded *Fluorescein angiography facilitates the in vivo study of the retinal circulation and is particularly useful in the management of diabetic retinopathy and macular degeneration, two leading causes of blindness.*

(Continued)

Procedure	Description	*(Continued)*

THERAPEUTIC PROCEDURES

Clinical

orthoptic training
or-THŎP-tĭk
TRĀ-nĭng
 	
   orth: straight
   opt: eye, vision
   -ic: pertaining to, relating to
	Exercises intended to improve eye movements or visual tracking that use training glasses, prism glasses, or tinted or colored lenses

Surgical

blepharectomy
blĕf-ă-RĔK-tō-mē
 	
   blephar: eyelid
   -ectomy: excision, removal
	Excision of a lesion on the eyelid

blepharoplasty
BLĔF-ă-rō-plăs-tē
 	
   blephar/o: eyelid
   -plasty: surgical repair
	Cosmetic surgery that removes fatty tissue called "bags" above and below the eye, which commonly form as a result of the aging process or excessive exposure to the sun

cochlear implant
KŎK-lē-ăr ĬM-plănt
 	
   cochle: cochlea
   -ar: pertaining to, relating to
	Artificial hearing device that produces useful hearing sensations by electrically stimulating nerves inside the inner ear; also called *bionic ear*

cyclodialysis
sī-klō-dī-ĂL-ĭ-sĭs
 	
   cycl/o: ciliary body of eye; circular, cycle
   dia: through, across
   -lysis: separation; destruction; loosening
	Formation of an opening between the anterior chamber and the suprachoroidal space for the draining of aqueous humor in glaucoma

enucleation ē-nū-klē-Ā-shŭn	Removal of the eyeball from the orbit *Enucleation is performed to treat cancer of the eye when the tumor is large and fills most of the structure.*
evisceration ē-vĭs-ĕr-Ā-shŭn	Removal of the contents of the eye while leaving the sclera and cornea *Evisceration is performed when the blind eye is painful or unsightly. The eye muscles are left intact, and a prothesis is fitted over the shell.*

Procedure	Description
keratotomy kĕr-ă-TŎT-ō-mē *kerat/o:* horny tissue; hard; cornea *-tomy:* incision	Incision of the cornea
radial	Surgical treatment for nearsightedness *In radial keratotomy, hairline radial incisions of the outer portion of the cornea allow it to flatten, thus correcting nearsightedness.*
mastoid antrotomy MĂS-toyd ăn-TRŎT-ō-mē	Surgical opening of a cavity within the mastoid process
otoplasty Ō-tō-plăs-tē *ot/o:* ear *-plasty:* surgical repair	Corrective surgery for a deformed or excessively large or small pinna *Otoplasty is also performed to rebuild new ears for those who lost them through burns or other trauma or were born without them.*
phacoemulsification făk-ō-ē-MŬL-si-fi-kā-shŭn	Method of treating cataracts by using ultrasonic waves to disintegrate the cloudy lens, which is then aspirated and removed
sclerostomy sklē-RŎS-tō-mē *scler/o:* hardening; sclera (white of eye) *-stomy:* forming an opening (mouth)	Surgical formation of an opening in the sclera *Sclerostomy is commonly performed in conjunction with surgery for glaucoma.*
tympanoplasty tĭm-păn-ō-PLĂS-tē *tympan/o:* tympanic membrane (eardrum) *-plasty:* surgical repair	Reconstruction of the eardrum, commonly due to a perforation; also called *myringoplasty*

 Pharmacology

Disorders of the eyes and ears are commonly treated with instillation of drops onto the surface of the eye or into the cavity of the ear. The eyes and ears are commonly irrigated with liquid solution to remove foreign objects and to provide topical applications of medications. Pharmacological agents used to treat eye disorders include antibiotics for bacterial eye infections, beta blockers and carbonic anhydrase inhibitors for glaucoma, and ophthalmic decongestants and moisturizers for irritated eyes. Mydriatics and miotics are used, not only to treat eye disorders but also to dilate (mydriatics) and contract (miotics) the pupil during eye examinations. Ear medications include antiemetics to relieve nausea associated with inner ear infections, products to loosen and remove wax buildup in the ear canal, and local anesthetics to relieve pain associated with ear infections. (See Table 15–1.)

Table 15-1   DRUGS USED TO TREAT SENSORY DISORDERS

This table lists common drug classifications used to treat eye and ear disorders, their therapeutic actions, and selected generic and trade names.

Classification	Therapeutic Action	Generic and Trade Names
Eye		
antibiotics, ophthalmic	Inhibit the growth of microorganisms that infect the eye *Ophthalmic antibiotics are dispensed as topical ointments and solutions to treat various bacterial eye infections such as conjunctivitis (pinkeye).*	**erythromycin base** ĕ-rith-rō-MĬ-sin 　*Del-Mycin, Ilotycin Ophthalmic, Staticin*
antiglaucoma agents	Treat glaucoma *Antiglaucoma agents include beta blockers and carbonic anhydrase inhibitors. Beta blockers block the production of aqueous humor to decrease intraocular pressure and are administered topically as eyedrops. Carbonic anhydrase inhibitors decrease the production of aqueous humor by blocking the enzyme carbonic anhydrase and are given orally.*	**betaxolol** bĕ-TĂK-sō-lŏl 　*Kerlone* **timolol** TĪ-mō-lŏl 　*Betimol, Blocadren, Timoptic* **acetazolamide** ăs-ĕt-ă-ZŌL-ă-mĭd 　*AK-Zol, Dazamide, Diamox*
mydriatics	Dilate the pupil (mydriasis) and paralyze the muscles of accommodation (cycloplegia) *Mydriatics dilate the eye for internal examination and to treat inflammatory conditions of the uveal tract and iris.*	**atropine sulfate** ĂT-rō-pēn　SŬL-fāt 　*Atropine-Care Ophthalmic, Atropisol Ophthalmic*
ophthalmic decongestants	Constrict the small arterioles of the eye, decreasing redness and relieving conjunctival congestion *Ophthalmic decongestants are over-the-counter products that temporarily relieve the itching and minor irritation commonly associated with allergy.*	**tetrahydrozoline** tĕt-ră-hi-DRŎZ-ō-lēn 　*Murine, Visine*
ophthalmic moisturizers	Soothe dry eyes due to environmental irritants and allergens *Ophthalmic moisturizers are administered topically and may also be used to facilitate ophthalmoscopic examination in gonioscopy and ophthalmoscopy.*	**buffered isotonic solutions** BŬ-fĕrd　ī-sō-TŎN-ĭk sō-LŪ-shŭnz 　*Akwa Tears, Refresh Plus, Moisture Eyes*

Table 15–1   DRUGS USED TO TREAT SENSORY DISORDERS

Classification	Therapeutic Action	Generic and Trade Names
Ear		
antiemetics	Treat and prevent nausea, vomiting, dizziness, and vertigo by reducing the sensitivity of the inner ear to motion or inhibiting stimuli from reaching the part of the brain that triggers nausea and vomiting *Antiemetics are commonly used to treat symptoms of labyrinthitis and vestibular neuritis, which irritate the inner ear and may cause vertigo.*	**meclizine** MĔK-lǐ-zēn *Antivert, Antrizine, Bonine, Meni-D*
otic analgesics	Provide temporary relief from pain and inflammation associated with otic disorders *Otic analgesics may be prescribed for otitis media, otitis externa, and swimmer's ear. Some otic analgesics are also wax emulsifiers.*	**antipyrine and benzocaine** ăn-ti-PI-rĕn, BĔN-zō-kān *Allergan Ear Drops, A/B Otic*
wax emulsifiers	Loosen and help remove impacted cerumen (ear wax) *When excessive wax blocks the canal and causes pain or loss of hearing, the physician may wash it out, vacuum it out, or remove it with special instruments. Alternatively, the physician may recommend various wax emulsifying drops to aid in wax removal.*	**carbamide peroxide** KĂR-bă-mǐd pĕr-ŎK-sǐd *Debrox Drops, Murine Ear Drops*

Abbreviations

This section introduces abbreviations related to the eye and ear along with their meanings.

Abbreviation	Meaning
EYE	
Acc	accommodation
ARMD, AMD	age-related macular degeneration
Ast	astigmatism
D	diopter (lens strength)
Em	emmetropia
EOM	extraocular movement

(Continued)

Abbreviation	Meaning	(Continued)
IOL	intraocular lens	
IOP	intraocular pressure	
mix astig	mixed astigmatism	
Myop	myopia	
*OD	right eye	
OD	Doctor of Optometry	
*OS	left eye	
*OU	both eyes	
PERRLA	pupils equal, round, and reactive to light and accommodation	
RK	radial keratotomy	
SICS	small incision cataract surgery	
ST	esotropia	
VA	visual acuity	
VF	visual field	
XT	exotropia	
EAR		
AC	air conduction	
*AD	right ear	
*AS	left ear	
*AU	both ears	
BC	bone conduction	
ENT	ears, nose, and throat	
NIHL	noise-induced hearing loss	
PE tube	pressure-equalizing tube (placed in the eardrum)	

*Although these abbreviations are currently found in medical records and clinical notes, the Joint Commission on Accreditation of Healthcare Organizations (JCAHO) requires their discontinuance. Instead, write out the meanings.

 It is time to review procedures, pharmacology, and abbreviations by completing Learning Activity 15–5.

LEARNING ACTIVITIES

The activities that follow provide review of the special senses terms introduced in this chapter. Complete each activity and review your answers to evaluate your understanding of the chapter.

Learning Activity 15-1

Identifying eye structures

Label the following illustration using the terms listed below.

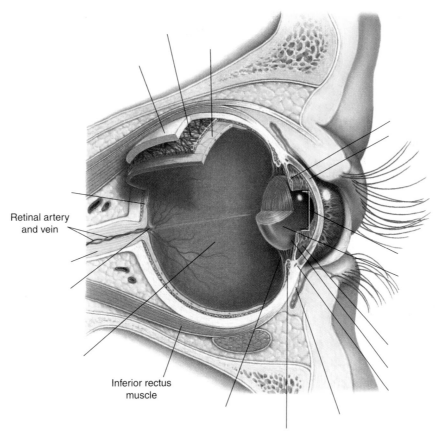

Retinal artery and vein

Inferior rectus muscle

anterior chamber	*fovea*	*pupil*
canal of Schlemm	*iris*	*retina*
choroid	*lens*	*sclera*
ciliary body	*optic disc*	*suspensory ligaments*
conjunctiva	*optic nerve*	*vitreous chamber*
cornea	*posterior chamber*	

Check your answers by referring to Figure 15–1 on page 459. Review material that you did not answer correctly.

Learning Activity 15–2

Identifying ear structures

Label the following illustration using the terms listed below.

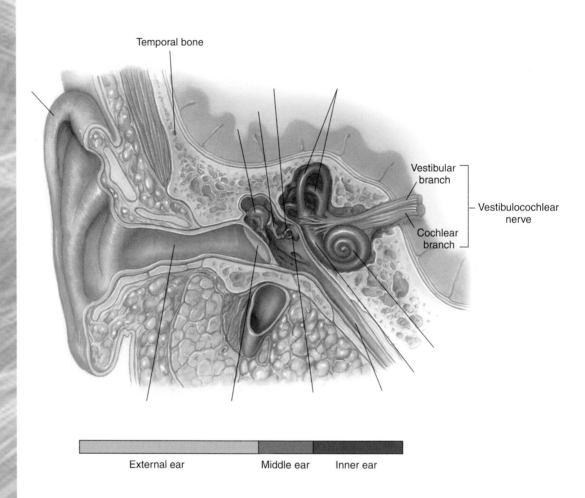

Temporal bone

Vestibular branch
Vestibulocochlear nerve
Cochlear branch

External ear   Middle ear   Inner ear

auricle	incus	stapes
cochlea	malleus	tympanic membrane
eustachian tube	oval window	vestibule
external auditory canal	semicircular canals	

 Check your answers by referring to Figure 15–3 on page 462. Review material that you did not answer correctly.

Learning Activity 15-3

Building medical words

Use **ophthalm/o** *(eye) to build words that mean:*

1. paralysis of the eye _____
2. study of the eye _____

Use **pupill/o** *(pupil) to build a word that means:*

3. examination of the pupil _____

Use **kerat/o** *(cornea) to build words that mean:*

4. softening of the cornea _____
5. instrument for measuring the cornea _____

Use **scler/o** *(sclera) to build words that mean:*

6. inflammation of the sclera _____
7. softening of the sclera _____

Use **irid/o** *(iris) to build words that mean:*

8. paralysis of the iris _____
9. herniation of the iris _____

Use **retin/o** *(retina) to build words that mean:*

10. disease of the retina _____
11. inflammation of the retina _____

Use **blephar/o** *(eyelid) to build words that mean:*

12. paralysis of the eyelid _____
13. prolapse of the eyelid _____

Use **ot/o** *(ear) to build a word that means:*

14. flow of pus from the ear _____

Use **audi/o** *(hearing) to build a word that means:*

15. instrument for measuring hearing _____

Use **myring/o** *(tympanic membrane [eardrum]) to build a word that means:*

16. instrument for cutting the eardrum _____

Use the suffix -opia (vision) to build words that mean:

17. dim or dull vision _____

18. excessive (far-sighted) vision _____

Use the suffix -acusis (hearing) to build words that mean:

19. without hearing _____

20. excessive (sensitivity to) hearing _____

Build surgical words that mean:

21. removal of the stapes _____

22. incision of the labyrinth _____

23. removal of the mastoid process _____

24. surgical repair of the eardrum _____

25. incision of the cornea _____

Check your answers in Appendix A. Review material that you did not answer correctly.

CORRECT ANSWERS _____ × **4** = _____ **% SCORE**

Learning Activity 15–4

Matching pathological, diagnostic, symptomatic, and related terms

Match the following terms with the definitions in the numbered list.

achromatopsia	epiphora	retinoblastoma
amblyopia	exotropia	strabismus
anacusis	gonioscopy	tinnitus
cataract	Ménière disease	tonometer
chalazion	neovascular	vertigo
diopter	nyctalopia	visual field
enucleation	otitis externa	

1. _____ opacity that forms on the lens and impairs vision
2. _____ complete color blindness
3. _____ inability to see well in dim light
4. _____ examination that determines the angle where the cornea meets the iris
5. _____ deafness
6. _____ infection of the external auditory canal
7. _____ measurement of refractive errors
8. _____ instrument that measures the internal pressure of the eye
9. _____ area in which objects are seen when the eye is in a fixed position
10. _____ abnormal overflow of tears
11. _____ a condition in which one eye is misaligned with the other eye; also called *heterotropia*
12. _____ disorder of the labyrinth that leads to progressive hearing loss
13. _____ refers to the wet form of macular degeneration
14. _____ feeling of dizziness or spinning
15. _____ outward deviation of the eye
16. _____ removal of the eye
17. _____ tumor of the eyelid
18. _____ "lazy-eye" syndrome
19. _____ neoplastic disease of the eye found primarily in children
20. _____ perception of ringing in the ears with no external stimuli

✓ Check your answers in Appendix A. Review any material that you did not answer correctly.

CORRECT ANSWERS _____ × 5 = _____ **% SCORE**

Learning Activity 15–5

Matching procedures, pharmacology, and abbreviations

Match the following terms with the definitions in the numbered list.

audiometry	evisceration	ophthalmoscopy	ST
beta blockers	fluorescein angiography	otic analgesics	tonometry
caloric stimulation test	gonioscopy	otoplasty	visual acuity test
cochlear implant	mydriatics	otoscopy	wax emulsifiers
enucleation	ophthalmic decongestants	radial keratotomy	XT

1. _____ test that uses different temperatures to assess the vestibular portion of the nerve

2. _____ visual examination of the interior of the eye

3. _____ artificial device that produces hearing sensations by electrically stimulating nerves inside the inner ear

4. _____ assesses blood vessels and retinal circulation using a colored dye while photographs are taken

5. _____ corrective surgery for large, small, or deformed ears

6. _____ agents that dilate the pupils and paralyze the eye muscles of accommodation

7. _____ measurement of the intraocular pressure for detecting glaucoma

8. _____ determines the smallest letters that can be read on a standardized chart

9. _____ removal of the contents of the eyeball, leaving the sclera and cornea

10. _____ antiglaucoma agents that block aqueous humor production

11. _____ loosen and help remove impacted cerumen

12. _____ removal of the entire eyeball from its orbit

13. _____ esotropia

14. _____ constrict small arterioles of the eye to decrease redness and conjunctival congestion

15. _____ exotropia

16. _____ examination of the angle of the anterior chamber of the eye

17. _____ visual examination of the external auditory canal

18. _____ measurement of hearing acuity at various frequencies

19. _____ surgical treatment for nearsightedness that uses small incisions to flatten the cornea

20. _____ provide temporary relief from earache

Check your answers in Appendix A. Review any material that you did not answer correctly.

CORRECT ANSWERS _____ × 5 = _____ **% SCORE**

MEDICAL RECORD ACTIVITIES

The two medical records included in the following activities use common clinical scenarios to show how medical terminology is used to document patient care. Complete the terminology and analysis sections for each activity to help you recognize and understand terms related to the eye and ear.

Medical Record Activity 15–1

Retained foreign bodies

Terminology

The terms listed in the chart come from the medical record *Retained Foreign Bodies* that follows. Use a medical dictionary such as *Taber's Cyclopedic Medical Dictionary*, the appendices of this book, or other resources to define each term. Then review the pronunciations for each term and practice by reading the medical record aloud.

Term	Definition
bilateral bī-LĂT-ĕr-ăl	
cerumen sĕ-ROO-mĕn	
perforation pĕr-fō-RĀ-shŭn	
supine sū-PĪN	
tympanostomy tĭm-pă-NŎS-tō-mē	

RETAINED FOREIGN BODIES

PREOPERATIVE DIAGNOSIS: Foreign body, ears

POSTOPERATIVE DIAGNOSIS: Foreign body, ears

ANESTHESIA: General

OPERATIVE INDICATIONS: The patient is a 9-year-old girl who presents with bilateral retained tympanostomy tubes. The tubes had been placed for more than 2.5 years.

OPERATIVE FINDINGS: Retained tympanostomy tubes, bilateral

PROCEDURE: Removal of foreign bodies from ears with placement of paper patches.

The risks and alternatives were explained to the mother, and she consented to the surgery. In the supine position under satisfactory general anesthesia via mask, the patient was draped in a routine fashion.

The operating microscope was used to inspect the right ear. A previously placed tympanostomy tube was found to be in position and was surrounded with hard cerumen. The cerumen and the tube were removed, resulting in a very large perforation. The edges of the perforation were freshened sharply with a pick, and a paper patch was applied. The patient tolerated the surgery very well, and was sent to recovery.

Analysis

Review the medical record *Retained Foreign Bodies* to answer the following questions.

1. Did the patient's surgery involve one or both ears?

   _____

2. What was the nature of the foreign body in the patient's ears?

   _____

3. What ear structure was involved?

   _____

4. What instrument was used to locate the tubes?

   _____

5. What was the material in which the tubes were embedded?

   _____

Medical Record Activity 15–2

Phacoemulsification and lens implant

Terminology

The terms listed in the chart come from the medical record *Phacoemulsification and Lens Implant* that follows. Use a medical dictionary such as *Taber's Cyclopedic Medical Dictionary*, the appendices of this book, or other resources to define each term. Then review the pronunciations for each term and practice by reading the medical record aloud.

Term	Definition
anesthesia ăn-ĕs-THĒ-zē-ă	
blepharostat BLĔF-ă-rō-stăt	
capsulorrhexis kăp-sū-lō-RĔK-sĭs	
cataract KĂT-ă-răkt	
conjunctival kŏn-jŭnk-TĪ-văl	
diopter dī-ŎP-tĕr	
intravenous ĭn-tră-VĒ-nŭs	
keratome KĔR-ă-tōm	
peritomy pĕr-ĬT-ō-mē	
phacoemulsification făk-ō-ē-MŬL-sĭ-fĭ-kā-shŭn	
posterior chamber pŏs-TĒ-rē-or CHĂM-bĕr	
retrobulbar block rĕt-rō-BŬL-băr BLŎK	
sutures SŪ-chūrz	
TobraDex TŌ-bră-dĕks	

PHACOEMULSIFICATION AND LENS IMPLANT

PREOPERATIVE DIAGNOSIS: Right eye cataract

POSTOPERATIVE DIAGNOSIS: Right eye cataract

PROCEDURE: Phacoemulsification, Rt eye, with posterior chamber lens implantation.

This 68-year-old male was brought to the operating suite on 8/4/xx as an outpatient. Intravenous anesthesia and retrobulbar block to the right eye were administered. The rt eye was prepped in the usual manner. A blepharostat was inserted and a surgical microscope was positioned. Conjunctival peritomy was performed. Using a keratome, the anterior chamber was entered at the 12 o'clock position. A capsulorrhexis was performed. The cataract was removed by phacoemulsification.

After confirming the 20.5 diopters on the package, the implant was easily inserted into the capsular bag. The wound was observed and shown to be fluid tight. The incision required no sutures. TobraDex ointment was applied and a sterile patch was taped into place. The patient was monitored until stable. Postoperative care was reviewed, and he was released with instructions to return to the office the following day.

Analysis

Review the medical record *Phacoemulsification and Lens Implant* to answer the following questions.

1. What technique was used to destroy the cataract?

   _____

2. In what portion of the eye was the implant placed?

   _____

3. What anesthetics were used for surgery?

   _____

4. What was the function of the blepharostat?

   _____

5. What was the function of the keratome?

   _____

6. Where was the implant inserted?

   _____

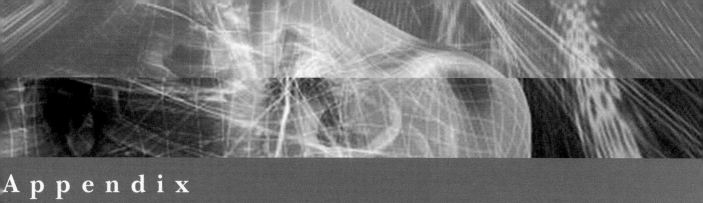

Appendix

A

Answer Key

CHAPTER 1 — Basic Elements of a Medical Word

LEARNING ACTIVITY 1–1

Understanding medical word elements

Fill in the following blanks to complete the sentences correctly.
 1. root, combining form, suffix, and prefix.
 2. teach

Identify the following statements as true or false. If false, rewrite the statement correctly in the space provided.
 3. False—A combining vowel is usually an "o."
 4. False—A combining form links a suffix that begins with a consonant.
 5. True
 6. True
 7. False—To define a medical word, first define the suffix or the end of the word. Second, define the first part of the word. Third, define the middle of the word.
 8. True

Underline the word root in each of following combining forms.
 9. splen/o
 10. hyster/o
 11. enter/o
 12. neur/o
 13. ot/o
 14. dermat/o
 15. hydr/o

LEARNING ACTIVITY 1–2

Identifying word roots and combining forms

Underline the word roots in the following terms.
 1. nephritis
 2. arthrodesis
 3. phlebotomy
 4. dentist
 5. gastrectomy
 6. chondritis
 7. hepatoma
 8. cardiologist
 9. gastria
 10. osteoma

Underline the elements below that are combining forms.
 11. nephr
 12. cardi/o
 13. arthr
 14. oste/o/arth
 15. cholangi/o

LEARNING ACTIVITY 1–3

Identifying suffixes and prefixes

Analyze each term and write the element from each that is a suffix.
 1. -tomy
 2. -scope
 3. -itis
 4. -itis
 5. -ectomy

Analyze each term and write the element from each that is a prefix.
 6. micro-
 7. hyper-
 8. macro-
 9. intra-
 10. a-

LEARNING ACTIVITY 1–4

Defining and building medical words

Use the three basic steps to define the following words.

Term	Definition
1. **gastritis** găs-TRĪ-tĭs	inflammation of the stomach
2. **nephritis** nĕf-RĪ-tĭs	inflammation of the kidneys
3. **gastrectomy** găs-TRĔK-tō-mē	excision of the stomach
4. **osteoma** ŏs-tē-Ō-mă	tumor of bone
5. **hepatoma** hĕp-ă-TŌ-mă	tumor of the liver
6. **hepatitis** hĕp-ă-TĪ-tĭs	inflammation of the liver

Write the number for the rule that applies to each listed term as well as a short summary of the rule.

Term	Rule	Summary of the Rule
7. **arthr/itis** ăr-THRĪ-tĭs	1	A WR links a suffix that begins with a vowel.
8. **scler/osis** sklĕ-RŌ-sĭs	1	A WR links a suffix that begins with a vowel.
9. **arthr/o/centesis** ăr-thrō-sĕn-TĒ-sĭs	2	A CF links a suffix that begins with a consonant.
10. **colon/o/scope** kō-LŎN-ō-skōp	2	A CF links a suffix that begins with a consonant.
11. **chondr/itis** kŏn-DRĪ-tĭs	1	A WR links a suffix that begins with a vowel.
12. **chondr/oma** kŏn-DRŌ-mă	1	A WR links a suffix that begins with a vowel.
13. **oste/o/chondr/itis** ŏs-tē-ō-kŏn-DRĪ-tĭs	3	A CF links multiple roots to each other. This rule holds true even if the next word root begins with a vowel.
	1	A WR links a suffix that begins with a vowel.
14. **muscul/ar** MŬS-kū-lăr	1	A WR links a suffix that begins with a vowel.
15. **oste/o/arthr/itis** ŏs-tē-ō-ăr-THRĪ-tĭs	3	A CF links multiple roots to each other. This ŏs-tē-ō-ăr-rule holds true even if the next word root begins with a vowel.
	1	A WR links a suffix that begins with a vowel.

LEARNING ACTIVITY 1–5

Understanding pronunciations

Review the pronunciation guidelines (located inside the front cover of this book) and then underline the correct answer in each of the following statements.

1. macron
2. breve
3. long
4. short
5. k
6. n
7. is
8. eye
9. second
10. separate

CHAPTER 2 — Suffixes

LEARNING ACTIVITY 2–1

Completing and building surgical words

1. episiotomy
2. colectomy
3. arthrocentesis
4. splenectomy
5. colostomy
6. osteotome
7. tympanotomy
8. tracheostomy
9. mastectomy
10. lithotomy
11. hemorrhoidectomy
12. colostomy
13. colectomy
14. osteotome
15. arthrocentesis
16. lithotomy
17. mastectomy
18. tympanotomy
19. tracheostomy
20. splenectomy

LEARNING ACTIVITY 2–2

Completing and building more surgical words

1. arthrodesis
2. rhinoplasty
3. tenoplasty
4. myorrhaphy
5. mastopexy
6. cystorrhaphy
7. osteoclasis
8. lithotripsy
9. enterolysis
10. neurotripsy
11. rhinoplasty
12. arthrodesis
13. myorrhaphy
14. mastopexy
15. cystorrhaphy
16. tenoplasty
17. osteoclasis
18. lithotripsy
19. enterolysis
20. neurotripsy

LEARNING ACTIVITY 2–3

Selecting a surgical suffix

1. lithotripsy
2. arthrocentesis
3. splenectomy
4. colostomy
5. dermatome
6. tracheostomy
7. lithotomy
8. mastectomy
9. hemorrhoidectomy
10. tracheotomy
11. mastopexy
12. colectomy
13. gastrorrhaphy
14. hysteropexy
15. rhinoplasty
16. arthrodesis
17. osteoclasis
18. neurolysis
19. myorrhaphy
20. tympanotomy

LEARNING ACTIVITY 2–4

Selecting diagnostic, pathological, and related suffixes

1. hepatoma
2. neuralgia
3. bronchiectasis
4. carcinogenesis
5. dermatosis
6. nephromegaly
7. otorrhea
8. hysterorrhexis

9. blepharospasm
10. cystocele
11. hemorrhage
12. lithiasis
13. hemiplegia
14. myopathy
15. dysphagia
16. osteomalacia
17. aphasia
18. leukemia
19. erythropenia
20. pelvimetry

LEARNING ACTIVITY 2–5

Building pathological and related words

1. bronchiectasis
2. cholelith
3. carcinogenesis
4. osteomalacia
5. hepatomegaly
6. cholelithiasis

7. hepatocele
8. neuropathy
9. dermatosis
10. hemiplegia
11. dysphagia
12. aphasia
13. cephalalgia
14. blepharospasm
15. hyperplasia, hypertrophy

LEARNING ACTIVITY 2–6

Selecting adjective, noun, and diminutive suffixes

1. thoracic
2. gastric, gastral
3. bacterial
4. aquatic
5. axillary
6. cardiac, cardial
7. spinal, spinous

8. membranous
9. internist
10. leukemia
11. sigmoidoscopy
12. alcoholism
13. senilism
14. allergist
15. mania
16. arteriole
17. ventricle
18. venule

LEARNING ACTIVITY 2–7

Forming plural words

Singular	Plural	Rule
1. diagnosis	diagnoses	Drop *is* and add *es.*
2. fornix	fornices	Drop *ix* and add *ices.*
3. vertebra	vertebrae	Retain *a* and add *e.*
4. keratosis	keratoses	Drop *is* and add *es.*
5. bronchus	bronchi	Drop *us* and add *i.*
6. spermatozoon	spermatozoa	Drop *on* and add *a.*
7. septum	septa	Drop *um* and add *a.*
8. coccus	cocci	Drop *us* and add *i.*
9. ganglion	ganglia	Drop *on* and add *a.*
10. prognosis	prognoses	Drop *is* and add *es.*
11. thrombus	thrombi	Drop *us* and add *i.*
12. appendix	appendices	Drop *ix* and add *ices.*
13. bacterium	bacteria	Drop *um* and add *a.*
14. testis	testes	Drop *is* and add *es.*
15. nevus	nevi	Drop *us* and add *i.*

CHAPTER 3 — Prefixes

LEARNING ACTIVITY 3–1

Identifying and defining prefixes

Word	Definition of Prefix
1. inter/dental	*between*
2. hypo/dermic	under, below, deficient
3. epi/dermis	above, upon
4. retro/version	backward, behind
5. sub/lingual	under, below
6. trans/vaginal	through, across
7. infra/costal	under, below
8. post/natal	after, behind
9. quadri/plegia	four
10. hyper/calcemia	excessive, above normal
11. primi/gravida	first
12. micro/scope	small
13. tri/plegia	three
14. poly/dipsia	many, much
15. ab/duction	from, away from
16. an/esthesia	without, not
17. macro/cyte	large
18. intra/muscular	in, within
19. supra/pelvic	above, excessive, superior
20. dia/rrhea	through, across
21. circum/duction	around
22. ad/duction	toward
23. peri/odontal	around
24. brady/cardia	slow
25. tachy/pnea	rapid
26. dys/tocia	bad, painful, difficult
27. eu/pnea	good, normal
28. hetero/graft	different
29. mal/nutrition	bad
30. pseudo/cyesis	false

LEARNING ACTIVITY 3–2

Matching prefixes of position, number and measurement, and direction

1. retroversion
2. hypodermic
3. prenatal
4. subnasal
5. postoperative
6. intercostal
7. pseudocyesis
8. periodontal
9. diarrhea
10. ectogenous
11. suprarenal
12. hemiplegia
13. quadriplegia
14. macrocyte
15. polyphobia

LEARNING ACTIVITY 3–3

Matching other prefixes

1. dyspepsia
2. heterosexual
3. panarthritis
4. antibacterial
5. bradycardia
6. malnutrition
7. amastia
8. anesthesia
9. eupnea
10. syndactylism
11. tachycardia
12. contraception
13. homosexual
14. dystocia
15. homograft

CHAPTER 4 — Body Structure

LEARNING ACTIVITY 4–3

Matching body cavity, spine, and directional terms

1. h.   ventral cavity that contains digestive, reproductive, and excretory structures
2. k.   movement toward the median plane
3. j.   part of the spine known as the neck
4. b.   tailbone
5. m.   away from the surface of the body; internal
6. f.   turning outward
7. l.   away from the head; toward the tail or lower part of a structure
8. i.   turning inward or inside out

9. n.   part of the spine known as the loin
10. a.   pertaining to the sole of the foot
11. o.   near the back of the body
12. e.   lying horizontal with face downward

13. g.   nearer to the center (trunk of the body)
14. d.   toward the surface of the body
15. c.   ventral cavity that contains heart, lungs, and associated structures

LEARNING ACTIVITY 4–4

Matching word elements

1. kary/o
2. dist/o
3. -graphy
4. -gnosis
5. leuk/o
6. viscer/o
7. jaund/o
8. hist/o
9. -genesis
10. infra-
11. ultra-
12. caud/o
13. dors/o
14. poli/o
15. eti/o
16. morph/o
17. xer/o
18. idi/o
19. ad-
20. somat/o

LEARNING ACTIVITY 4–5

Matching diagnostic and therapeutic terms and procedures

1. radiology
2. Doppler
3. ultrasonography
4. thoracoscopy
5. punch biopsy
6. endoscopy
7. nuclear scan
8. fluoroscopy
9. morbid
10. radionuclide
11. febrile
12. resection
13. suppurative
14. cauterize
15. ablation

MEDICAL RECORD ACTIVITY 4–1

Radiologic consultation: Cervical and lumbar spine

1. Why was the x-ray film taken of the cervical spine?
    To determine cervical curvature
2. Did the patient appear to have experienced any type of recent injury to the spine?
    No, there was no evidence of recent body disease or injury.
3. What cervical vertebrae form the atlantoaxial joint?
    The first cervical vertebra (atlas) and the second cervical vertebra (axis)
4. Was the odontoid process fractured?
    No, the odontoid process was intact.
5. What did the radiologist believe was the possible cause of the minimal scoliosis?
    Muscle spasm

MEDICAL RECORD ACTIVITY 4–2

Radiographic consultation: Injury of left wrist and hand

1. What is the abbreviation for anteroposterior?
    AP
2. What caused the soft tissue deformity?
    Fracture caused damage to surrounding tissue.
3. Why was an AP view of the humerus taken?
    To determine whether the elbow was fractured
4. Where are the left wrist fractures located?
    The distal shafts of the radius and ulna
5. Did the radiologist take any side views of the left elbow?
    Single view of the left elbow was obtained in the lateral projection.

CHAPTER 5 — Integumentary System

LEARNING ACTIVITY 5–2

Building medical words

1. adipoma, lipoma
2. adipocele, lipocele
3. adipoid, lipoid
4. adipocyte, lipocyte
5. dermatitis
6. dermatotome
7. onychoma
8. onychomalacia
9. onychosis
10. onychomycosis
11. onychocryptosis
12. onychopathy
13. trichopathy
14. trichomycosis
15. dermatology
16. dermatologist
17. adipectomy, lipectomy
18. onychectomy
19. onychotomy
20. dermatoplasty, dermoplasty

LEARNING ACTIVITY 5–4

Matching burn and oncology terms

1. i.   redness of skin
2. e.   no evidence of primary tumor
3. h.   cancerous; may be life-threatening
4. g.   heals without scar formation
5. f.   determines degree of abnormal cancer cells compared with normal cells
6. a.   develops from keratinizing epidermal cells
7. b.   noncancerous
8. j.   primary tumor size, small with minimal invasion
9. c.   no evidence of metastasis
10. d.   extensive damage to underlying connective tissue

LEARNING ACTIVITY 5–5

Matching diagnostic, symptomatic, procedure, and pharmacology terms

1. pediculosis
2. vitiligo
3. tinea
4. scabies
5. impetigo
6. urticaria
7. chloasma
8. ecchymosis
9. petechiae
10. alopecia
11. antifungals
12. fulguration
13. corticosteroids
14. dermabrasion
15. parasiticides
16. keratolytics
17. intradermal test
18. patch test
19. autograft
20. xenograft

MEDICAL RECORD ACTIVITY 5–1

Pathology report of skin lesion

1. In the specimen section, what does "skin on dorsum left wrist" mean?
   Skin was obtained from the back or posterior surface of the left wrist.
2. What was the inflammatory infiltrate?
   Lymphocytic inflammatory infiltrate in the papillary dermis
3. What was the pathologist's diagnosis for the left forearm?
   Nodular and infiltrating basal cell carcinoma near the elbow
4. Provide a brief description of Bowen disease, the pathologist's diagnosis for the left wrist.
   Bowen disease is a form of intraepidermal carcinoma (squamous cell), characterized by red-brown scaly or crusted lesions that resemble a patch of psoriasis or dermatitis.

MEDICAL RECORD ACTIVITY 5–2

Patient referral letter: Onychomycosis

1. What pertinent disorders were identified in the past medical history?
   History of hypertension and cancer
2. What pertinent surgery was identified in the past surgical history?
   Mastectomy
3. Did the doctor identify any problems in the vascular system or nervous system?
   Vascular and neurological systems were intact.
4. What was the significant finding in the laboratory results?
   Alkaline phosphatase was elevated.
5. What treatment did the doctor employ for the onychomycosis?
   Debridement and medication or Sporanox PulsePak
6. What did the doctor recommend regarding the abnormal laboratory finding?
   The doctor recommended a repeat of the liver enzymes in approximately 4 weeks.

CHAPTER 6 — Digestive System

LEARNING ACTIVITY 6–3

Building medical words

1. esophagodynia, esophagalgia
2. esophagospasm
3. esophagostenosis
4. gastritis
5. gastrodynia, gastralgia
6. gastropathy
7. jejunectomy
8. duodenal
9. ileitis
10. jejunoileal
11. enteritis
12. enteropathy
13. colitis
14. colorectal
15. coloenteritis, enterocolitis
16. coloptosis
17. colopathy
18. proctostenosis, rectostenosis
19. rectocele, proctocele
20. proctoplegia, proctoparalysis
21. cholecystitis
22. cholelithiasis
23. hepatoma
24. hepatomegaly
25. pancreatitis

LEARNING ACTIVITY 6–4

Building surgical words

1. gingivectomy
2. glossectomy
3. esophagoplasty
4. gastrectomy
5. gastrojejunostomy
6. esophagectomy
7. gastroenterocolostomy
8. enteroplasty
9. enteropexy
10. choledochorrhaphy
11. colostomy
12. hepatopexy
13. proctoplasty, rectoplasty
14. cholecystectomy
15. choledochoplasty

LEARNING ACTIVITY 6–5

Matching pathological, diagnostic, symptomatic, and related terms

1. hematemesis
2. dysphagia
3. fecalith
4. halitosis
5. anorexia
6. dyspepsia
7. cirrhosis
8. cachexia
9. obstipation
10. lesion

LEARNING ACTIVITY 6–6

Matching procedures, pharmacology, and abbreviations

1. pc, pp
2. bilirubin
3. emetics
4. bid
5. choledochoplasty
6. lower GI series
7. gastroscopy
8. stomatoplasty
9. intubation
10. anastomosis
11. stool guaiac
12. endoscopy
13. laxatives
14. antacids
15. ultrasonography
16. liver function tests
17. qid
18. stat
19. proctosigmoidoscopy
20. upper GI series

MEDICAL RECORD ACTIVITY 6–1

GI evaluation

1. While referring to Figure 6–3, describe the location of the gallbladder in relation to the liver.
   Posterior and inferior portion of the right lobe of the liver
2. Why did the patient undergo the cholecystectomy?
   To treat cholecystitis and cholelithiasis
3. List the patient's prior surgeries.
   Tonsillectomy, appendectomy, and cholecystectomy
4. How does the patient's most recent postoperative episode of discomfort (pain) differ from the initial pain she described?
   Continuous deep right-sided pain, which took a crescendo pattern and then a decrescendo pattern—the initial pain was intermittent and sharp.

MEDICAL RECORD ACTIVITY 6–2

Esophagogastroduodenoscopy with biopsy

1. What caused the hematemesis?
   Etiology was unknown. Inflammation of the mucosa in the stomach and duodenum was noted.
2. What procedures were carried out to determine the cause of bleeding?
   During x-ray tomography using the videoendoscope, biopsies were taken of the stomach and duodenum. It was also noted that previously the patient had esophageal varices.
3. How much blood did the patient lose during the procedure?
   None
4. Were there any ulcerations or erosions found during the exploratory procedure that might account for the bleeding?
   No
5. What type of sedation was used during the procedure?
   Demerol and Versed administered intravenously
6. What did the doctors find when they examined the stomach and duodenum?
   Diffuse and punctate erythema

CHAPTER 7 — Respiratory System

LEARNING ACTIVITY 7–2

Building medical words

1. rhinorrhea
2. rhinitis
3. laryngoscopy
4. laryngitis
5. laryngostenosis
6. bronchiectasis
7. bronchopathy
8. bronchospasm
9. pneumothorax
10. pneumonitis
11. pulmonologist
12. pulmonary, pulmonic
13. dyspnea
14. bradypnea
15. tachypnea
16. apnea
17. rhinoplasty
18. thoracocentesis, thoracentesis
19. pulmonectomy, pneumonectomy
20. tracheostomy

LEARNING ACTIVITY 7–3

Matching pathological, diagnostic, symptomatic, and related terms

1. atelectasis
2. empyema
3. surfactant
4. consolidation
5. ascites
6. anosmia
7. hypoxemia
8. tubercles
9. apnea
10. emphysema
11. compliance
12. epistaxis
13. pulmonary edema
14. rale, crackle
15. deviated nasal septum
16. coryza
17. pneumonoconiosis
18. pleurisy
19. stridor
20. pertussis

LEARNING ACTIVITY 7–4

Matching procedures, pharmacology, and abbreviations

1. lung scan
2. polysomnography
3. radiography
4. antral lavage
5. antihistamines
6. antitussives
7. sweat test
8. oximetry
9. AFB
10. aerosol therapy
11. decongestants
12. Mantoux test
13. ABGs
14. expectorants
15. throat culture
16. pulmonary function studies
17. laryngoscopy
18. septoplasty
19. pneumectomy
20. rhinoplasty

MEDICAL RECORD ACTIVITY 7–1

Respiratory evaluation

1. What symptom caused the patient to seek medical help?
   Shortness of breath
2. What was the patient's previous history?
   Difficult breathing, high blood pressure, chronic obstructive pulmonary disease, and peripheral vascular disease
3. What were the findings of the physical examination?
   Bilateral wheezes and rhonchi heard anteriorly and posteriorly
4. What changes were noted from the previous film?
   Interstitial vascular congestion with possible superimposed inflammatory change and some pleural reactive change
5. What is the present Dx?
   Acute exacerbation of chronic obstructive pulmonary disease; heart failure; hypertension; peripheral vascular disease
6. What new diagnosis was made that did not appear in the previous medical history?
   Heart failure

MEDICAL RECORD ACTIVITY 7–2

Chronic interstitial lung disease

1. When did the patient notice SOB?
   With activity
2. Other than the respiratory system, what other body systems are identified in the history of present illness?
   Cardiovascular, urinary, and nervous system
3. What were the findings regarding the neck?
   Supple and no evidence of thyromegaly or adenomegaly
4. What was the finding regarding the spine?
   Mild kyphosis without scoliosis
5. What appears to be the likely cause of the chronic interstitial lung disease?
   Combination of pulmonary fibrosis and heart failure
6. Define the following abbreviations: ABGs, Po_2, Pco_2, and pH.
   ABGs, arterial blood gasses; Po_2, partial pressure of oxygen; Pco_2, carbon dioxide partial pressure; pH, degree of alkalinity and acidity
7. What is the therapeutic action of Lasix?
   Diuretic

CHAPTER 8 — Cardiovascular System

LEARNING ACTIVITY 8–2

Building medical words

1. atheroma
2. atherosclerosis
3. phlebitis
4. phlebothrombosis
5. venous
6. venospasm
7. cardiologist
8. cardiorrhexis
9. cardiotoxic
10. cardiomegaly
11. angiomalacia
12. angioma
13. thrombogen, thrombogenesis
14. thrombosis
15. aortostenosis
16. aortography
17. cardiocentesis
18. arteriorrhaphy
19. embolectomy
20. thrombolysis

LEARNING ACTIVITY 8–3

Matching pathological, diagnostic, symptomatic, and related terms

1. infarct
2. angina
3. incompetent
4. vegetations
5. varices
6. bruit
7. catheter
8. palpitation
9. lumen
10. aneurysm
11. embolus
12. arrhythmia
13. arrest
14. thrombolysis
15. stent
16. hypertension
17. hyperlipidemia
18. primary
19. secondary
20. perfusion

LEARNING ACTIVITY 8–4

Matching procedures, pharmacology, and abbreviations

1. Holter monitor test
2. echocardiography
3. coronary angiography
4. nitrates
5. statins
6. diuretics
7. cardiac enzyme studies
8. scintigraphy
9. stress test
10. ligation and stripping
11. commissurotomy
12. arterial biopsy
13. catheter ablation
14. embolization
15. angioplasty
16. PTCA
17. CABG
18. atherectomy
19. venipuncture
20. thrombolysis

MEDICAL RECORD ACTIVITY 8–1

Acute myocardial infarction

1. How long had the patient experienced chest pain before she was seen in the hospital?
   Approximately 2 hours
2. Did the patient have a previous history of chest pain?
   Yes
3. What are the cardiac enzymes that are tested to confirm the diagnosis of MI?
   Tropinin T, tropinin I, creatine, creatinine kinase
4. Initially, what medications were administered to stabilize the patient?
   Streptokinase and heparin
5. During the current admission, what part of the heart was damaged?
   The lateral front side of the heart (anterior of heart)
6. Was the location of damage to the heart for this admission the same as for the initial MI?
   No, in the earlier admission, the damage was to the lower part of the heart.

MEDICAL RECORD ACTIVITY 8–2

Operative report: Rule out temporal arteritis

1. Why was the right temporal artery biopsied?
   Rule out arteritis
2. In what position was the patient placed?
   Supine
3. What was the incision area?
   Right preauricular area
4. How was the temporal artery described in the report?
   Palpable
5. How was the dissection carried out?
   Down through the subcutaneous tissue and superficial fascia
6. What was the size of the specimen?
   Approximately 1.5 cm

CHAPTER 9 — Blood, Lymph, and Immune Systems

LEARNING ACTIVITY 9–2

Building medical words

1. erythrocytosis
2. leukocytosis
3. lymphocytosis
4. reticulocytosis
5. erythropenia
6. leukopenia
7. thrombocytopenia, thrombopenia
8. lymphocytopenia
9. hemopoiesis, hematopoiesis
10. leukopoiesis, leukocytopoiesis
11. thrombocytopoiesis
12. immunologist
13. immunology
14. splenocele
15. splenolysis
16. splenectomy
17. thymectomy
18. thymolysis
19. splenotomy
20. splenopexy

LEARNING ACTIVITY 9–3

Matching pathological, diagnostic, symptomatic, and related terms

1. exacerbations
2. hemoglobinopathy
3. bacteremia
4. hemostasis
5. active
6. Kaposi sarcoma
7. normocytic
8. lymphadenopathy
9. immunocompromised
10. hemophilia
11. infectious mononucleosis
12. myelogenous
13. passive
14. artificial
15. hemolysis
16. hematoma
17. graft rejection
18. anisocytosis
19. titer
20. septicemia

LEARNING ACTIVITY 9–4

Matching procedures, pharmacology, and abbreviations

1. aspiration
2. hematocrit
3. Monospot
4. anticoagulants
5. WBC
6. homologous
7. lymphangiectomy
8. RBC indices
9. Shilling
10. lymphadenography
11. autologous
12. hemostatics
13. RBC
14. thrombolytics
15. differential

MEDICAL RECORD ACTIVITY 9–1

Discharge summary: Sickle cell crisis

1. What blood product was administered to the patient?
   Two units of packed red blood cells
2. Why was this blood product given to the patient?
   The patient was anemic due to sickle cell anemia.

MEDICAL RECORD ACTIVITY 9–2

Discharge summary: PCP and HIV

1. How do you think the patient acquired the HIV infection?
   Through her husband, who died of HIV
2. What were the two diagnoses of the husband?
   Multifocal leukoencephalopathy (PMN) and Kaposi sarcoma

3. Why was a CT scan performed on the patient?
   To determine the cause of abdominal pain
4. What were the three findings of the CT scan?
   Ileus in the small bowel, dilated small bowel loops, and abnormal enhancement pattern in the kidney
5. Why should the patient see his regular doctor?
   To follow up on the renal abnormality

3. What four disorders in the medical history are significant for HIV?
   Several episodes of diarrhea, sinusitis, thrush, and vaginal candidiasis
4. What was the x-ray finding?
   Diffuse lower lobe infiltrates
5. What two procedures are going to be performed to confirm the diagnosis of PCP pneumonia?
   Bronchoscopy and alveolar lavage

CHAPTER 10 — Musculoskeletal System

LEARNING ACTIVITY 10–4

Building medical words

1. osteocytes
2. ostealgia, osteodynia
3. osteoarthropathy
4. osteogenesis
5. cervical
6. cervicobrachial
7. cervicofacial
8. myelocele
9. myelosarcoma
10. myelomalacia
11. myeloid
12. suprasternal
13. sternoid
14. chondroblast
15. arthritis
16. osteoarthritis
17. pelvimeter
18. myospasm
19. myopathy
20. myorrhexis
21. phalangectomy
22. thoracotomy
23. vertebrectomy
24. arthrodesis
25. myoplasty

LEARNING ACTIVITY 10–5

Matching pathological, diagnostic, symptomatic, and related terms

1. subluxation
2. rickets
3. spondylolisthesis
4. claudication
5. muscular dystrophy
6. talipes
7. sequestrum
8. myasthenia gravis
9. prosthesis
10. ganglion cyst
11. hypotonia
12. Ewing sarcoma
13. greenstick fracture
14. kyphosis
15. osteoporosis
16. scoliosis
17. chondrosarcoma
18. comminuted fracture
19. spondylitis
20. gout
21. hematopoiesis
22. pyogenic
23. necrosis
24. ankylosis
25. phantom limb

LEARNING ACTIVITY 10–6

Matching procedures, pharmacology, and abbreviations

1. myelography
2. open reduction
3. gold salts
4. CTS
5. laminectomy
6. arthrography
7. arthrodesis
8. amputation
9. HNP
10. salicylates
11. arthroscopy
12. sequestrectomy
13. ACL
14. relaxants
15. closed reduction

MEDICAL RECORD ACTIVITY 10–1

Right knee arthroscopy and medial meniscectomy

1. Describe the meniscus and identify its location.
   The meniscus is the curved, fibrous cartilage in the knees and other joints.
2. What is the probable cause of the tear in the patient's meniscus?
   The continuous pressure on the knees from jogging on a hard surface, such as the pavement
3. What does normal ACL and PCL refer to in the report?
   The anterior and posterior cruciate ligaments appeared to be normal.
4. Explain the McMurray sign test.
   Rotation of the tibia on the femur is used to determine injury to meniscal structures. An audible click during manipulation of tibia with the leg flexed is an indication that the meniscus has been injured.
5. Because Lachman and McMurray tests were negative (normal), why was the surgery performed?
   The medial compartment of the knee showed an inferior surface posterior and midmedial meniscal tear that was flipped up on top of itself. The surgeon resected the tear, and the remaining meniscus was contoured back to a stable rim.

MEDICAL RECORD ACTIVITY 10–2

Radiographic consultation: Tibial diaphysis nuclear scan

1. Where was the pain located?
   Middle 1/3 of the left tibia
2. What medication was the patient taking for pain and did it provide relief?
   He finds no relief with NSAIDs.
3. How was the blood flow to the affected area described by the radiologist?
   There is focal, increased blood flow and blood pooling.
4. How was the radiotracer accumulation described?
   The radiotracer accumulated within the left mid-posterior tibial diaphysis was delayed.
5. What will be the probable outcome with continued excessive repetitive stress?
   The rate of resorption will exceed the rate of bone replacement.
6. What will happen if resorption continues to exceed replacement?
   A stress fracture will occur.

CHAPTER 11 — Genitourinary System

LEARNING ACTIVITY 11–3

Building medical words

1. nephrolith
2. nephropyosis, pyonephrosis
3. hydronephrosis, nephrohydrosis
4. pyelectasis, pyelectasia
5. pyelopathy
6. ureterectasis, ureterectasia
7. ureterolith
8. cystitis
9. cystoscope
10. vesicocele
11. vesicoprostatic
12. urethrostenosis
13. urethrotome
14. urography
15. uropathy
16. dysuria
17. oliguria

18. orchidopathy, orchiopathy
19. orchialgia, orchiodynia, orchidalgia
20. balanorrhea
21. orchidectomy, orchiectomy

22. balanoplasty
23. vasectomy
24. pyelotomy
25. cystopexy

LEARNING ACTIVITY 11–4

Matching pathological, diagnostic, symptomatic, and related terms

1. urgency
2. fistula
3. anorchism
4. anuria
5. azotemia
6. orchiopexy
7. benign prostatic hypertrophy
8. hesitancy
9. oliguria
10. nephrotic syndrome
11. phimosis
12. sterility
13. epispadias
14. aspermia
15. pyuria
16. herniorrhaphy
17. nocturia
18. enuresis
19. hydrocele
20. balanitis

LEARNING ACTIVITY 11–5

Matching procedures, pharmacology, and abbreviations

1. KUB
2. semen analysis
3. cystoscopy
4. antibiotics
5. C&S
6. diuretics
7. urethrotomy
8. ESWL
9. peritoneal dialysis
10. resection
11. vasectomy
12. orchiectomy
13. circumcision
14. androgens
15. potassium supplements

MEDICAL RECORD ACTIVITY 11–1

Operative report: Ureterocele

1. Why did the doctor perform a cystoscopy?
   To examine the bladder
2. What was the name and size of the urethral sound used in the procedure?
   #26 French Van Buren
3. What is the function of the urethral sound?
   Dilate the urethra
4. In what direction was the ureterocele incised?
   Longitudinally
5. Was fulguration required? Why or why not?
   Fulguration was not required because there was no bleeding.

MEDICAL RECORD ACTIVITY 11–2

Operative report: Extracorporeal shockwave lithotripsy

1. What previous procedures were performed on the patient?
   ESWL and double-J stent placement
2. Why is this current procedure being performed?
   To fragment the remaining calculus and remove the double-J stent
3. What imaging technique was used for positioning the patient to ensure that the shockwaves would strike the calculus?
   Fluoroscopy
4. In what position was the patient placed in the cystoscopy suite?
   Dorsal lithotomy
5. How was the double-J stent removed?
   Using grasping forceps and removing it as the scope was withdrawn

CHAPTER 12 — Female Reproductive System

LEARNING ACTIVITY 12–3

Building medical words

1. gynecopathy
2. gynecologist
3. cervicovaginitis
4. cervicovesical
5. colposcope
6. colposcopy
7. vaginitis
8. vaginocele
9. hysteromyoma
10. hysteropathy
11. hysterosalpingography
12. metrorrhagia
13. parametritis
14. uterocele
15. uterocervical
16. uterovesical
17. oophoritis
18. oophorosalpingitis
19. salpingocele
20. salpingography
21. oophoropexy, ovariopexy
22. hystero-oophorectomy
23. episiorrhaphy, perineorrhaphy
24. hysterosalpingo-oophorectomy
25. amniocentesis

LEARNING ACTIVITY 12–4

Matching pathological, diagnostic, symptomatic, and related terms

1. pyosalpinx
2. primipara
3. gestation
4. chancre
5. retroversion
6. congenital
7. dystocia
8. atresia
9. Down syndrome
10. pruritus vulvae
11. asymptomatic
12. metrorrhagia
13. menarche
14. leiomyoma
15. oligomenorrhea
16. parturition
17. eclampsia
18. viable
19. condylomas
20. primigravida

LEARNING ACTIVITY 12–5

Matching procedures, pharmacology, and abbreviations

1. Pap test
2. hysterosalpingography
3. amniocentesis
4. antifungals
5. colpocleisis
6. D&C
7. total abdominal hysterectomy (TAH)
8. tubal ligation
9. OCPs
10. laparoscopy
11. episiotomy
12. ultrasonography
13. chorionic villus sampling
14. estrogens
15. oxytocins
16. cryocautery
17. IUD
18. cordocentesis
19. lumpectomy
20. prostaglandins

MEDICAL RECORD ACTIVITY 12–1

Primary herpes 1 infection

1. Did the patient have any discharge? If so, describe it.
   A brownish discharge
2. What type of discomfort was the patient experiencing around the vulvar area?
   She was experiencing severe itching (pruritus) and pain.
3. Has the patient been taking her oral contraceptive pills regularly?
   Yes
4. Where was the viral culture obtained?
   Ulcerlike lesion on the right labia
5. Even though her partner used a condom, how do you think the patient became infected with herpes?
   She probably got infected from the cold sore when having oral-genital sex.

MEDICAL RECORD ACTIVITY 12–2

Menometrorrhagia

1. How many pregnancies did this woman have? How many viable infants did she deliver?
   Two pregnancies and one viable birth
2. What is a therapeutic abortion?
   An abortion performed when the pregnancy endangers the mother's mental or physical health or when the fetus has a known condition incompatible with life
3. Why did the physician propose to perform a hysterectomy?
   Patient desires definitive treatment for menometrorrhagia and has declined palliative treatment
4. What is a vaginal hysterectomy?
   Surgical removal of the uterus through the vagina
5. Does the surgeon plan to remove one or both ovaries and fallopian tubes?
   The surgeon plans to perform a bilateral (relates to two sides) salpingo-oophorectomy.
6. Why do you think the physician will use the laparoscope to perform the hysterectomy?
   To permit visualization of the abdominal cavity as the ovaries and fallopian tubes are removed through the vagina

CHAPTER 13 — Endocrine System

LEARNING ACTIVITY 13–2

Building medical words

1. hyperglycemia
2. hypoglycemia
3. glycogenesis
4. pancreatitis
5. pancreatolysis
6. pancreatopathy
7. thyroiditis
8. thyromegaly
9. parathyroidectomy
10. adrenalectomy

LEARNING ACTIVITY 13–3

Matching pathological, diagnostic, symptomatic, and related terms

1. virile
2. myxedema
3. diuresis
4. hirsutism
5. cretinism
6. insulin
7. Addison disease
8. exophthalmic goiter
9. hyperkalemia
10. pheochromocytoma
11. type 1 diabetes
12. hyponatremia
13. glycosuria
14. Cushing syndrome
15. type 2 diabetes

LEARNING ACTIVITY 13–4

Matching procedures, pharmacology, and abbreviations

1. FBS
2. RAIU
3. corticosteroids
4. growth hormone
5. thyroid scan
6. T_4
7. oral antidiabetics
8. GTT
9. antithyroids
10. protein-bound iodine
11. T_3
12. magnetic resonance imaging (MRI)
13. exophthalmometry
14. computed tomography (CT) scan
15. Humulin

MEDICAL RECORD ACTIVITY 13–1

Hyperparathyroidism

1. What is an adenoma?
   Benign tumor of a gland
2. What does the physician suspect caused the patient's hyperparathyroidism?
   Possible parathyroid adenoma

3. What type of laboratory findings revealed parathyroid disease?
   Elevated calcium level
4. What is hypercalciuria?
   Excessive amount of calcium in the urine
5. If the patient smoked 548 packs of cigarettes per year, how many packs did she smoke in an average day?
   Approximately 1.5 packs per day

MEDICAL RECORD ACTIVITY 13–2

Diabetes mellitus

1. How long has this patient been experiencing voracious eating?
   For the past 10 days
2. Was the patient's obesity due to overeating or metabolic imbalance?
   Overeating

3. Why did the doctor experience difficulty in examining the patient's abdomen?
   Because she was so obese
4. Was the patient's blood glucose above or below normal on admission?
   Above normal
5. What is the reference range for fasting blood glucose?
   The range for fasting blood glucose is 70/110 mg/dL.

CHAPTER 14 — Nervous System

LEARNING ACTIVITY 14–2

Building medical words

1. encephalopathy
2. encephalocele
3. encephalography
4. cerebropathy
5. cerebritis
6. craniocele
7. craniometer
8. neuralgia, neurodynia
9. neurologist
10. neurotripsy
11. myelocele
12. myeloplegia
13. psychotic, psychic
14. psychosis
15. bradykinesia
16. dyskinesia
17. hemiplegia
18. quadriplegia
19. dysphasia
20. aphasia
21. neurolysis
22. craniotomy
23. cranioplasty
24. neurorrhaphy
25. encephalotomy

LEARNING ACTIVITY 14–3

Matching pathological, diagnostic, symptomatic, and related terms

1. hemiparesis
2. dysrhythmias
3. Alzheimer disease
4. bulimia nervosa
5. clonic spasm
6. Guillain-Barré syndrome
7. phobias
8. bipolar disorder
9. leptomeningitis
10. asthenia
11. shingles
12. lethargy
13. paraplegia
14. poliomyelitis
15. stroke
16. transient ischemic attack (TIA)
17. autism
18. Parkinson disease
19. multiple sclerosis
20. concussion

LEARNING ACTIVITY 14–4

Matching procedures, pharmacology, and abbreviations

1. NVC
2. psychostimulants
3. antipsychotics
4. general anesthetics
5. echoencephalography
6. cryosurgery
7. myelography
8. cerebral angiography
9. CSF analysis
10. electromyography
11. analgesics
12. PET
13. tractotomy
14. hypnotics
15. trephination

MEDICAL RECORD ACTIVITY 14–1

Subarachnoid hemorrhage

1. In what part of the head did the patient feel pain?
   Occipital, the back part of the head
2. What imaging tests were performed, and what was the finding in each test?
   CT scan showed blood in the cisterna subarachnoidalis and mild acute hydrocephalus. Cerebral angiogram and MRI showed no aneurysm.
3. How does meningismus differ from meningitis?
   Meningismus is irritation of the brain and spinal cord with symptoms simulating meningitis but without actual inflammation. Meningitis is an inflammation of the membranes of the spinal cord or brain.
4. Did the lumbar puncture rule out or confirm a second subarachnoid hemorrhage?
   It confirmed subarachnoid hemorrhage.

MEDICAL RECORD ACTIVITY 14–2

Consultation report: Acute onset paraplegia

1. What was the original cause of the patient's current problems and what treatments were provided?
   Fall at work about 15–20 years ago, and she had four subsequent lumbar surgeries
2. Why was the patient admitted to the hospital?
   Pain management
3. What intravenous medications did the patient receive and why was each given?
   Clonidine for hypertension and methadone for pain
4. What was the cause of bladder retention?
   Administration of clonidine
5. What occurred after the catheter was removed?
   Subacute onset of paresis, paresthesias, and pain in the legs approximately $2\frac{1}{2}$ to 3 hours later
6. What three disorders were listed in the differential diagnosis?
   Subarachnoid hemorrhage, epidural abscess, and transverse myelitis

CHAPTER 15 — Special Senses

LEARNING ACTIVITY 15–3

Building medical words

1. ophthalmoplegia, ophthalmoparalysis
2. ophthalmology
3. pupilloscopy
4. keratomalacia
5. keratometer
6. scleritis
7. scleromalacia
8. iridoplegia, iridoparalysis
9. iridocele
10. retinopathy
11. retinitis
12. blepharoplegia
13. blepharoptosis
14. otopyorrhea
15. audiometer
16. myringotome
17. amblyopia
18. hyperopia
19. anacusis
20. hyperacusis
21. stapedectomy
22. labyrinthotomy
23. mastoidectomy
24. myringoplasty, tympanoplasty
25. keratotomy

LEARNING ACTIVITY 15–4

Matching pathological, diagnostic, symptomatic, and related terms

1. cataract
2. achromatopsia
3. nyctalopia
4. gonioscopy
5. anacusis
6. otitis externa
7. diopter
8. tonometer
9. visual field
10. epiphora
11. strabismus
12. Ménière disease
13. neovascular
14. vertigo
15. exotropia
16. enucleation
17. chalazion
18. amblyopia
19. retinoblastoma
20. tinnitus

LEARNING ACTIVITY 15–5

Matching procedures, pharmacology, and abbreviations

1. caloric stimulation test
2. ophthalmoscopy
3. cochlear implant
4. fluorescein angiography
5. otoplasty
6. mydriatics
7. tonometry
8. visual acuity test
9. evisceration
10. beta blockers
11. wax emulsifiers
12. enucleation
13. ST
14. ophthalmic decongestants
15. XT
16. gonioscopy
17. otoscopy
18. audiometry
19. radial keratotomy
20. otic analgesics

MEDICAL RECORD ACTIVITY 15–1

Retained foreign bodies

1. Did the patient's surgery involve one or both ears?
   Bilateral, it involved both ears.
2. What was the nature of the foreign body in the patient's ears?
   Retained tympanostomy tubes
3. What ear structure was involved?
   Eardrum, or tympanum
4. What instrument was used to locate the tubes?
   Operating microscope
5. What was the material in which the tubes were embedded?
   Earwax, or cerumen

MEDICAL RECORD ACTIVITY 15–2

Phacoemulsification and lens implant

1. What technique was used to destroy the cataract?
   Phacoemulsification, an ultrasound technique
2. In what portion of the eye was the implant placed?
   Posterior chamber
3. What anesthetics were used for surgery?
   Intravenous and retrobulbar block
4. What was the function of the blepharostat?
   To separate the eyelids during surgery
5. What was the function of the keratome?
   A knife used to incise the cornea
6. Where was the implant inserted?
   In the capsular bag

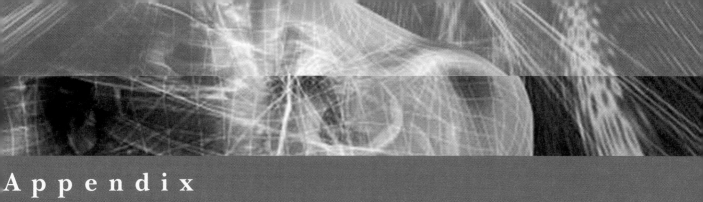

Appendix

B

Abbreviations

Abbreviation	Meaning	Abbreviation	Meaning
AAA	abdominal aortic aneurysm	AST	angiotensin sensitivity test; aspartate aminotransferase (cardiac enzyme, formerly called *SGOT*)
AB, ab	abortion, antibodies		
ABC	aspiration biopsy cytology		
ABG	arterial blood gas		
ABO	blood groups A, AB, B, and O	Ast	astigmatism
		ATN	acute tubular necrosis
ac	before meals	*AU	both ears
AC	air conduction	AV	atrioventricular, arteriovenous
Acc	accommodation		
ACL	anterior cruciate ligament	Ba	barium
ACTH	adrenocorticotropic hormone	BaE	barium enema
		baso	basophil (type of white blood cell)
AD	Alzheimer disease		
*AD	right ear	BBB	bundle branch block
ADH	antidiuretic hormone (vasopressin)	BC	bone conduction
		BCC	basal cell carcinoma
AE	above the elbow	BE	below the elbow
AF	atrial fibrillation	BEAM	brain electrical activity mapping
AFB	acid-fast bacillus (TB organism)		
		bid	twice a day
AGN	acute glomerulonephritis	BK	below the knee
AI	artificial insemination	BM	bowel movement
AIDS	acquired immunodeficiency syndrome	BMR	basal metabolic rate
		BNO	bladder neck obstruction
AK	above the knee	BP	blood pressure
alk phos	alkaline phosphatase	BPH	benign prostatic hyperplasia; benign prostatic hypertrophy
ALL	acute lymphocytic leukemia		
ALS	amyotrophic lateral sclerosis; also called *Lou Gehrig disease*	BSE	breast self-examination
		BUN	blood urea nitrogen
		Bx, bx	biopsy
ALT	alanine aminotransferase (elevated in liver and heart disease); formerly *SGPT*	C&S	culture and sensitivity
		C1, C2, and so on	first cervical vertebra, second cervical vertebra, and so on
AML	acute myelogenous leukemia	CA	cancer; chronological age; cardiac arrest
ANS	autonomic nervous system	Ca	calcium; cancer
ant	anterior	CABG	coronary artery bypass graft
AP	anteroposterior		
APTT	activated partial thromboplastin time	CAD	coronary artery disease
		cath	catheterization; catheter
ARDS	acute respiratory distress syndrome	CBC	complete blood count
		CC	cardiac catheterization
ARF	acute renal failure	CCU	coronary care unit
ARMD, AMD	age-related macular degeneration	CDH	congenital dislocation of the hip
AS	aortic stenosis	CHD	coronary heart disease
*AS	left ear	CHF	congestive heart failure
ASD	atrial septal defect	Chol	cholesterol
ASHD	arteriosclerotic heart disease	CK	creatine kinase (cardiac enzyme)

Abbreviation	Meaning	Abbreviation	Meaning
CLL	chronic lymphocytic leukemia	ED	erectile dysfunction; emergency department
cm	centimeter	EEG	electroencephalogram; electroencephalography
CML	chronic myelogenous leukemia	EGD	esophagogastroduo-denoscopy
CNS	central nervous system		
CO₂	carbon dioxide	Em	emmetropia
COPD	chronic obstructive pulmonary disease	EMG	electromyography
		ENT	ears, nose, and throat
CP	cerebral palsy	EOM	extraocular movement
CPD	cephalopelvic disproportion	eos	eosinophil (type of white blood cell)
CPR	cardiopulmonary resuscitation	ERCP	endoscopic retrograde cholangiopancreatography
CS, C-section	cesarean section		
CSF	cerebrospinal fluid	ESR, sed rate	erythrocyte sedimentation rate; sedimentation rate
CT	computed tomography		
CT scan, CAT scan	computed tomography scan	ESRD	end-stage renal disease
CTS	carpal tunnel syndrome	ESWL	extracorporeal shockwave lithotripsy
CV	cardiovascular		
CVA	cerebrovascular accident	EU	excretory urography; also called *intravenous pyelography (IVP)* or *intravenous urography (IVU)*
CVS	chorionic villus sampling		
CWP	childbirth without pain		
CXR	chest x-ray, chest radi-ograph		
		FECG; FEKG	fetal electrocardiogram
cysto	cystoscopy	FHR	fetal heart rate
D	diopter (lens strength)	FHT	fetal heart tone
D&C	dilatation (dilation) and curettage	FS	frozen section
		FSH	follicle-stimulating hormone
*DC	discharge	FTND	full-term normal delivery
decub	decubitus (ulcer); bedsore	FVC	forced vital capacity
derm	dermatology	Fx	fracture
DI	diabetes insipidus; diagnostic imaging	G	gravida (pregnant)
		GB	gallbladder
diff	differential count (white blood cells)	GBS	gallbladder series
		GC	gonorrhea
DJD	degenerative joint disease	GER	gastroesophageal reflux
DKA	diabetic ketoacidosis	GERD	gastroesophageal reflux disease
DM	diabetes mellitus		
DOE	dyspnea on exertion	GH	growth hormone
DPT	diphtheria, pertussis, tetanus	GI	gastrointestinal
DRE	digital rectal examination	GU	genitourinary
DSA	digital subtraction angiography	GVHR	graft-versus-host reaction
		GYN	gynecology
DUB	dysfunctional uterine bleeding	HAV	hepatitis A virus
		Hb, Hgb	hemoglobin
DVT	deep vein thrombosis	HBV	hepatitis B virus
Dx	diagnosis	HCT, Hct	hematocrit
EBV	Epstein-Barr virus	HCV	hepatitis C virus
ECG, EKG	electrocardiogram	HD	hemodialysis; hip disarticulation; hearing distance
ECHO	echocardiogram; echoencephalogram		

Abbreviation	Meaning	Abbreviation	Meaning
HDL	high-density lipoprotein	K	potassium (an electrolyte)
HDN	hemolytic disease of the newborn	KD	knee disarticulation
		KUB	kidney, ureter, bladder
HDV	hepatitis D virus	L1, L2, and so on	first lumbar vertebra, second lumbar vertebra, and so on
HEV	hepatitis E virus		
HF	heart failure		
HIV	human immunodeficiency virus	LAT, lat	lateral
		LBW	low birth weight
HMD	hyaline membrane disease	LD	lactate dehydrogenase; lactic acid dehydrogenase (cardiac enzyme)
HNP	herniated nucleus pulposus (herniated disk)		
HP	hemipelvectomy	LDL	low-density lipoprotein
HPV	human papillomavirus	LH	luteinizing hormone
HRT	hormone replacement therapy	LLQ	left lower quadrant
		LMP	last menstrual period
*hs	at bedtime	LOC	loss of consciousness
HSG	hysterosalpingography	LP	lumbar puncture
HSV	herpes simplex virus	LSO	left salpingo-oophorectomy
I&D	incision and drainage	lt	left
IBS	irritable bowel syndrome	LUQ	left upper quadrant
ICP	intracranial pressure	lymphos	lymphocytes
ID	intradermal	MCH	mean corpuscular hemoglobin; mean cell hemoglobin (average amount of hemoglobin per cell)
IDDM	insulin-dependent diabetes mellitus		
Igs	immunoglobulins		
I.M., IM	intramuscular; infectious mononucleosis		
		MCHC	mean cell hemoglobin concentration (average concentration of hemoglobin in a single red cell)
IMP	impression (*diagnosis*)		
IOL	intraocular lens		
IOP	intraocular pressure		
IPPB	intermittent positive-pressure breathing	MCV	mean cell volume (average volume or size of a single red blood cell; high MCV = macrocytic cells; low MCV = microcytic cells)
IRDS	infant respiratory distress syndrome		
IS	intracostal space		
ITP	idiopathic thrombocytopenia purpura		
IUD	intrauterine device	MEG	magnetoencephalog- raphy
IUGR	intrauterine growth rate; intrauterine growth retardation	MG	myasthenia gravis
		MI	myocardial infarction
I.V., IV	intravenous	mix astig	mixed astigmatism
IVF-ET	in vitro fertilization and embryo transfer	mL, ml	milliliters
		MRA	magnetic resonance angiogram; magnetic resonance angiography
IVP	intravenous pyelography; also called *excretory urography (EU)* or *intravenous urography (IVU)*		
		MRI	magnetic resonance imaging
		MRI scan	magnetic resonance imaging scan
IVU	intravenous urography (IVU); also called *excretory urography (EU)* or *intravenous pyelography (IVP)*	MS	musculoskeletal; multiple sclerosis; mental status; mitral stenosis

Abbreviation	Meaning	Abbreviation	Meaning
MSH	melanocyte-stimulating hormone	pH	symbol for degree of acidity or alkalinity
MVP	mitral valve prolapse	PID	pelvic inflammatory disease
Myop	myopia	PMP	previous menstrual period
Na+	sodium (an electrolyte)	PMS	premenstrual syndrome
NB	newborn	PND	paroxysmal nocturnal dyspnea
NCV	nerve conduction velocity		
NG	nasogastric	po	by mouth (per os)
NIDDM	non-insulin-dependent diabetes mellitus	Po_2	partial pressure of oxygen
		poly, PMN, PMNL	polymorphonuclear leukocyte
NIHL	noise-induced hearing loss		
NMTs	nebulized mist treatments	post	posterior
NPH	neutral protamine Hagedorn (insulin)	PRL	prolactin
		prn	as required
npo	nothing by mouth	PSA	prostate-specific antigen
NSAIDs	nonsteroidal anti-inflammatory drugs	PT	prothrombin time, physical therapy
O_2	oxygen	PTCA	percutaneous transluminal coronary angioplasty
OB	obstetrics		
OCPs	oral contraceptive pills	PTH	parathyroid hormone; also called *parathormone*
*OD	right eye		
OD	Doctor of Optometry	PTT	partial thromboplastin time
ORTH, ortho	orthopedics	PUD	peptic ulcer disease
*OS	left eye	PVC	premature ventricular contraction
*OU	both eyes		
P	phosphorous; pulse	q2h	every 2 hours
PA	posteroanterior; pernicious anemia	qam, qm	every morning
		*qd	every day
PAC	premature atrial contraction	qh	every hour
Pap	Papanicolaou smear	qid	four times a day
para 1, 2, 3	unipara, bipara, tripara (number of viable births)	*qod	every other day
		qpm, qn	every night
		R/O	rule out
PAT	paroxysmal atrial tachycardia	RA	rheumatoid arthritis
pc, pp	after meals (postprandial)	RAI	radioactive iodine
PCL	posterior cruciate ligament	RAIU	radioactive iodine uptake
PCNL	percutaneous nephrolithotomy	RBC, rbc	red blood cell, red blood count
Pco_2	partial pressure of carbon dioxide	RD	respiratory distress
		RDS	respiratory distress syndrome
PCP	*Pneumocystis carinii* pneumonia	RF	rheumatoid factor
		RK	radial keratotomy
PCV	packed cell volume	RLQ	right lower quadrant
PE tube	pressure-equalizing tube (placed in the eardrum)	ROM	range of motion
		RP	retrograde pyelography
PERRLA	pupils equal, round, and reactive to light and accommodation	RSO	right salpingo-oophorectomy
		rt	right
		RUQ	right upper quadrant
PET	positron emission tomography	RV	residual volume; right ventricle
PFT	pulmonary function tests	SA	sinoatrial
PGH	pituitary growth hormone	Sao_2	arterial oxygen saturation

Abbreviation	Meaning	Abbreviation	Meaning
SD	shoulder disarticulation	TIA	transient ischemic attack
segs	segmented neutrophils	*tid	three times a day
SICS	small incision cataract surgery	TKA	total knee arthroplasty
		TKR	total knee replacement
SIDS	sudden infant death syndrome	TPR	temperature, pulse, and respiration
SLE	systemic lupus erythematosus	TSE	testicular self-examination
SNS	sympathetic nervous system	TSH	thyroid-stimulating
SOB	shortness of breath	hormone	
sono	sonogram	TURP	transurethral resection of the prostate (for prostatectomy)
sp. gr.	specific gravity		
SPECT	single photon emission computed tomography		
		TVH	total vaginal hysterectomy
ST	esotropia	Tx	treatment
stat	immediately	U&L, U/L	upper and lower
STD	sexually transmitted disease	UA	urinalysis
		UC	uterine contractions
Sub-Q, subQ	subcutaneous (injection)	ung	ointment
Sx	symptom	URI	upper respiratory infection
T&A	tonsillectomy and adenoidectomy	US	ultrasound
		VA	visual acuity
T₃	triiodothyronine (thyroid hormone)	VC	vital capacity
		VCUG	voiding cystourethrography
T₄	thyroxine (thyroid hormone)	VD	venereal disease
		VF	visual field
TAH	total abdominal hysterectomy	VSD	ventricular septal defect
		VT	ventricular tachycardia
TB	tuberculosis	WBC, wbc	white blood cell, white blood count
TFT	thyroid function test		
THA	total hip arthroplasty	XP, XDP	xeroderma pigmentosum
THR	total hip replacement	XT	exotropia

*Although these abbreviations are currently found in medical records and clinical notes, the Joint Commission on Accreditation of Healthcare Organizations (JCAHO) requires their discontinuance. Instead, write out the meanings.

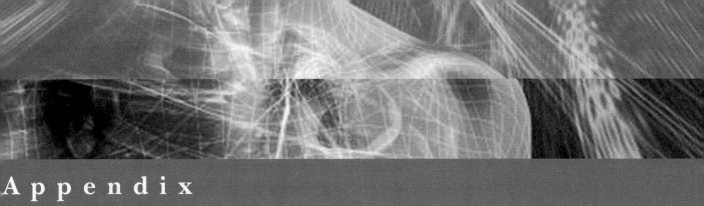

C

Glossary of Medical Word Elements

Medical Word Elements

Medical Word Element	Meaning
A	
a-	without, not
ab-	from, away from
abdomin/o	abdomen
abort/o	to miscarry
-ac	pertaining to, relating to
acous/o	hearing
acr/o	extremity
acromi/o	acromion (projection of scapula)
-acusis	hearing
-ad	toward
ad-	toward
aden/o	gland
adenoid/o	adenoids
adip/o	fat
adren/o	adrenal glands
adrenal/o	adrenal glands
aer/o	air
af-	toward
agglutin/o	clumping, gluing
agora-	marketplace
-al	pertaining to, relating to
albin/o	white
albumin/o	albumin (protein)
-algesia	pain
-algia	pain
allo-	other, differing from the normal
alveol/o	alveolus (plural, alveoli)
ambly/o	dull, dim
amni/o	amnion (amniotic sac)
an-	without, not
an/o	anus
ana-	against; up; back
andr/o	male
aneurysm/o	a widening, a widened blood vessel
angi/o	vessel (usually blood or lymph)
aniso-	unequal, dissimilar
ankyl/o	stiffness; bent, crooked
ante-	before, in front of

Medical Word Element	Meaning
anter/o	anterior, front
anthrac/o	black, coal
anti-	against
aort/o	aorta
append/o	appendix
appendic/o	appendix
aque/o	water
-ar	pertaining to, relating to
-arche	beginning
arteri/o	artery
arteriol/o	arteriole
arthr/o	joint
-ary	pertaining to, relating to
asbest/o	asbestos
-asthenia	weakness, debility
astr/o	star
-ate	having the form of, possessing
atel/o	incomplete; imperfect
ather/o	fatty plaque
-ation	process (of)
atri/o	atrium
audi/o	hearing
audit/o	hearing
aur/o	ear
auricul/o	ear
auto-	self, own
ax/o	axis, axon
azot/o	nitrogenous compounds
B	
bacteri/o	bacteria
balan/o	glans penis
bas/o	base (alkaline, opposite of acid)
bi-	two
bi/o	life
-blast	embryonic cell
blast/o	embryonic cell
blephar/o	eyelid
brachi/o	arm
brady-	slow
bronch/o	bronchus (plural, bronchi)
bronchi/o	bronchus (plural, bronchi)

Medical Word Element	Meaning
bronchiol/o	bronchiole
bucc/o	cheek

C

Medical Word Element	Meaning
calc/o	calcium
calcane/o	calcaneum (heel bone)
-capnia	carbon dioxide (CO_2)
carcin/o	cancer
cardi/o	heart
-cardia	heart condition
carp/o	carpus (wrist bones)
cata-	down
caud/o	tail
cauter/o	heat, burn
-cele	hernia, swelling
-centesis	surgical puncture
cephal/o	head
-ception	conceiving
cerebell/o	cerebellum
cerebr/o	cerebrum
cervic/o	neck; cervix uteri (neck of uterus)
chalic/o	limestone
cheil/o	lip
chem/o	chemical; drug
chlor/o	green
chol/e	bile, gall
cholangi/o	bile vessel
cholecyst/o	gallbladder
choledoch/o	bile duct
chondr/o	cartilage
chori/o	chorion
choroid/o	choroid
chrom/o	color
chromat/o	color
-cide	killing
cine-	movement
cinemat/o	things that move
circum-	around
cirrh/o	yellow
-cision	a cutting
-clasia	to break; surgical fracture
-clasis	to break; surgical fracture

Medical Word Element	Meaning
-clast	to break; surgical fracture
clavicul/o	clavicle (collar bone)
-cleisis	closure
clon/o	clonus (turmoil)
-clysis	irrigation, washing
coccyg/o	coccyx (tailbone)
cochle/o	cochlea
col/o	colon
colon/o	colon
colp/o	vagina
condyl/o	condyle
coni/o	dust
conjunctiv/o	conjunctiva
-continence	to hold back
contra-	against, opposite
core/o	pupil
corne/o	cornea
cor/o	pupil
corp/o	body
corpor/o	body
cortic/o	cortex
cost/o	ribs
crani/o	cranium (skull)
crin/o	secrete
-crine	secrete
cruci/o	cross
cry/o	cold
crypt/o	hidden
culd/o	cul-de-sac
-cusia	hearing
-cusis	hearing
cutane/o	skin
cyan/o	blue
cycl/o	ciliary body of eye; circular, cycle
-cyesis	pregnancy
cyst/o	bladder
cyt/o	cell
-cyte	cell

D

Medical Word Element	Meaning
dacry/o	tear; lacrimal apparatus (duct, sac, or gland)
dacryocyst/o	lacrimal sac

Medical Word Element	Meaning
dactyl/o	fingers; toes
de-	cessation
dendr/o	tree
dent/o	teeth
derm/o	skin
-derma	skin
dermat/o	skin
-desis	binding, fixation (of a bone or joint)
di-	double
dia-	through, across
dipl-	double
dipl/o	double
dips/o	thirst
-dipsia	thirst
dist/o	far, farthest
dors/o	back (of body)
duct/o	to lead; carry
-duction	act of leading, bringing, conducting
duoden/o	duodenum (first part of small intestine)
dur/o	dura mater; hard
-dynia	pain
dys-	bad; painful; difficult

E

Medical Word Element	Meaning
-eal	pertaining to, relating to
ec-	out, out from
echo-	a repeated sound
-ectasis	dilation, expansion
ecto-	outside, outward
-ectomy	excision, removal
-edema	swelling
ef-	away from
electr/o	electricity
-ema	state of; condition
embol/o	plug
-emesis	vomiting
-emia	blood condition
emphys/o	to inflate
end-	in, within

Medical Word Element	Meaning
encephal/o	brain
end-	within
endo-	in, within
enter/o	intestine (usually small intestine)
eosin/o	dawn (rose-colored)
epi-	above, upon
epididym/o	epididymis
epiglott/o	epiglottis
episi/o	vulva
erythem/o	red
erythemat/o	red
erythr/o	red
eschar/o	scab
-esis	condition
eso-	inward
esophag/o	esophagus
esthes/o	feeling
-esthesia	feeling
eti/o	cause
eu-	good, normal
ex-	out, out from
exo-	outside, outward
extra-	outside

F

Medical Word Element	Meaning
faci/o	face
fasci/o	band, fascia (fibrous membrane supporting and separating muscles)
femor/o	femur (thigh bone)
-ferent	to carry
fibr/o	fiber, fibrous tissue
fibul/o	fibula (smaller bone of lower leg)
fluor/o	luminous, fluorescence
frotteur/o	to rub

G

Medical Word Element	Meaning
galact/o	milk
gangli/o	ganglion (knot or knotlike mass)

Medical Word Element	Meaning
gastr/o	stomach
-gen	forming, producing, origin
gen/o	forming, producing, origin
-genesis	forming, producing, origin
gingiv/o	gum(s)
glauc/o	gray
gli/o	glue; neuroglial tissue
-glia	glue; neuroglial tissue
-globin	protein
glomerul/o	glomerulus
gloss/o	tongue
glott/o	glottis
gluc/o	sugar, sweetness
glucos/o	sugar, sweetness
glyc/o	sugar, sweetness
-gnosis	knowing
gonad/o	gonads, sex glands
goni/o	angle
-graft	transplantation
-gram	record, writing
granul/o	granule
-graph	instrument for recording
-graphy	process of recording
-gravida	pregnant woman
gyn/o	woman, female
gynec/o	woman, female

H

Medical Word Element	Meaning
hallucin/o	hallucination
hedon/o	pleasure
hem/o	blood
hemangi/o	blood vessel
hemat/o	blood
hemi-	one half
hepat/o	liver
hetero-	different
hidr/o	sweat
hist/o	tissue
histi/o	tissue
homeo-	same, alike
homo-	same

Medical Word Element	Meaning
humer/o	humerus (upper arm bone)
hydr/o	water
hyper-	excessive, above normal
hypn/o	sleep
hypo-	under, below, deficient
hyster/o	uterus (womb)

I

Medical Word Element	Meaning
-ia	condition
-iac	pertaining to, relating to
-iasis	abnormal condition (produced by something specified)
iatr/o	physician; medicine; treatment
-iatry	medicine; treatment
-ic	pertaining to, relating to
-ical	pertaining to, relating to
-ice	noun ending
ichthy/o	dry, scaly
-ician	specialist
-icle	small, minute
-icterus	jaundice
idi/o	unknown, peculiar
-ile	pertaining to, relating to
ile/o	ileum (third part of small intestine)
ili/o	ilium (lateral, flaring portion of hip bone)
im-	not
immun/o	immune, immunity, safe
in-	in, not
-ine	pertaining to, relating to
infer/o	lower, below
infra-	under, below
inguin/o	groin
insulin/o	insulin
inter-	between
intra-	in, within
-ion	the act of
-ior	pertaining to, relating to
irid/o	iris
-is	noun ending

Medical Word Element	Meaning
isch/o	to hold back
ischi/o	ischium (lower portion of hip bone)
-ism	condition
iso-	same, equal
-ist	specialist
-isy	state of; condition
-itic	pertaining to, relating to
-itis	inflammation
-ive	pertaining to, relating to
-ization	process (of)

J

jaund/o	yellow
jejun/o	jejunum (second part of small intestine)

K

kal/i	potassium (an electrolyte)
kary/o	nucleus
kerat/o	horny tissue; hard; cornea
kern/o	kernel (nucleus)
ket/o	ketone bodies (acids and acetones)
keton/o	ketone bodies (acids and acetones)
kinesi/o	movement
-kinesia	movement
kinet/o	movement
klept/o	to steal
kyph/o	hill, mountain

L

labi/o	lip
labyrinth/o	labyrinth (inner ear)
lacrim/o	tear; lacrimal apparatus (duct, sac, or gland)
lact/o	milk
-lalia	speech, babble
lamin/o	lamina (part of vertebral arch)
lapar/o	abdomen
laryng/o	larynx (voice box)

Medical Word Element	Meaning
later/o	side, to one side
lei/o	smooth
leiomy/o	smooth muscle (visceral)
-lepsy	seizure
lept/o	thin, slender
leuk/o	white
lex/o	word, phrase
lingu/o	tongue
lip/o	fat
lipid/o	fat
-lith	stone, calculus
lith/o	stone, calculus
lob/o	lobe
log/o	study of
-logist	specialist in study of
-logy	study of
lord/o	curve, swayback
-lucent	to shine; clear
lumb/o	loins (lower back)
lymph/o	lymph
lymphaden/o	lymph gland (node)
lymphangi/o	lymph vessel
-lysis	separation; destruction; loosening

M

macro-	large
mal-	bad
-malacia	softening
mamm/o	breast
-mania	state of mental disorder, frenzy
mast/o	breast
mastoid/o	mastoid process
maxill/o	maxilla (upper jaw bone)
meat/o	opening, meatus
medi-	middle
medi/o	middle
medull/o	medulla
mega-	enlargement
megal/o	enlargement
-megaly	enlargement

Medical Word Element	Meaning	Medical Word Element	Meaning
melan/o	black	neur/o	nerve
men/o	menses, menstruation	neutr/o	neutral; neither
mening/o	meninges (membranes covering brain and spinal cord)	nid/o	nest
		noct/o	night
		nucle/o	nucleus
meningi/o	meninges (membranes covering brain and spinal cord)	nulli-	none
		nyctal/o	night
ment/o	mind	**O**	
meso-	middle		
meta-	change, beyond	obstetr/o	midwife
metacarp/o	metacarpus (hand bones)	ocul/o	eye
metatars/o	metatarsus (foot bones)	odont/o	teeth
-meter	instrument for measuring	-oid	resembling
metr/o	uterus (womb); measure	-ole	small, minute
metri/o	uterus (womb)	olig/o	scanty
-metry	act of measuring	-oma	tumor
mi/o	smaller, less	omphal/o	navel (umbilicus)
micr/o	small	onc/o	tumor
micro-	small	onych/o	nail
mono-	one	oophor/o	ovary
morph/o	form, shape, structure	-opaque	obscure
muc/o	mucus	ophthalm/o	eye
multi-	many, much	-opia	vision
muscul/o	muscle	-opsia	vision
mut/a	genetic change	-opsy	view of
my/o	muscle	opt/o	eye, vision
myc/o	fungus	optic/o	eye, vision
mydr/o	widen, enlarge	or/o	mouth
myel/o	bone marrow; spinal cord	orch/o	testis (plural, testes)
myos/o	muscle	orchi/o	testis (plural, testes)
myring/o	tympanic membrane (eardrum)	orchid/o	testis (plural, testes)
		-orexia	appetite
myx/o	mucus	orth/o	straight
N		-ory	pertaining to, relating to
		-osis	abnormal condition; increase (used primarily with blood cells)
narc/o	stupor; numbness; sleep		
nas/o	nose		
nat/o	birth	-osmia	smell
natr/o	sodium (an electrolyte)	oste/o	bone
necr/o	death, necrosis	ot/o	ear
neo-	new	-ous	pertaining to, relating to
nephr/o	kidney	ovari/o	ovary

Medical Word Element	Meaning
ox/i	oxygen
-oxia	oxygen
ox/o	oxygen
oxy-	quick, sharp

P

Medical Word Element	Meaning
pachy-	thick
palat/o	palate (roof of mouth)
pan-	all
pancreat/o	pancreas
-para	to bear (offspring)
para-	near, beside; beyond
parathyroid/o	parathyroid glands
-paresis	partial paralysis
patell/o	patella (kneecap)
path/o	disease
-pathy	disease
pector/o	chest
ped/i	foot; child
ped/o	foot; child
pedicul/o	a louse
pelv/i	pelvis
pelv/o	pelvis
pen/o	penis
-penia	decrease, deficiency
-pepsia	digestion
per-	through
peri-	around
perine/o	perineum
peritone/o	peritoneum
-pexy	fixation (of an organ)
phac/o	lens
phag/o	swallowing, eating
-phage	swallowing, eating
-phagia	swallowing, eating
phalang/o	phalanges (bones of fingers and toes)
pharmaceutic/o	drug, medicine
pharyng/o	pharynx (throat)
-phasia	speech
phe/o	dusky, dark
-phil	attraction for

Medical Word Element	Meaning
phil/o	attraction for
-philia	attraction for
phim/o	muzzle
phleb/o	vein
-phobia	fear
phon/o	voice, sound
-phonia	voice, sound
-phoresis	carrying, transmission
-phoria	feeling (mental state)
phot/o	light
phren/o	diaphragm; mind
-phylaxis	protection
-physis	growth
pil/o	hair
pituitar/o	pituitary gland
-plakia	plaque
plas/o	formation, growth
-plasia	formation, growth
-plasm	formation, growth
-plasty	surgical repair
-plegia	paralysis
pleur/o	pleura
-plexy	stroke
-pnea	breathing
pneum/o	air; lung
pneumon/o	air; lung
pod/o	foot
-poiesis	formation, production
poikil/o	varied, irregular
poli/o	gray; gray matter (of brain or spinal cord)
poly-	many, much
polyp/o	small growth
-porosis	porous
post-	after, behind
poster/o	back (of body), behind, posterior
-potence	power
-prandial	meal
pre-	before, in front of
presby/o	old age
primi-	first

Medical Word Element	Meaning	Medical Word Element	Meaning
pro-	before, in front of	-rrhexis	rupture
proct/o	anus, rectum	rube/o	red
prostat/o	prostate gland		
proxim/o	near, nearest	**S**	
pseudo-	false	sacr/o	sacrum
psych/o	mind	salping/o	tube (usually fallopian or eustachian [auditory] tubes)
ptyal/o	saliva		
-ptosis	prolapse, downward displacement	-salpinx	tube (usually fallopian or eustachian [auditory] tubes)
-ptysis	spitting		
pub/o	pelvis bone (anterior part of pelvic bone)	sarc/o	flesh (connective tissue)
		scapul/o	scapula (shoulder blade)
pulmon/o	lung	-sarcoma	malignant tumor of connective tissue
pupill/o	pupil		
py/o	pus	-schisis	a splitting
pyel/o	renal pelvis	schiz/o	split
pylor/o	pylorus	scler/o	hardening; sclera (white of eye)
pyr/o	fire		
		scoli/o	crooked, bent
Q		-scope	instrument for examining
quadri-	four	-scopy	visual examination
		scot/o	darkness
R		seb/o	sebum, sebaceous
rachi/o	spine	semi-	one half
radi/o	radiation, x-ray; radius (lower arm bone on thumb side)	sept/o	septum
		sequestr/o	a separation
		ser/o	serum
radicul/o	nerve root	sial/o	saliva, salivary gland
rect/o	rectum	sider/o	iron
ren/o	kidney	sigmoid/o	sigmoid colon
reticul/o	net, mesh	silic/o	flint
retin/o	retina	sin/o	sinus, cavity
retro-	backward, behind	sinus/o	sinus, cavity
rhabd/o	rod-shaped (striated)	-sis	state of; condition
rhabdomy/o	striated (skeletal) muscle	-social	society
rhin/o	nose	somat/o	body
rhytid/o	wrinkle	somn/o	sleep
roentgen/o	x-rays	son/o	sound
-rrhage	bursting forth (of)	-spadias	slit, fissure
-rrhagia	bursting forth (of)	-spasm	involuntary contraction, twitching
-rrhaphy	suture		
-rrhea	discharge, flow	sperm/o	spermatozoa, sperm cells

Medical Word Element	Meaning
spermat/o	spermatozoa, sperm cells
sphygm/o	pulse
-sphyxia	pulse
spin/o	spine
spir/o	breathe
splen/o	spleen
spondyl/o	vertebrae (backbone)
squam/o	scale
staped/o	stapes
-stasis	standing still
steat/o	fat
sten/o	narrowing, stricture
-stenosis	narrowing, stricture
stern/o	sternum (breastbone)
steth/o	chest
sthen/o	strength
stigmat/o	a point
stomat/o	mouth
-stomy	forming an opening (mouth)
sub-	under, below
sudor/o	sweat
super-	upper, above
supra-	above; excessive; superior
sym-	union, together, joined
syn-	union, together, joined
synapt/o	synapsis, point of contact
synov/o	synovial membrane, synovial fluid

T

Medical Word Element	Meaning
tachy-	rapid
tax/o	order, coordination
-taxia	order, coordination
ten/o	tendon
tend/o	tendon
tendin/o	tendon
-tension	to stretch
test/o	testis (plural, testes)
thalam/o	thalamus
thalass/o	sea
thec/o	sheath (usually refers to meninges)
thel/o	nipple

Medical Word Element	Meaning
therapeut/o	treatment
-therapy	treatment
therm/o	heat
thorac/o	chest
-thorax	chest
thromb/o	blood clot
thym/o	thymus gland
-thymia	mind; emotion
thyr/o	thyroid gland
thyroid/o	thyroid gland
tibi/o	tibia (larger bone of lower leg)
-tic	pertaining to, relating to
till/o	to pull
-tocia	childbirth, labor
tom/o	to cut
-tome	instrument to cut
-tomy	incision
ton/o	tension
tonsill/o	tonsils
tox/o	poison
-toxic	poison
toxic/o	poison
trabecul/o	trabecula (supporting bundles of fibers)
trache/o	trachea (windpipe)
trans-	through, across
tri-	three
trich/o	hair
trigon/o	trigone (triangular region at base of bladder)
-tripsy	crushing
-trophy	development, nourishment
-tropia	turning
-tropin	stimulate
tubercul/o	a little swelling
tympan/o	tympanic membrane (eardrum)

U

Medical Word Element	Meaning
-ula	small, minute
-ule	small, minute
uln/o	ulna (lower arm bone on opposite side of thumb)

Medical Word Element	Meaning	Medical Word Element	Meaning
ultra-	excess, beyond	ventricul/o	ventricle (of heart or brain)
-um	structure, thing	-version	turning
umbilic/o	umbilicus, navel	vertebr/o	vertebrae (backbone)
ungu/o	nail	vesic/o	bladder
uni-	one	vesicul/o	seminal vesicle
ur/o	urine	vest/o	clothes
ureter/o	ureter	viscer/o	internal organs
urethr/o	urethra	vitr/o	vitreous body (of eye)
-uria	urine	vitre/o	glassy
urin/o	urine	vol/o	volume
-us	condition; structure	voyeur/o	to see
uter/o	uterus (womb)	vulv/o	vulva
uvul/o	uvula		

V

vagin/o	vagina		
valv/o	valve		
varic/o	dilated vein		
vas/o	vessel; vas deferens; duct		
vascul/o	vessel		
ven/o	vein		
ventr/o	belly, belly side		

X

xanth/o	yellow
xen/o	foreign, strange
xer/o	dry
xiph/o	sword

Y

-y	condition; process

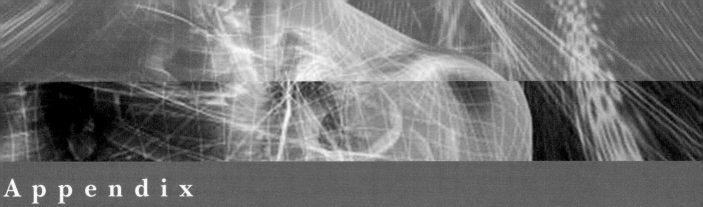

Appendix

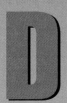

Index of Genetic Disorders

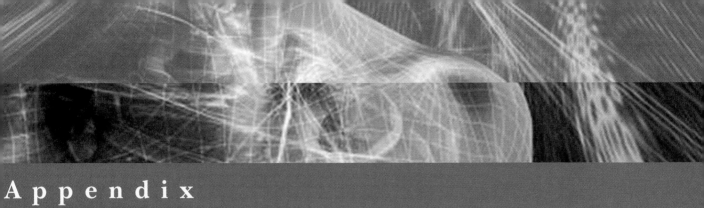

Appendix

E

Index of Diagnostic Imaging Procedures

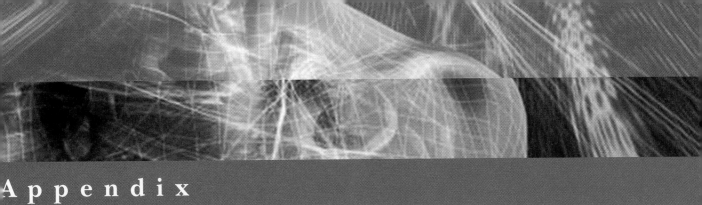

F

Index of Pharmacology

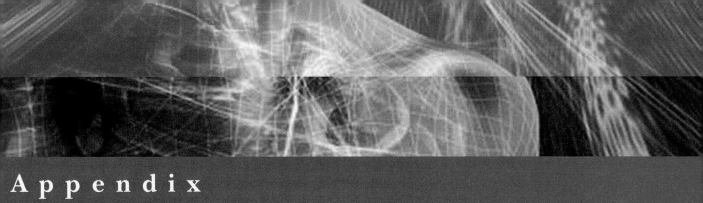

G

Index of Oncological Terms

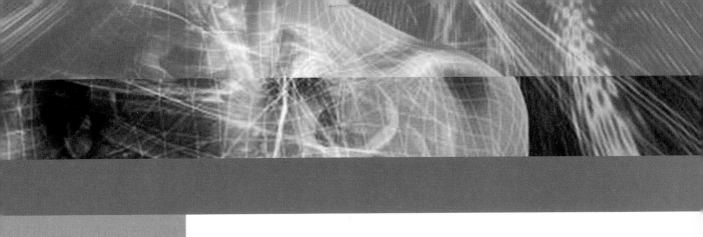

Index